Successful aging

European Network on Longitudinal Studies on Individual Development (ENLS)

The European Science Foundation (ESF) is an association of 50 research councils and scientific academies in 18 European countries. The member organizations represent all scientific disciplines – in natural sciences, in medical and biosciences, in social sciences, and in humanities. One of its main modes of operation is establishing scientific networks.

In this framework the European Network on Longitudinal Studies on Individual Development (ENLS) was established. By organizing a series of workshops on substantive and methodological topics the network has brought together several hundred scientists from very different fields – criminology, developmental biology, epidemiology, pediatrics, psychiatry, psychology, sociology, statistics, and others – all actively involved in longitudinal research. By distributing fellowships to young researchers and twinning grants to researchers for planning common projects and by the development and administration of an inventory covering all major longitudinal projects in Europe, the ENLS has further supported and stimulated longitudinal research.

Chairman: David Magnusson
Coordination Committee Members: Paul Baltes, Paul Casaer, Alex Kalverboer, Jostein Mykletun, Anik de Ribaupierre, Michael Rutter, Fini Schulsinger, and Martti Takala

Previous ESF books published by Cambridge University Press
Michael Rutter, ed., *Studies of psychosocial risk: the power of longitudinal data*
Anik de Ribaupierre, ed., *Transition mechanisms in child development: the longitudinal perspective*
David Magnusson and Lars R. Bergman, eds., *Data quality in longitudinal research*

Successful aging

Perspectives from the behavioral sciences

Edited by

PAUL B. BALTES
Max Planck Institute for Human Development and Education, Berlin

MARGRET M. BALTES
Free University of Berlin

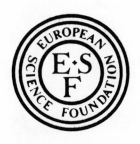

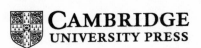

CAMBRIDGE
UNIVERSITY PRESS

Published by the Press Syndicate of the University of Cambridge
The Pitt Building, Trumpington Street, Cambridge CB2 1RP
40 West 20th Street, New York, NY 10011-4211, USA
10 Stamford Road, Oakleigh, Victoria 3166, Australia

First published 1990
Reprinted 1991
First paperback edition 1993

Printed in Canada

Library of Congress Cataloging-in-Publication Data

Successful aging: perspectives from the behavioral sciences / edited
by Paul B. Baltes and Margret M. Baltes.
p.   cm.
Includes bibliographical references.
ISBN 0-521-37454-5
1. Aged – Longitudinal studies.   2. Aging – Psychological aspects –
Longitudinal studies.   3. Aged – Health and hygiene – Longitudinal
studies.   I. Baltes, Paul B.   II. Baltes, Margret M.
HQ1061.S845
305.26–dc20   90–34827
                                                                    CIP

British Library Cataloguing in Publication Data

Successful aging: perspectives from the behavioral
sciences.
1. Adults. Development & ageing
I. European Network on Longitudinal Studies on Individual
Development   II. Baltes, Paul B.   III. Baltes, Margret M.
155.6

ISBN 0-521-37454-5 hardback
ISBN 0-521-43582-X paperback

Contents

Contributors

Lars Bäckman (Chapter 5), Stockholm Gerontology Research Center, Karolinska Institute, Dalagatan 9–11, S-113 82 Stockholm, Sweden

Margret M. Baltes (Chapter 1), Free University of Berlin, Department of Gerontopsychiatry, Ulmenallee 32, 1000 Berlin 19, FRG

Paul B. Baltes (Chapter 1), Max Planck Institute for Human Development and Education, Lentzeallee 94, 1000 Berlin 33, FRG

Bernhard Baltes-Götz (Chapter 7), Department of Psychology, University of Trier, Postfach 3825 – Tarforst, 5500 Trier, FRG

Jochen Brandtstädter (Chapter 7), Department of Psychology, University of Trier, Postfach 3825 – Tarforst, 5500 Trier, FRG

Lorna Champion (Chapter 10), MRC Child Psychiatry Unit, Institute of Psychiatry, De Crespigny Park, Denmark Hill, London SE5 8AF, England

K. Anders Ericsson (Chapter 6), Department of Psychology, Muenzinger Psychology Building, University of Colorado at Boulder, Boulder, CO 80309-0345, USA

David L. Featherman (Chapter 3), Social Science Research Council, 605 Third Avenue, New York, NY 10158, USA

James F. Fries (Chapter 2), Health Research and Policy Building, Immunology 109C, Stanford University Medical Center, Stanford, CA 94305, USA

Jennifer R. Harris (Chapter 12), Department of Environmental Hygiene, Karolinska Institute, P.O. Box 60400, S-104 01 Stockholm, Sweden

Agneta Herlitz (Chapter 5), Stockholm Gerontology Research Center, Karolinska Institute, Dalagatan 9–11, S-113 82 Stockholm, Sweden

Timo Mäntylä (Chapter 5), Stockholm Gerontology Research Center, Karolinska Institute, Dalagatan 9–11, S-113 82 Stockholm, Sweden

Barbara Maughan (Chapter 10), MRC Child Psychiatry Unit, Institute of Psychiatry, De Crespigny Park, Denmark Hill, London SE5 8AF, England

Nancy L. Pedersen (Chapter 12), Department of Environmental Hygiene, Karolinska Institute, P.O. Box 60400, S-104 01 Stockholm, Sweden

James G. Peterson (Chapter 3), University of Southern California, Department of Industrial and Systems Engineering, Los Angeles, CA 90089-0191, USA

Georg Rudinger (Chapter 9), Institute of Psychology, University of Bonn, Römerstrasse 164, 5300 Bonn 1, FRG

K. Warner Schaie (Chapter 4), Department of Human Development and Family Studies, The Pennsylvania State University, 110 Henderson Building South, University Park, PA 16802, USA

Roxane Cohen Silver (Chapter 8), Department of Psychology, University of California at Irvine, Irvine, CA 92717, USA

Jacqui Smith (Chapter 3), Max Planck Institute for Human Development and Education, Lentzeallee 94, 1000 Berlin 33, FRG

Hans Thomae (Chapter 9), Institute of Psychology, University of Bonn, Römerstrasse 164, 5300 Bonn 1, FRG

George E. Vaillant (Chapter 11), Dartmouth College, Medical School, Hanover, NH 03756, USA

Camille B. Wortman (Chapter 8), Department of Psychology, State University of New York at Stony Brook, Stony Brook, NY 11794-2500, USA

Foreword

For a long time, research on developmental issues in the biological and social sciences was mostly concerned with the early parts of life, such as infancy and adolescence. Studies paying full attention to people after they had passed through late adolescence were rare even though we all know that humans continue to develop. The dynamics of adult life can be as forceful and full of transitory states as is life before 20. Individual development is a lifelong process: from the moment of conception to the moment of death. Recently, more and more researchers have turned their attention to the problems of development and aging in later periods of life. This increased interest is caused partly by growing social demands from the aged generations in many Western countries and partly by the fact that longitudinal research endeavors have now started to yield impressive results concerning life-span development.

Developmental problems cannot be very well investigated and understood in all their facets without a solid longitudinal methodology. Therefore, the European Network on Longitudinal Studies on Individual Development (ENLS), established by the European Science Foundation, decided to devote special attention to the issues of aging. One tangible indication of the network's commitment to this area of research is the volume you are now holding in your hands. This volume contains a number of contributions from prominent European and American scientists actively involved in research on aging, providing us with stimulating insights into and a new understanding of the multifaceted and highly complex process of life-span development.

It is my firm conviction that such knowledge will entail a deeper comprehension of what courses of events direct individual development toward health or disease, optimal or bad functioning, happiness or misery, in the final phases of human life.

> David L. Magnusson, Chairman
> Coordination Committee for the
> European Network on Longitudinal Studies
> on Individual Development

Preface

This book is the outgrowth of a workshop sponsored in 1987 by the European Science Foundation (ESF) and its European Network on Longitudinal Studies on Individual Development (David L. Magnusson, Chairman). The workshop had two interrelated purposes. The first was to explore the nature of successful aging, its conditions, and its variations. The second was to highlight the importance of longitudinal and cohort-sequential studies in gaining an adequate understanding of the factors, causes, and contexts of successful aging.

There is a dearth of longitudinal research primarily designed to understand the precursors and conditions of "successful" aging. Nevertheless, we believed that it should be possible to select authors who in all probability would be able to draw on their longitudinal data sources and reanalyze them with such a purpose in mind. We are grateful to the authors for their efforts to respond imaginatively to the challenge posed and for their commitment to improving their chapters on the basis of stimulating conference discussions.

The workshop chapters were also revised after extensive reviews. Thus, also on behalf of the chapter authors, we would like to acknowledge with gratitude the constructive criticisms of the reviewers: Ronald P. Abeles, Lars Bäckman, Alan Baddeley, Vern L. Bengtson, Hans-Peter Blossfeld, Jochen Brandtstädter, Phame M. Camarena, Paul Casaer, Lorna Champion, Neil Charness, Brian Cooper, Steven W. Cornelius, Paul T. Costa, Jr., Fergus I. M. Craik, Dale Dannefer, Nancy W. Denney, Freya Dittmann-Kohli, K. Anders Ericsson, L. Erlenmeyer-Kimling, David L. Featherman, James F. Fries, Jürgen Guthke, Dennis P. Hogan, William J. Hoyer, David F. Hultsch, Scott Johnson, Marja Jylhä, Alex F. Kalverboer, Donald H. Kausler, Reinhold Kliegl, Albert Kozma, Gisela Labouvie-Vief, Margie E. Lachman, Ellen J. Langer, M. Powell Lawton, Eleonore Lehr, Richard M. Lerner, Peter M. Lewinsohn, Michael Linden, Ulman Lindenberger, David Magnusson, Karl Ulrich Mayer, Elizabeth Maylor, Jack J. McArdle, John R. Nesselroade, Susan Nolen-Hoeksema, Nancy L. Pedersen, Anne C. Petersen, Anik de Ribaupierre, Michael Rutter, John M. Rybash, Carol D. Ryff, Hans-Gerhard Sack, Timothy A. Salthouse, K. Warner Schaie, Klaus A. Schneewind, Carmi Schooler, Yvonne Schütze, Rainer K. Silbereisen, Ellen A. Skinner, Thorkild I. A. Sørensen, Elisabeth Steinhagen-Thiessen, Martti Takala, Shelly E. Taylor, Linda Teri, Laura A. Thompson, George E. Vaillant, Michael Wagner, Richard A. Weinberg, Susan Krauss Whitbourne, Camille B. Wortman, and Susanne Zank.

Several other institutions and people contributed in different ways to the preparation and editing of this book in addition to the European Science Foundation and the European Network on Longitudinal Studies on Individual Development. First, there was the general support provided by our two home institutions: the Berlin Max Planck Institute for Human Development and Education (P. B. Baltes) and the Free University of Berlin (M. M. Baltes). Second, we express special gratitude to our editorial and secretarial staff, both at the Berlin Max Planck Institute and at the Free University: Irmgard Pahl assisted us ably and reliably in format editing and proofreading; Helga Kaiser, Stephanie Shanks, and Jutta Urban provided excellent secretarial support; Helga Kaiser and Stephanie Shanks were also responsible for the administrative coordination of the workshop itself, which, incidentally, took place at the lovely conference center of the Max Planck Society located in the Bavarian Alps (Schloss Ringberg, Tegernsee). The present book owes much to the atmosphere of that conference center and the collegial support created by our staff.

In our introductory chapter we offer our conceptual insights into the nature of successful aging. As we wrote this chapter and commented as editors on the others, it became increasingly clear to us that the topic of successful aging poses a challenge that is highly complex and subject to continuous individual and societal reevaluation. Not only is there a lack of adequate concepts and data, but also the perspectives offered by the various disciplines are not always congruent. Each discipline, on the one hand, offers valuable contributions to the whole. On the other hand, each discipline produces information and views that question what researchers from other disciplines so firmly believe in. This is perhaps the nature and challenge of interdisciplinary discourse.

Considering the complexity and recency of the topic, it is not surprising that a book such as the present one cannot offer definite or comprehensive knowledge on the conditions and variations of successful aging. The content is selective, and other researchers and lines of scholarship could have been considered. Despite these limitations, we are hopeful that the book offers new insights and a good selection of what current behavioral and social research into the nature of successful aging has to offer.

Paul B. Baltes
Margret M. Baltes

1 Psychological perspectives on successful aging: The model of selective optimization with compensation

PAUL B. BALTES AND MARGRET M. BALTES

The purpose of this chapter is twofold. First, we review research on the nature of psychological aging in terms of seven propositions. Second, we present a psychological model for the study of successful aging that, we contend, is consistent with the propositional framework. The approach advanced is based on the premise that successful, individual development (including aging) is a process involving three components: selection, optimization, and compensation. How these components of adaption are realized depends on the specific personal and societal circumstances individuals face and produce as they age.

Introduction

Two scientific concepts have had a major impact on our thinking about successful aging: interindividual *variability* and intraindividual *plasticity* (M. Baltes & P. Baltes, 1982; P. Baltes & M. Baltes, 1980; P. Baltes & Schaie, 1976). Reflection on the theoretical and policy-related implications of both concepts has suggested to us that there is much opportunity for the continual optimization of human development (see also Brim & Kagan, 1980; Labouvie-Vief, 1981; Lerner, 1984). Over the years, we have begun to believe that systematic age-related shifts in the extent of variability and plasticity are cornerstones for a developmental theory of human adaptation. Initial evidence for this perspective is available in our first attempt to formulate an agenda for successful aging (P. Baltes & M. Baltes, 1980). After reviewing research on variability and plasticity, we laid the groundwork for a prototheory of successful aging as an adaptive process involving the components of selection, optimization, and

1

compensation. The present chapter builds on this earlier effort and the contributions of others (Brim, 1988; Featherman, Smith, & Peterson, this volume) who have followed similar lines of reasoning and worked toward similar goals.

Because this is the opening chapter of this volume, we begin with some general introductory observations. In these observations, we comment first on the role of beliefs about old age. We suggest that optimism about old age influences research and personal action by directing it toward the search for positive aspects of aging. For this purpose, we invoke the Roman philosopher Cicero. Second, we comment on the general nature of criteria of successful aging and the question of subjective versus objective modes of assessment. Thereafter, we shift to the main focus of this chapter: the presentation of several propositions about the nature of aging and an exposition of one possible model of successful aging.

A precursor: Cicero's *De Senectute*

It was the Roman philosopher and statesman Cicero (106–43 B.C.) who produced perhaps the first powerful statement on the nature of good aging with his essay *De Senectute* (44 B.C./1979). Cicero wrote this essay in his early sixties to show that old age is not a phase of decline and loss. Instead, Cicero argued that old age, if approached properly, harbors many opportunities for positive change and productive functioning.

In our view, in *De Senectute* Cicero implicitly proceeds from the assumption that aging is a variable and plastic phenomenon and offers a persuasive demonstration of the power of the individual mind in constructing a positive image of old age and aging. Applying principles of stoicism (a school of philosophy that emphasized the virtues of the mind and argued that the body is often a negative force in achieving willful behavior), Cicero extols the potential strengths of old age for exactly the same reasons that others have viewed old age as a phase of loss and decline. Cicero contends, from a stoicist perspective, that in old age it is *finally* possible for the individual to focus on further development and enjoyment of the mind and not to be distracted by bodily needs and pleasures: "Nothing [is] more directly destructive to the dignity of man than the pursuit of bodily pleasure" (p. 82).

Cicero's essay is full of supporting arguments and creative observations about old age, many of which pass the test of modern psychological gerontology. Unfortunately, a few examples must suffice. In his philosophical journey toward the stoicist conclusion that old age offers the capstone experience of the human mind, Cicero refutes a number of expectations that cloud everyday views of old age. For example, Cicero introduces the distinction between "normal" and "sick" old age and argues that we should not confuse old age with illness. Illness is a condition that, for some people, is added on to old age. Furthermore, Cicero discusses various negative expectations about old age such as failing memory. If older persons had a failing memory, he queries, how could they reach the highest level of mindful performance? Cicero's rejoinder has two parts. First, he rejects memory loss as a general phenomenon and concludes that only those older persons who also suffer from a brain disease have memory deficits. Second, he emphasizes that memory loss is selective. Older persons forget only those facts and cognitive skills in which they are no longer interested and, therefore, do not care to practice in their everyday lives. Cicero's witty example speaks for itself: "Have you heard of an old man who forgot where he hid his treasure?"

As an effective human being and as a good practical philosopher, Cicero is highly confident about the value of his propositions on old age and about the advice he offers his young students. Using himself as an example for the effectiveness of his discourse on aging, Cicero reports having attained a new view on his own impending old age. Fears and anxieties about old age made way for new feelings of harmony and satisfaction. Surely Cicero's account of old age is optimistic, a psychological utopia based on the power of the human mind to design and control thoughts, feelings, and aspirations beyond the constraints of one's biology. However, utopias are powerful vehicles to help us think in ways that reality would not suggest to us: "Utopias have their value – nothing so wonderfully expands imaginative horizons of human potentialities" (Berlin, 1988, p. 16).

Cicero's essay provides an encouragement for efforts to explore the nature of successful aging. Even so, current efforts are unlikely to be fully consistent with Cicero's approach. In our own case, for instance, we will propose a model of successful aging that departs from Cicero's view in one very significant aspect: It does not ignore the biology of the aging body. Thus, although we adapt Cicero's optimism and stoicist belief in the power of the human mind and will (see also Langer, 1989, for a current version of this position), we propose a model in which the aging body, with its reduced reserves and increased vulnerability to illness, is part of the story.

The concept of successful aging

The concept of successful aging dates back several decades (e.g., Havig-hurst, 1963; Palmore, 1979; Williams & Wirths, 1965), although it has

only recently been forcefully promoted as a guiding theme in gerontological research and as a challenge for the design of social policy (M. Baltes,
1987; Butt & Beiser, 1987; Rowe & Kahn, 1987; Ryff, 1982). The fact that
the theme of successful aging has attracted much attention recently is due
not only to the catchword-like qualities of the term itself and the importance of issues of aging in a modern world. It most likely also reflects a
newfound optimism in the field of gerontology itself (e.g., P. Baltes, 1987;
Birren & Bengtson, 1988; Labouvie-Vief, 1981; Langer, 1989; Lehr, 1987;
Riley, 1983). For example, there is an increasing body of knowledge about
untapped reserves of the elderly and their potential for change. Thus, a
discussion about successful aging converges with the search for factors
and conditions that help us to understand the potential of aging and, if
desirable, to identify ways to modify the nature of human aging as it exists
today. Whether in the long run the concept of successful aging will remain
a scientifically viable topic is perhaps less significant than its power in
identifying and organizing questions and research directions that reflect
the current dynamics of the field.

At first glance, aging and success seem to represent a contradiction:
Aging conjures a picture of loss, decline, and approaching death, whereas
success connotes gains, winning the game, and a positive balance. Thus,
the association of aging with success seems intellectually and emotionally
a paradox. There is also the possible critique that the notion of successful
aging may be a latent vestige of social Darwinism, a rampant competitive
spirit, and one of the less desirable excesses of Western capitalist traditions. Even the last phase of life, critics can argue, is about to be captured
by the view that success, defined by standards external to the individual,
is a necessary part of the good life.

At second glance, however, the association of aging with success might
indicate that the apparent contradiction is intended to provoke a probing
analysis of the nature of old age as it exists today. We are asked not only to
reflect upon but also to participate in the creation of aging, instead of
passively experiencing it as a given reality that is "natural" only for the
reason that it exists. In this sense, the concept of successful aging suggests
a vigorous examination of what might in principle be possible. Moreover,
a critical but constructive analysis of the concept may indeed serve to
articulate the idea that forms and vehicles of "success" in old age may be
different from those in earlier phases of life.

The problem of indicators

Defining the nature of success is elusive. Even in such areas as sports, for
instance, consensus about the definition of success is difficult to achieve.

In gerontology, length of life is most often proposed as the prototypical indicator of successful aging.

Which criteria?

To live as long as possible, to be the oldest living human, is a dream or desire that, to some, is a persuasive criterion of success. Yet, there is no need to call upon Darwin's often-used notion of "survival of the fittest" bestowing success upon a world-record holder for the number of years lived, because there is another side to this coin. The world-record holder in length of life will also have experienced many undesirable events. He or she also might be the one who has most often lost friends, most often stood at open graves, and perhaps most often endured illness. The first motto of the Gerontological Society of America illustrates this two-sided view. This motto in 1955 called for "adding life to years, not just more years to life."

As this example emphasizes, the search for indicators of successful aging is a complex endeavor. It is not possible to solve this problem without invoking values and without a systemic view. Quantitative and qualitative aspects of life need to be balanced. A first step toward identifying an all-encompassing definition of successful aging is to think in terms of multiple criteria. From such a *multicriteria approach*, the following characteristics frequently appear either as concurrent or as outcome criteria in the literature (Bengtson & Kuypers, 1985; Palmore, 1979; Rowe & Kahn, 1987; Ryff, 1982):

- length of life
- biological health
- mental health
- cognitive efficacy
- social competence and productivity
- personal control
- life satisfaction

Existing research on successful aging reflects this multicriteria approach, although a consensus on their interrelationship or relative importance has not been achieved. In general, it seems fair to conclude that the criteria mentioned exhibit a positive manifold. However, the positive interrelations are not of sufficient magnitude so that a single latent dimension is indicated. Moreover, at least in psychological gerontology, research has not yet reached a point where there is good "causal" evidence about predictor variables or about the role of risk and protective factors.

Integrating subjective and objective criteria

In addition to the question of dimensionality and relative weight of the criteria, a further issue concerns the categorization of criteria along yet another dimension, namely, *subjective versus objective* indicators. In psychological and social science research, there is a preponderance of the use of subjective criteria such as measures of life satisfaction, self-concept, and self-esteem and, more recently, measures of perceived or personal control. This emphasis on subjective indicators reflects the assumption that a certain parallelism exists between the subjective and objective world and also the view that, for the social scientist, reality is in part socially and personally constructed. It also reflects the value judgment that the perceiving self ought to be the litmus test for the quality of life (Bengtson, Reedy, & Gordon, 1985; Schwartz, 1974).

The usefulness of subjective criteria is somewhat undermined, in our view, by the fact that the human psyche is extraordinarily plastic, adaptive, and able to compensate (see also Brim, 1988; Epstein, 1981; Filipp & Klauer, 1986; Greenwald, 1980; Markus & Wurf, 1987). By the use of various psychological mechanisms, humans are able to "successfully" adapt their subjective assessments to objectively quite diverse conditions. It is astonishing, for instance, how little difference has been found in life satisfaction between people who live in objectively adverse life conditions (such as during wartime or in prisons or slums) and those who live under normal or even superior life conditions.

Consequently, we submit that subjective indicators are possibly overweighted in typical definitions of successful aging. They are necessary but not sufficient conditions for an adequate definition of successful aging. Moreover, we contend that subjective assessments of well-being might even be misleading if used as the only indicators. For example, because of the mind's power to transform reality and in the extreme even to ignore it, the sole use of subjective indicators is likely to underestimate both the existence of behavioral and ecological deficiencies and the potential for further progress. Thus, for the planning of environments aimed at the optimization of individual development, it seems essential to supplement subjective criteria with objective ones.

The search for objective criteria for life quality seems to proceed generally along two avenues. The first is based on a *normative* definition of an ideal state. Such a normative definition describes developmental outcomes (such as mental health) and goals (life goals and patterns) that are used as a standard for success. Erikson's theory of lifelong personality development, with generativity and wisdom as the central themes of later life, is an example of such an approach (Erikson, Erikson, & Kivnick,

1986; Ryff, 1984). Achieving generativity and wisdom, then, becomes the yardstick for successful aging. The fundamental objection to such models is that they start, as the label *normative* suggests, with the assumption of a highly standardized society. In addition, the standards chosen often reflect the priorities and values of the middle and upper classes. Successful aging should not be a phenomenon restricted to a given social class.

The second avenue leading toward a specification of objective measures of successful aging is based on the concept of *adaptivity* (or *behavioral plasticity*). This approach seems more general because it does not imply a single outcome, specific contents, or life goals. Rather, its focus is on the measurement of the efficacy of a system. Adaptivity or behavioral plasticity is a measure of potential and preparedness for dealing with a variety of demands (M. Baltes, 1987; P. Baltes, 1987; Coper, Jänicke, & Schulze, 1986; Shock, 1977). Illustrations of adaptivity in the psychological realm are the quality of one's memory and cognition and the quality of one's ability to cope with stressful events. Taken together, such measures are expected to yield indicators of the adaptive plasticity and potential of a person.

In summary, an encompassing definition of successful aging requires a value-based, systemic, and ecological perspective. Both subjective and objective indicators need to be considered within a given cultural context with its particular contents and ecological demands. However, both the objective aspects of medical, psychological, and social functioning and the subjective aspects of life quality and life meaning seem to form a Gordian knot that no one is prepared to untie at the present time. Our suggested solution is to use multiple subjective and objective criteria and to explicitly recognize individual and cultural variations.

A framework of propositions

In the following, seven propositions about the nature of human aging are presented from a psychological point of view. It is argued that a conception of successful aging needs to be placed into the context of this framework. Subsequently, we will derive one prototheoretical model of successful aging that in our view is consistent with this framework.

Proposition 1: There are major differences between normal, optimal, and sick (pathological) aging

The first proposition concerns the differentiation among normal, optimal, and sick aging (Cicero, 44 B.C./1979; Rowe & Kahn, 1987; Whitbourne, 1985). Normal aging refers to aging without biological or mental pathology. It thus concerns the aging process that is dominant within a society for persons who are not suffering from a manifest illness. Optimal aging refers to a kind of utopia, namely, aging under development-enhancing and age-friendly environmental conditions. Finally, sick or pathological aging characterizes an aging process determined by medical etiology and syndromes of illness. A classical example is dementia of the Alzheimer type.

This distinction among normal, optimal, and pathological aging is not unequivocal, but it is useful as a heuristic. Whether there is aging without pathology is an open question. Fries (this volume), for example, argues that it is possible, in principle, to either reduce or postpone the occurrence of chronic diseases such that the "natural and fixed" biological life span can run its course into old age before illness becomes overtly manifest. Death would end life before disease hampers daily living, similar to a clock that suddenly stops ticking without warning or any appearance of damage. Whether this futuristic propositon of Fries will become reality is not essential to the basic argument. The important point is that it is pathological incidents that primarily produce a qualitatively different organism in old age and not aging itself.

Proposition 2: There is much heterogeneity (variability) in aging

The second proposition is that aging is characterized by large interindividual variability in level, rate, and direction of change. Aging is a very individual and differential process with regard to mental, behavioral, and social outcome variables. There are 70-year-olds who look and think like 50-year-olds and vice versa.

Why is there so much variability in aging? Three sources seem to produce this effect. First, there are differences in genetic factors and environmental conditions that act cumulatively over ontogenetic time. For example, some genetic effects may be augmented over the life span, and there are also late-life genes (Plomin & Thompson, 1986). Second, there are individualizing effects resulting from the way each person influences his or her own life course (Brandtstädter, 1984; Brandtstädter, Krampen, & Heil, 1986; Lerner, 1984). Finally, and especially in the late decades of life, variability may increase because the course of normal aging can be modulated by a variety of different patterns of pathologies (Proposition 1).

The notion of interindividual variability or heterogeneity of aging receives much support from longitudinal studies on adulthood and old age (Maddox, 1987; Thomae, 1979, 1987). In our assessment, five longitudinal projects are of particular significance. Historically, the Kansas City

Studies of Adult Life conducted by Havighurst, Henry, Neugarten, and associates opened the way for a differential perspective (Neugarten, 1968, 1987). Subsequently, the Duke Longitudinal Studies (Busse & Maddox, 1985; Maddox, 1987), the Baltimore Longitudinal Study on Aging (Costa & Andres, 1986; Shock et al., 1984), the Bonn Longitudinal Study of Aging (Lehr & Thomae, 1987; Thomae, 1979), and Schaie's Seattle Longitudinal Study of Intellectual Aging (Schaie, 1979, 1983) produced converging evidence. Each of these longitudinal studies documented that aging was not a general and uniform process. Instead, individuals were shown to age very differently.

Research on the sociology (Dannefer, 1984; Featherman, 1983; Maddox, 1987; Riley, 1985) and the biology of aging (Finch, 1988; Fries & Crapo, 1981; Rowe & Kahn, 1987) further strengthened the view that aging in Western societies is a highly heterogeneous process. A general perspective on aging evolved and took hold. This perspective stated that human biology and human culture set the "genotypic" stage for a remarkable degree of "phenotypic" individuality and variability.

Although large heterogeneity in old age is a widely accepted fact, nevertheless, there is disagreement about whether interindividual variability increases with age (Bornstein & Smircina, 1982). Aside from the empirical evidence in current data, there is a new theoretical issue associated with future changes in length of life. If more and more people approach their "maximum" biological life span, as Fries (1983) suggests, the unifying force of a common biological program of aging and dying may actually contribute to a reduction of interindividual variability in future cohorts of very old persons.

Proposition 3: There is much latent reserve

The concept of plasticity provides a conceptual foundation for this proposition and emerges in conjunction with another kind of longitudinal research, that is, gerontological intervention studies. When individuals were subjected to targeted interventions, whether in the area of self-care, social behavior, or perceived control or in the domain of cognitive functioning, evidence for a sizable amount of intraindividual plasticity was obtained. Studies repeatedly demonstrated that most old people, like young people, possess sizable reserves that can be activated via learning, exercise, or training. As a result, the focus has been on the concept of *reserve capacity*, a concept whose utility in clinical diagnosis was advanced, for example, as early as 1934 by Vygotsky (see Guthke, 1972, 1982; Roether, 1983; Schmidt, 1971).

In operant-experimental research on dependent versus independent behavior, for instance, many different types of dependent behavior have been examined (for reviews see M. Baltes & Barton, 1979; Mosher-Ashley, 1986–87; Wisocki, 1984). Using diverse reinforcement and stimulus control procedures, researchers have demonstrated substantial behavioral plasticity in the elderly. These laboratory-type findings support the possibility of behavioral optimization and corrective compensation in old age. The important role of environmental conditions in determining the emittance of either dependent or independent behavior has been validated by observational studies in the field (see M. Baltes, 1988; M. Baltes & Wahl, 1987). The findings appear to represent a dependence–support script: The social environment (the social partners) of the elderly reinforces dependent behavior and ignores independent behavior. Consequently, it is likely that the reserve capacities of older persons are not fully activated in their everyday lives.

Similar evidence for substantial reserve capacity also exists in the domain of cognitive functioning. Here, the data show that healthy elderly people in the age range between 60 and 80 benefit from practice (like younger adults do) and show an increase in performance on the specific abilities trained that is comparable in its magnitude to the aging decline found in untrained persons in longitudinal studies (P. Baltes & Lindenberger, 1988; Schaie & Willis, 1986). Moreover, it has been shown that a variety of cognitive interventions can be effective, even ones that involve a minimum amount of instruction and practice (Denney, 1984; Labouvie-Vief, 1985; Roether, 1986; Willis, 1987).

For example, when comparing the effects of tutor-guided and self-guided practice for fluid intelligence (this cluster of intellectual abilities shows consistent aging loss), P. Baltes, Sowarka, and Kliegl (1989) found that healthy older adults were able to generate, by themselves, levels of performance that hitherto were attributed to guided instruction by others (Figure 1.1). In addition, it has been shown that healthy old people are able to learn new cognitive skills, for instance, by becoming memory experts (Kliegl, J. Smith, & P. Baltes, 1989). Such findings suggest that for many older adults the mechanics of the cognitive system continue to function during old age in the same general way as they do during earlier phases of the life course. Thus, older adults are able to use their cognitive mechanics to acquire new forms of declarative and procedural knowledge.

The fact that older adults have the cognitive reserves to acquire new forms of factual and procedural knowledge is important because it suggests that cognitive aging does not only consist of the maintenance of past functioning. Based on the fact that *new learning* is possible, one can argue that older adults may continue to produce new forms of adaptive capacity

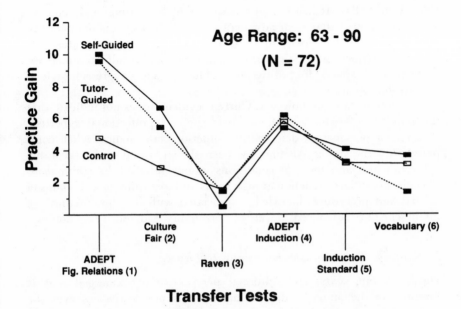

Figure 1.1. Pattern of transfer gains following training in one fluid ability (figural relations) for two training groups (tutor-guided, self-guided) and a control group (data from P. Baltes, Sowarka, & Kliegl, 1989). The results show that older adults have the capacity for self-directed learning involving certain domains of fluid intelligence.

(P. Baltes, 1987; Charness, 1985; Dixon & P. Baltes, 1986; Featherman, 1986; Hoyer, 1985; Labouvie-Vief, 1981; Perlmutter, in press; Roether, 1983; Rybash, Hoyer, & Roodin, 1986). This is relevant, for instance, regarding the acquisition, maintenance, and transformation of expertise in the professional world.

The capacity for new learning has implications for domains of life that have been identified for late-life growth, as perhaps most forcefully argued on the conceptual level by Labouvie-Vief (1981). Wisdom, in particular, has been singled out as a candidate (P. Baltes & J. Smith, 1990; Holliday & Chandler, 1986; Meacham, 1982; Perlmutter, in press; J. Smith, Dixon, & P. Baltes, 1989; Sternberg, in press). Indeed, in cross-sectional studies on wisdom and life knowledge, it has been shown that some older adults are in the group showing top levels of performance (P. Baltes & J. Smith, 1990; J. Smith & P. Baltes, 1990; Sowarka, 1989; Staudinger, 1989). In addition, scholars have argued for positive (desirable) late-life changes in certain aspects of personality such as a movement toward interiority, less dominance, social generativity, and emotional integrity (Gutmann, 1987; Henry, 1988; Labouvie-Vief, 1981,

1986; Ryff, 1984). It has been proposed (e.g., by Gutmann, Labouvie-Vief, and Henry) that such advances in psychological functioning may even be facilitated by losses or transformations in biological status. For instance, a reduction of male hormones in men could result in an increase in the reserve capacity for positive change toward a less aggressive style of human functioning.

One note of caution, however: Current evidence does not indicate that the majority of older adults, in areas such as professional expertise, wisdom, or personality, demonstrate superior performances when compared with the young. All that has been shown is that under favorable environmental and medical conditions, many older adults continue to have the potential to function at high levels and to acquire new domains of factual and procedural knowledge associated with the "pragmatics" of intelligence or "advanced" levels of personality and social functioning.

Proposition 4: There is an aging loss near limits of reserve

During recent years, an additional perspective has emerged that is essential to the understanding of aging. This perspective involves the search for *limits* to behavioral plasticity or adaptivity. Consequently, a *Janus-like*, dual view on plasticity and its limits has resulted (P. Baltes, 1987; Kliegl & P. Baltes, 1987).

Despite sizable reserve capacities in the old, evidence is mounting that shows, at the same time, aging-correlated limits to the magnitude and scope of cognitive reserve capacity. Similar to biological and physical functioning (M. Baltes & Kindermann, 1985; Coper et al., 1986; Stones & Kozma, 1985; Whitbourne, 1985), psychological researchers have now begun to examine this issue more closely. The key test is whether under conditions most favorable to optimal performance, older adults can reach the same levels of top performance as the young. Testing-the-limits is a methodological strategy to estimate levels of current and future reserve capacity. The three levels to be explored are baseline performance, baseline reserve capacity, and developmental reserve capacity (Table 1.1).

Evidence for the contention that there is definite aging loss in cognitive reserve capacity is available from long-term training studies involving reaction time and other speed-related indicators of information-processing capacity (Craik, 1983; Salthouse, 1985). For example, it does not appear possible for older adults to reach the same level of top performance as younger adults in reaction time on either simple- or complex-choice reaction tasks. This aging loss at limits is most evident for abilities characterized as part of the "mechanics" of the mind (P. Baltes, 1987; Hunt, 1978; Kliegl & P. Baltes, 1987).

Table 1.1. *Three tiers of reserve capacity*

Baseline performance	Assessment of performance under standardized conditions without intervention
Baseline reserve capacity	Assessment of current maximum performance potential by strategies aimed at optimization through variation of performance factors (context, instruction, motivation, etc.)
Developmental reserve capacity	Assessment of future performance potential by means of development-enhancing interventions

Note: Modified from P. Baltes, Dittmann-Kohli, & Dixon, 1984; Kliegl & Baltes, 1987.

In the cognitive laboratory of the Berlin Max Planck Institute, this approach has been extended using a testing-the-limits paradigm in the area of memory functioning. Applying principles of cognitive psychology as well as theoretical suggestions from research on memory experts (Ericsson, 1985), we engineer high levels of a cognitive expertise, such as a mnemonic skill, in the laboratory and have subjects of different adult ages practice these skills for extended periods of time. To date, the evidence indicates that older adults, despite their sizable reserve capacity, are not able to reach the same level of performance in such memory skills as young adult subjects of comparable IQ levels. Results from a study by Kliegl, J. Smith, and P. Baltes (1989) are shown in Figure 1.2 to illustrate this finding.

Further research (P. Baltes & Kliegl, 1989; Kliegl, 1989) has demonstrated that the aging loss apparent at limits of performance cannot be fully eliminated even when older adults participate in extended programs of practice. In addition, this result has been obtained even when older adults are selected based on their history of professional accomplishments. For instance, healthy, older graphic designers who, because of their professional specializations, excel in some of the skills that are part of the memory system to be trained are unable to reach the same level of performance as younger, adult graphic designers (Lindenberger, 1990).

Evidence from testing-the-limits research on maximum levels of performance adds a new dimension to past research on reserve capacity (see also Ericsson, this volume, who explores a similar question for middle adulthood). On the one hand, it provides further support for the existence of a substantial reserve capacity (Proposition 3). Most older adults can reach high levels of cognitive performance and exhibit new forms of cognitive skills. On the other hand, age differences are magnified when performances are studied at levels that approximate limits of performance

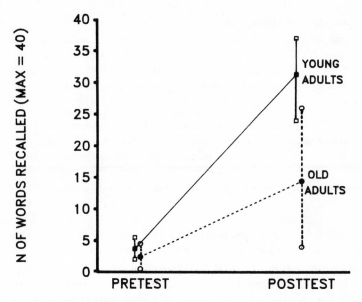

Figure 1.2. Plasticity and limits to plasticity in testing-the-limits research on memory functioning. Bar lines indicate range of scores (data from Kliegl, J. Smith, & P. Baltes, 1989).

potential. In fact, in the study of expert memory (see Figure 1.2), age-group differences were so large at posttest that almost none of the elderly persons could operate at the same level as many young adults.

This series of initial studies seems to suggest almost unchangeable or fixed limits to the efficiency of the mechanics of intelligence and memory. Obviously, much more work is needed to substantiate this claim. Nevertheless, if considered in conjunction with other theoretical positions associated with the concept of limited capacity (Craik, 1977, 1983; Salthouse, 1985), available evidence is highly suggestive of the conclusion that the magnitude of cognitive reserve capacity is reduced in old age and that this reduction is conspicuous when limits of performance and developmental reserve are tested. It is our prediction that a similar reduction would be found if energy-related, motivational resources were studied. Older adults report having less energy, and animal studies with old rats (Coper et al., 1986), for example, seem to demonstrate less physical vigor on energy-intensive tasks, such as running in a drum-wheel.

Is a reduced range of cognitive and motivational reserve capacity relevant for everyday behavior? It depends. In two cases the answer is affirmative. First, reduced reserve capacity affects behavior on any task that requires levels of functioning beyond the limits available. In everyday life such instances may be rare and only experienced when the range (limits) of reserve capacity has dropped extensively (e.g., onset of Alzheimer's disease). Second, the consequences of a reduced reserve capacity may accumulate over a series of tasks. Thus, it is likely that elderly adults are able to perform fewer strenuous behaviors within a given time unit, such as an hour, a day, or a week, without exhausting their reserve capacity.

Proposition 5: Knowledge-based pragmatics and technology can offset age-related decline in cognitive mechanics

Propositions 3 and 4 offer somewhat contradictory evidence: evidence for latent potential (reserve capacity) but also aging-related losses in the range of such latent potential. Proposition 5 addresses the dynamics between the processes associated with these two propositions. We illustrate the important role of knowledge (and technology) in offsetting certain losses in reserve capacity using the area of intellectual functioning as a sample case.

The domain of intellectual functioning encompasses two major, distinct categories: the fluid, cognitive mechanics and the crystallized, cognitive pragmatics (P. Baltes, 1987; Cattell, 1971; Horn, 1970). Consideration of the interplay between cognitive mechanics and pragmatics offers an important avenue for understanding how successful aging is possible. The suggestion is that cognitive pragmatics can compensate for losses (differences) in cognitive mechanics. This conclusion is based on the view that any given intellectual product such as performance on a given test of intelligence or remembering a long poem or story is the outcome of a *multitude* of component skills involving both the mechanics and the knowledge-based pragmatics as building blocks.

Knowledge is a powerful enricher and modulator of the mind. The amount and quality of factual and procedural knowledge available determine to a very large extent what can be achieved with a particular set of cognitive mechanics. Thus, even if some individuals have "worse" cognitive mechanics, if their task-related knowledge is "better," these persons will excel in performance on that task (Staudinger, Cornelius, & P. Baltes, 1989). The effects of knowledge and of associated strategies of cognitive engineering can be quite large indeed, as illustrated in the work on expert memory summarized earlier. Individuals from most walks of life (including the elderly) can become memory experts by using and practicing mnemonic techniques, which essentially comprise the acquisition of factual and procedural knowledge.

From the perspective of the aging individual, therefore, a loss in

cognitive mechanics can be overcome to a large degree by the development of pragmatic knowledge. The powerful compensatory and enriching
effect of knowledge is perhaps best demonstrated by research that has
focused on adults in real life who excel in their performance (i.e., experts).
This research takes advantage of the practice, training, and knowledge
acquisition that occur in natural settings and over extended periods of
time. For example, in a creatively designed study, Salthouse (1984)
examined the performance of younger and older good typists. He found
that tapping speed, a component skill involved in typing, was significantly
slower in the older typists. However, some older typists exhibited superior
typing performance. How was this possible? The findings of Salthouse's
study made it possible to argue that older typists likely compensated for
the decline in tapping speed by reading farther ahead in the text to be
typed. In our interpretation, tapping speed is an indicator of cognitive
mechanics, whereas reading of text is a measure of the knowledge-based
pragmatics. Older typists can overcome their deficit in tapping speed by
developing a strategy that is based on what psychologists call declarative
and procedural knowledge (Brown, 1982; Mandl & Spada, 1988; Weinert,
1986).

Knowledge, of course, is available not only as an "internal component"
of an individual's mind but also as a cultural product. Therefore, technology and other support systems can facilitate the enrichment and compensation of individual differences in cognitive and motivational reserve
capacities. Society is challenged to invest some of its resources with the
particular goal of generating pragmatic knowledge and technical support
systems to compensate for losses due to aging (e.g., cognitive mechanics,
physical vigor).

Proposition 6: With aging the balance between gains and losses becomes less positive

The essence of Proposition 6 is a summary statement about the relative
balance of positive and negative changes with development. The proposition proceeds from the view that development at any life period reflects a
dynamic interplay between gains and losses. We contend that this dynamic becomes one involving an increasingly less positive balance in old age.
This trend toward a less positive balance is evident on the level of both
subjective expectations as well as objective behavioral assessment.

There are two major causes for this phenomenon. The first is inherent
in any developmental process because development is never only a gain.
This is so because every developmental change is an adaptive specialization (P. Baltes, 1987; Featherman et al., this volume; Greenough, 1986;

Labouvie-Vief, 1981; Singer, 1987). Because of this specialization, any given developmental process that entails a positive change in some kind of adaptive capacity also contains the loss of other developmental capacities and future options.

This point is illustrated well by examples in social, cognitive, and biological domains. Professional career development, for instance, involves a decreasing probability of alternative career lines. Another example is the fact that becoming a multilingual speaker always involves the possibility of positive and negative transfer regarding the acquisition of additional languages. Likewise in the cognitive domain, as children become experts in highly regulated forms of logical thinking, they are likely to lose some of their capacity for fantasy and playfulness. Finally, similar perspectives are part of developmental biology (e.g., canalization): The differentiation of certain neuronal developmental paths occurs at the cost of other possible developmental pathways. Thus, every realized developmental process is not merely progress in adaptive capacity but also implies at the same time some degree of loss.

The second cause is unique to aging and is associated with an aging-related loss in adaptivity or plasticity. Why should the balance between gains and losses become less and less positive in old age? We propose that a change in the balance between gains and losses toward a less positive balance is a necessary product of the aging-related reduction in the scope of cognitive and motivational reserve capacity (Proposition 4). Therefore, life tasks exceed more easily the limits of reserve capacity. Such a shift in the balance between gains and losses could be avoided or minimized only if societies were structured in a way that their age-related allocation of resources would fully compensate for the aging loss in "biological" reserve capacity.

The phenomenon of an increasingly negative balance between gains and losses is also part of subjective expectations about old age. Proceeding from the existence of a negative aging stereotype, Heckhausen, Dixon, and P. Baltes (1989), for example, predicted that adults would attribute an increasingly larger number of losses to the later periods of the life span. A gain was defined as an expectation of a change with age that was desirable (such as becoming more intelligent); a loss was defined as an expected change that was undesirable (such as becoming less healthy).

In this study, adults were asked about the desirability of changes expected to occur throughout adulthood from ages 20 to 90 on a large number of attributes. On the average, subjects reported less desirable change expectations for attributes having an expected onset of change at older ages (see Figure 1.3). If one aggregates all expectations, the balance between expected gains and losses shifts toward a less and less positive

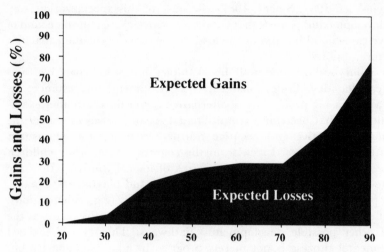

Figure 1.3. Age-related pattern involving 163 psychological attributes: expected gains (increase in desirable attributes) and losses (increase in undesirable attributes) across the adult life span (data from Heckhausen, Dixon, & P. Baltes, 1989).

pattern with age. At the same time, even in very old age, some positive changes were expected. For instance, there was the expectation that wisdom and dignity emerge during late life.

Proposition 7: The self remains resilient in old age

Proposition 7 addresses the aging self. Research has yielded counterintuitive evidence on this topic that is critical for an adequate conception of mastery in old age. Because of a negative aging stereotype (Harris, 1975), one might easily expect that older persons would hold less positive views of themselves and their efficacy to control their own lives. Contradictory to this expectation, however, old people on the average do not differ from young people in reports of their subjective life satisfaction or on self-related measures such as personal control or self-efficacy (M. Baltes & P. Baltes, 1986; Butt & Beiser, 1987; Felton, 1987; Filipp & Klauer, 1986; Lachman, 1986; Veroff, Douvan, & Kulka, 1981).

Three factors are probably responsible for the fact that older adults do not differ from younger adults when asked about their own views of self and life satisfaction. First, there is the phenomenon of multiple selves. Research suggests that people hold more than one view of the self (Filipp & Klauer, 1986; Markus & Nurius, 1986; Neisser, 1988). We all have a number of quite different images of who we are, who we were, who we want to be, or who we could be. The existence of multiple selves and the images connected to them are an effective mechanism for adjustment to diverse life situations. Second, it is possible that there is a change in goals and levels of aspiration (Abeles, 1987; Brandtstädter & Baltes-Götz, this volume; Brim, 1988). Based on experiences of failure and success as well as expectations about the nature of life stages with their own changing scenarios, individuals are quite capable of adjusting their expectations to new levels. Third, there is the process of social comparison. Adjustment to new goals and expectations, which is part of many major life transitions, is facilitated by life events and often leads to a change in one's reference groups (Schwarzer, Lange, & Jerusalem, 1982; Suls & Mullen, 1982; Wills, 1981; Wood, 1989). Old people, for instance, even if they are worse off than the rest of the population, tend to orient their comparison standards toward other old people in similar situations. The result is an adjusted assessment that allows one's own life situation and one's self to appear in a new frame of reference.

These observations on the relative resilience of views of self in old age do not imply that all older adults have intact selves and a high level of self-esteem or personal control. Of course, as is true for younger age-groups as well, there are sizable individual differences among the elderly in indicators of selfhood and the ability to adjust and cope. For example, Brandtstädter and Baltes-Götz (this volume) found in a longitudinal study on partnership relationships during adulthood that people differed markedly in their ability to adjust their individual and mutual developmental goals. Proposition 7 only suggests that, on the average, older adults do not appear to differ markedly from younger age-groups in indicators of what Brewster Smith (1978) has called "selfhood."

Strategies for successful aging

General principles

Based on this framework of propositions about the nature of aging, a series of general principles can be derived with regard to potential strategies for successful aging. Aside from the general optimism associated with these perspectives, these guidelines are not earthshaking if taken individually. However, as a pattern they suggest a coordinated and focused approach.

First, it seems desirable to engage in a healthy life-style in order to reduce the probability of pathological aging conditions (Proposition 1). Second, because of considerable heterogeneity in the onset, direction, and diversity of aging, it is important to avoid simple solutions and to encourage individual and societal flexibility (Proposition 2). Third, it is desirable to strengthen one's reserve capacities (Proposition 3) via educational, motivational, and health-related activities as well as the formation and nurturance of social convoys (Antonucci & Jackson, 1987; Kahn & Antonucci, 1980). The greater one's reserve capacities, be they physical, mental, or social reserves, the more likely successful aging will take place. This is also true because a larger reserve capacity facilitates the search for and creation of optimizing environments, as implied, for instance, in Lawton's conception of "environmental proactivity" (Lawton, 1988; Parmelee & Lawton, 1990). In order to enact these general strategies, the provision of societal resources and opportunities is a prerequisite. Development-enhancing societal opportunities and supports need to be offered.

Limits to reserve capacity (Proposition 4) and the enriching and compensatory role of knowledge and technology (Proposition 5) suggest another general strategic principle. Because of loss in adaptive capacity, particularly at limits of capacity, older adults will need special compensatory supports. A creative search is required for substitute and prosthetic devices, age-appropriate life-styles, and age-friendly environments (M. Baltes, 1987; Lawton, 1982, 1988; Lehr & Thomae, 1987; Thomae, 1987). This is perhaps the most underdeveloped part of our culture. Age-friendly environments refer to ecologies that, in addition to providing development-enhancing conditions, are less taxing on person's reserve capacities and, furthermore, contain prosthetic devices. Examples from diverse areas of life are environmental supports for the handicapped in traffic and public buildings, home health care systems, and day clinics for the elderly.

The changing balance in gain/loss ratios (Proposition 6) and the continued resilience of the self (Proposition 7) suggest the consideration of strategies that facilitate adjustments to "objective" reality without loss of selfhood. By definition, life-span development and aging cannot only be a "winning game" (P. Baltes & Kliegl, 1986; Brim, 1988). In terms of absolute criteria of functional capacity, losses will occur. The central task will be to assist individuals in acquiring effective strategies involving changes in aspirations and the scope of goals.

The facilitation of changes in aspirations and goals is complicated by the question of when to accept the fact of loss and reorient one's life. Brim (1988) has proposed a criterion of "performance standard/capacity ratio" associated with the notion of "just manageable difficulty." Using a performance standard/capacity ratio approach, it may be possible to specify when objective reality would mandate the acceptance of a loss. Acceptance of certain losses would be necessary, for example, when the same behaviors can be displayed only if a dysfunctionally high level of reserve capacity (performance standard/capacity ratio) is required for their execution; that is, if the target behavior overtaxes the system of mental, social, and motivational resources. Such a view is consistent with the position that dependency in old age can be an effective strategy for avoiding overtaxing or depletion of one's reserve (M. Baltes & Wahl, 1987).

Taken together, these perspectives underscore the theme of heterogeneity and variability (Proposition 2). Because aging is a highly individual process, societal input should be primarily geared toward the individualization of resources and opportunities. Because of large variability in aging, a parallel diversity of societal resources must be offered that would allow each person to find his or her personal form and expression of aging. It is likely that no single set of conditions and no single trajectory of aging would qualify as *the* form of successful or optimal aging.

The principle of selective optimization with compensation

Is it possible to specify a model that reflects this dynamic interplay between gains and losses, between development-oriented plasticity and age-related boundaries of such plasticity? Can we devise a model that could serve as a guideline for an individual's thoughts and actions and for social policy? Can we envision a prototypical strategy of effective aging that allows for self-efficacy and growth in the context of increasing biological vulnerability and reduced reserve capacity?

During the last decade we have begun to articulate such a prototypical strategy of successful aging and named it "selective optimization with compensation" (P. Baltes & M. Baltes, 1980; M. Baltes, 1987; P. Baltes, 1987; P. Baltes, Dittmann-Kohli, & Dixon, 1984; see also Featherman et al., this volume). Figure 1.4 summarizes the dynamics of this process of adaptation. In our view, the key concept, selective optimization with compensation, describes a *general* process of adaptation. Individuals are likely to engage in this process throughout life. We believe, however, that the process of selective optimization with compensation takes on a new significance and dynamic in old age because of the loss of biological, mental, and social reserves.

In the model of selective and compensatory optimization, there are three interacting elements and processes. First, there is the element of *selection*, which refers to an increasing restriction of one's life world to fewer domains of functioning because of an aging loss in the range of adaptive potential. It is the adaptive task of the person and society to concentrate on those domains that are of high priority and involve a convergence of environmental demands and individual motivations, skills, and biological

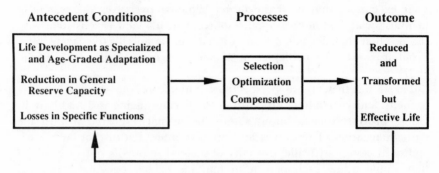

Figure 1.4. The ongoing dynamics of selective optimization with compensation. The process is a lifelong phenomenon, but it is amplified in old age. The essentials of the process are universal. Its phenotypic manifestation, however, varies widely between individuals.

capacity. Although selection connotes a reduction in the number of high-efficacy domains, it can also involve new or transformed domains and goals of life. Thus, the process of selection implies that an individual's expectations are adjusted to permit the subjective experience of satisfaction as well as personal control.

The second element, *optimization,* reflects the view that people engage in behaviors to enrich and augment their general reserves and to maximize their chosen life courses (and associated forms of behavior) with regard to quantity and quality. Intervention studies on plasticity have demonstrated that old people continue to be able to implement this optimizing process.

The third element, *compensation,* results also (like selection) from restrictions in the range of plasticity or adaptive potential. It becomes operative when specific behavioral capacities are lost or are reduced below a standard required for adequate functioning. This restriction is experienced particularly at a time when situations and goal characteristics require a wide range of activity and a high level of performance (e.g., mountain climbing, competitive sports, risky traffic situations, daily hassles, and situations that require quick thinking and memorization). The element of compensation involves aspects of the mind and technology. Psychological compensatory efforts include, for instance, the use of new mnemonic strategies (including external memory aids) when internal memory mechanics or strategies are insufficient. The use of a hearing aid would be an instance of compensation by means of technology.

Example: Cognitive functioning. Table 1.2 describes the process of selective optimization with compensation for the domain of intellectual aging. The

Table 1.2. *Selective optimization with compensation: A process prototypical of adaptive life-span development of cognitive functioning*

- A general feature of life-span development is an age-related increase in specialization (selection) of motivational and cognitive resources and skills.
- There are two main features of the aging of cognitive functions:
  (1) The reserve capacity for peak or maximum performances in fluid functioning (mechanics of intelligence) is reduced.
  (2) Some procedural and declarative knowledge systems (pragmatics of intelligence) can continue to evolve and function at peak levels.
- When and if limits of reserve capacity (especially in the mechanics) are exceeded during the course of aging for a given individual, the following developmental consequences result:
  (1) Increased selection (channeling) and further reduction of the number of high-efficacy domains.
  (2) Development of compensatory and/or substitute mechanisms.

Note: Modified from P. Baltes & M. Baltes, 1980.

example is drawn from a research program on the aging of intelligence (P. Baltes, 1987; Kliegl & P. Baltes, 1987; J. Smith et al., 1989; Staudinger et al., 1989; Thompson & Kliegl, 1989). In this research program, two large systems of intelligence are differentiated: the knowledge-free, fluid mechanics and the knowledge-rich, crystallized pragmatics. Using a computer analogy, this distinction is similar to the hardware–software distinction. With respect to the fluid cognitive mechanics, a loss with age in efficiency and speed is posited. At the same time, it is argued that select aspects of the crystallized pragmatics of intelligence can be maintained into old age, perhaps even evincing some further growth.

The interesting question involving the process of selective optimization with compensation refers to the interaction between these two cognitive systems and the use of pragmatics to prevent or balance the aging decline in the mechanics of intelligence. As discussed in Proposition 5, this can be accomplished, for instance, via optimization of knowledge systems and the acquisition of compensatory thinking and memory strategies. In that context, research on mnemonic training in old age and on expert older typists was presented.

Example: Nursing homes. The process of selective optimization with compensation can be further illustrated by reference to the design and use of age-friendly environments such as nursing homes. In this instance, the process is evident at both the macrolevel and the microlevel.

At the macrolevel, the intent of nursing homes is to create a special world that, by definition, includes aspects of increased selection, optimization, and compensation. Selection is expressed by the provision of a less demanding physical and social ecology, optimization by opportunities given for practice in domains targeted for further growth, and compensation by the availability of technological and medical systems to support functions with diminished reserve capacities. It is uncertain, of course, whether all these goals are sufficiently met.

On the microlevel, research by Margret Baltes and her colleagues (M. Baltes & Reisenzein, 1986; M. Baltes & Wahl, 1987, in press; M. Baltes, Kindermann, Reisenzein, & Schmid, 1987) demonstrates how the process of selective optimization with compensation operates within the nursing home in the social interactions between elderly residents and staff. Using detailed observations of the flow of interactional patterns between elderly residents and staff, this research demonstrates two phenomena that are consistent with a model of selective optimization with compensation on a microsocial level.

First, selection and compensation are evident in the fact that elderly residents and staff display a definite pattern (social script) of resident dependency that is followed by staff support for dependency. We argue that this script implies that dependent behaviors are judged to be appropriate, and that the weaknesses of the elderly are to be compensated for by the staff. This focus on the dependence–support script is so strong that when independent behavior on the part of the elderly occurs, such behavior is ignored by the staff (see Figure 1.5). Second, this concentration on the dependence–support script enables elderly residents, at the same time, to achieve optimization in another aspect, that is, social contact. After elderly residents engage in dependent behaviors (e.g., request for bodily care), these result in prompt and reliable consequences on the part of the staff involving not only care but also social attention. Therefore, although dependent behavior may result in a lack of and possibly a loss in self-care behavior, it gives elderly nursing home residents a strategy for exerting control over their social environment, gaining social contact, and, thereby, perhaps avoiding isolation (M. Baltes, 1988; M. Baltes & Wahl, 1987).

Other examples. Selective optimization with compensation allows the elderly to engage in life tasks that are important to them despite a reduction in energy or in biological and mental reserves. As such, the strategy of selective and compensatory adaptation is hypothesized to have general or universal application. The individualization of this prototypical strategy of mastery lies in the individual patterning, which may vary according to interests, health, preferences, and resources. In each case of successful aging, there is likely to be a creative, individualized, and societally appropriate combination of selection, optimization, and compensation.

Antecedent Behavior   **Consequent Behavior**

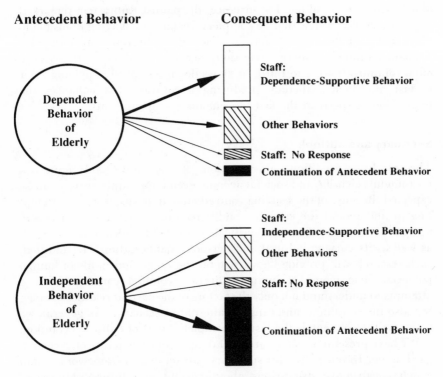

Figure 1.5. The dependence-support script in nursing homes. Dependent behavior of the elderly is firmly associated with the staff's offering of physical care. Independent behavior, however, is ignored (data from M. Baltes & Wahl, in press). A by-product is that physical care also offers the primary occasion for social contact.

Consider, for example, a person who has excelled as a marathon runner all of his or her adult life and wants to continue this activity into old age. If this runner wants to stay at the same performance level, more time and energy will need to be invested in running. As a consequence, the person will have to reduce or give up other activities (selection). At the same time, the runner will have to increase his or her training and knowledge about optimizing conditions such as the influence of daily rhythms and dieting (optimization), and finally he or she will have to become an expert in techniques aimed at reducing the impact of loss in functioning (compensation). Which shoes to use and how to treat injuries are examples of such compensatory strategies. By combining these elements of selection, optimization, and compensation, a high level of performance in marathon running might be retained into old age.

Similar selection and compensatory strategies can be imagined for almost any domain of life. For instance, the pianist Rubinstein remarked in a television interview that he conquers weaknesses of aging in his piano playing in the following manner: First, he reduces his repertoire and plays a smaller number of pieces (selection); second, he practices these more often (optimization); and third, he slows down his speed of playing prior to fast movements, thereby producing a contrast that enhances the impression of speed in the fast movements (compensation).

Summary and outlook

The search for conditions and variations of successful (good) aging is a meaningful scientific and societal agenda, even if no simple answer can be expected. Because of the seeming contradiction in terms, research attempting to understand the criteria, conditions, and variations of successful aging is likely to contribute to a critical analysis of the idea of success itself as well as its varying cultural and personal manifestations. In addition, such research will provide knowledge on the range and limits of human potential. The magic of human cultural evolution can be found in attempts to understand not only the factors of the current realities of aging but also the conditions and range of alternative scenarios. In general, we maintain that old age is the last "incomplete" part of cultural evolution.

We have presented a summary of findings about the nature of psychological aging. In our view, this summary can serve as a framework within which constructive discussions about current and future patterns of human aging can take place. Aside from the unresolved questions about appropriate criteria for successful aging, we have emphasized seven propositions or themes: (1) the distinction between normal, pathological, and optimal aging; (2) interindividual variability (heterogeneity); (3) plasticity and latent reserve capacity; (4) aging loss in the range of reserve capacity or adaptivity; (5) the enriching and compensatory role of individual and social knowledge, including technology; (6) aging-related changes toward an increasingly negative balance in gain-loss ratios; and finally (7) the phenomenon of a resilient self.

It is likely that there are several ways to derive models of successful aging from this framework of propositions (see the chapters by Featherman et al. and Fries in this volume for alternative but related conceptions). We have argued that a joint consideration of all propositions is essential for the identification of a prototypical strategy of successful aging.

One such prototypical strategy is the model of selective optimization with compensation. This model, which in its constituent features is implemented at any age, gains increasing importance in old age because of two empirical facts specific to old age: (1) The primary biological feature of normal aging is increased vulnerability and a concomitant reduction in general adaptability (reserve capacity) to environmental variation, and (2) the normal trajectory of psychological and biological development and aging is a continual evolution of specialized forms of adaptation, that is, increasing individualization of life trajectories. There are two other corollaries. First, individuals' subjective views of the self are constructed to deal well with such changes, and psychological mechanisms are available to adjust life goals and aspirations in the face of changing internal and external circumstances. Second, the process of selective optimization with compensation, although general in its "genotypic" characteristics, is quite diverse in its phenotypic manifestations. Depending on individual and societal conditions, it can take many forms in content and timing.

We contend that by using strategies of selection, optimization, and compensation, individuals can contribute to their own successful aging. On the one hand, then, it is correct that the biological nature of human aging limits more and more the overall range of possibilities in old age. On the other hand, however, the adaptive task of the aging individual is to select and concentrate on those domains that are of high priority and that involve a convergence of environmental demands and individual motivations, skills, and biological capacity. Under these conditions, Cicero's basic view may be useful after all. Although his stoicist optimism about the power of the human mind is certainly an oversimplification of the mind–body interface, forming a coalition between the human mind and society to outwit the limits of biological constraints in old age seems an obtainable and challenging goal for cultural evolution.

NOTE

In addition to the reviewers, we especially thank Steven W. Cornelius for extensive comments and helpful suggestions on an earlier draft of this chapter.

REFERENCES

Abeles, R. P. (Ed.). (1987). *Life-span perspectives and social psychology*. Hillsdale, NJ: Lawrence Erlbaum.

Antonucci, T. C., & Jackson, J. S. (1987). Social support, interpersonal efficacy, and health: A life course perspective. In L. L. Carstensen & B. A. Edelstein (Eds.), *Handbook of clinical gerontology* (pp. 291–311). New York: Pergamon Press.

Baltes, M. M. (1987). Erfolgreiches Altern als Ausdruck von Verhaltenskompetenz und Umweltqualität. In C. Niemitz (Ed.), *Der Mensch im Zusammenspiel von Anlage and Umwelt* (pp. 353–377). Frankfurt: Suhrkamp.

Baltes, M. M. (1988). The etiology and maintenance of dependency in the elderly: Three phases of operant research. *Behavior Therapy, 19,* 301–319.

Baltes, M. M., & Baltes, P. B. (1982). Microanalytic research on environmental factors and plasticity in psychological aging. In T. M. Field, A. Huston, H. C. Quay, C. Troll, & G. E. Finley (Eds.), *Review of human development* (pp. 524–539). New York: Wiley.

Baltes, M. M., & Baltes, P. B. (Eds.). (1986). *The psychology of control and aging.* Hillsdale, NJ: Lawrence Erlbaum.

Baltes, M. M., & Barton, E. M. (1979). Behavioral analysis of aging: A review of the operant model and research. *International Journal of Behavioral Development, 2,* 297–320.

Baltes, M. M., & Kindermann, T. (1985). Die Bedeutung der Plastizität für die klinische Beurteilung des Leistungsverhaltens im Alter. In D. Bente, H. Coper, & S. Kanowski (Eds.), *Hirnorganische Psychosyndrome im Alter: Vol. 2. Methoden zur Objektivierung pharmakotherapeutischer Wirkung* (pp. 171–184). Berlin: Springer Verlag.

Baltes, M. M., Kindermann, T., Reisenzein, R., & Schmid, U. (1987). Further observational data on the behavioral and social world of institutions for the aged. *Psychology and Aging, 2,* 390–403.

Baltes, M. M., & Reisenzein, R. (1986). The social world in long-term care institutions: Psychological control toward dependency. In M. M. Baltes & P. B. Baltes (Eds.), *The psychology of control and aging* (pp. 315–343). Hillsdale, NJ: Lawrence Erlbaum.

Baltes, M. M., & Wahl, H.-W. (1987). Dependency in aging. In L. L. Carstensen & B. A. Edelstein (Eds.), *Handbook of clinical gerontology* (pp. 204–221). New York: Pergamon Press.

Baltes, M. M., & Wahl, H.-W. (in press). The behavioral system of dependency in the elderly: Interaction with the social environment. In M. Ory & R. P. Abeles (Eds.), *Aging, health, and behavior.* Baltimore, MD: Johns Hopkins University Press.

Baltes, P. B. (1987). Theoretical propositions of life-span developmental psychology: On the dynamics between growth and decline. *Developmental Psychology, 23,* 611–626.

Baltes, P. B., & Baltes, M. M. (1980). Plasticity and variability in psychological aging: Methodological and theoretical issues. In G. E. Gurski (Ed.), *Determining the effects of aging on the central nervous system* (pp. 41–66). Berlin: Schering.

Baltes, P. B., Dittmann-Kohli, F., & Dixon, R. A. (1984). New perspectives on the development of intelligence in adulthood: Toward a dual-process conception and a model of selective optimization with compensation. In P. B. Baltes & O. G. Brim, Jr. (Eds.), *Life-span development and behavior* (Vol. 6, pp. 33–76). New York: Academic Press.

Baltes, P. B., & Kliegl, R. (1986). On the dynamics between growth and decline in the aging of intelligence and memory. In K. Poeck, H.-J. Freund, & H. Gänshirt (Eds.), *Neurology* (pp. 1–17). Heidelberg: Springer.

Baltes, P. B., & Kliegl, R. (1989). *Testing-the-limits research suggests irreversible aging loss in mental imagery.* Unpublished manuscript, Max Planck Institute for Human Development and Education, Berlin, Federal Republic of Germany.

Baltes, P. B., & Lindenberger, U. (1988). On the range of cognitive plasticity in old age as a function of experience: 15 years of intervention research. *Behavior Therapy, 19*, 283–300.

Baltes, P. B., & Schaie, K. W. (1976). On the plasticity of intelligence in adulthood and old age: Where Horn and Donaldson fail. *American Psychologist, 31*, 720–725.

Baltes, P. B., & Smith, J. (1990). Toward a psychology of wisdom and its ontogenesis. In R. J. Sternberg (Ed.), *Wisdom: Its nature, origins, and development* (pp. 87–120). New York: Cambridge University Press.

Baltes, P. B., Sowarka, D., & Kliegl, R. (1989). Cognitive training research on fluid intelligence in old age: What can older adults achieve by themselves? *Psychology and Aging, 4*, 217–221.

Bengtson, V. L., & Kuypers, J. A. (1985). The family support cycle: Psychosocial issues in the aging family. In J. M. A. Munnichs, P. Mussen, & E. Olbrich (Eds.), *Life-span and change in a gerontological perspective* (pp. 61–77). New York: Academic Press.

Bengtson, V. L., Reedy, M., & Gordon, C. (1985). Aging and self-concept: Personality processes and social contexts. In J. E. Birren & K. W. Schaie (Eds.), *Handbook of the psychology of aging* (2nd ed., pp. 544–593). New York: Van Nostrand Reinhold.

Berlin, I. (1988). On the pursuit of the ideal. *New York Review of Books, 35*, 16.

Birren, J. E., & Bengtson, V. L. (Eds.). (1988). *Emergent theories of aging.* New York: Springer.

Bornstein, R., & Smircina, M. T. (1982). The status of empirical support for the hypothesis of increased interindividual variability in aging. *Gerontologist, 22*, 258–260.

Brandtstädter, J. (1984). Personal and social control over development: Some implications of an action perspective in life-span developmental psychology. In P. B. Baltes & O. G. Brim, Jr. (Eds.), *Life-span development and behavior* (Vol. 6, pp. 1–32). New York: Academic Press.

Brandtstädter, J., Krampen, G., & Heil, F. E. (1986). Personal control and emotional evaluation of development in partnership relations during adulthood. In M. M. Baltes & P. B. Baltes (Eds.), *The psychology of control and aging* (pp. 265–296). Hillsdale, NJ: Lawrence Erlbaum.

Brim, O. G., Jr. (1988). Losing and winning: The nature of ambition in everyday life. *Psychology Today, 9*, 48–52.

Brim, O. G., Jr., & Kagan, J. (1980). Constancy and change: A view of the issues. In O. G. Brim, Jr., & J. Kagan (Eds.), *Constancy and change in human development* (pp. 1–25). Cambridge: Harvard University Press.

Brown, A. L. (1982). Learning and development: The problem of compatibility, access, and induction. *Human Development, 25*, 89–115.

Busse, E. W., & Maddox, G. L. (1985), *The Duke Longitudinal Studies of normal aging: 1955–1980.* New York: Springer.

Butt, D. S., & Beiser, M. (1987). Successful aging: A theme for international psychology. *Psychology and Aging, 2*, 87–94.

Cattell, R. B. (1971). *Abilities: Their structure, growth, and action.* Boston: Houghton Mifflin.

Charness, N. (Ed.). (1985). *Aging and human performance.* Chichester, England: John Wiley & Sons.

Cicero, M. T. (44 B.C.) *Cato major – De senectute.* (Original work translated by J.

Logan and published by B. Franklin 1744 as *Cato major; or, His discourse of old age*. Philadelphia, PA: Benjamin Franklin.) Reprinted by Arno Press, 1979.

Coper, H., Jänicke, B., & Schulze, G. (1986). Biopsychological research on adaptivity across the life span of animals. In P. B. Baltes, D. L. Featherman, & R. M. Lerner (Eds.), *Life-span development and behavior* (Vol. 7, pp. 207–232). Hillsdale, NJ: Lawrence Erlbaum.

Costa, P. T., Jr., & Andres, R. (1986). Patterns of age changes. In I. Rossman (Ed.), *Clinical geriatrics* (pp. 23–30). New York: Lippincott.

Craik, F. I. M. (1977). Age differences in human memory. In J. E. Birren & K. W. Schaie (Eds.), *Handbook of the psychology of aging* (pp. 384–420). New York: Van Nostrand Reinhold.

Craik, F. I. M. (1983). On the transfer of information from temporary to permanent memory. *Philosophical Transactions of the Royal Society of London, B-302*, 341–359.

Dannefer, D. (1984). Adult development and social theory: A paradigmatic reappraisal. *American Sociological Review, 49*, 100–116.

Denney, N. W. (1984). A model of cognitive development across the life span. *Developmental Review, 4*, 171–191.

Dixon, R. A., & Baltes, P. B. (1986). Toward life-span research on the functions and pragmatics of intelligence. In R. J. Sternberg & R. K. Wagner (Eds.), *Practical intelligence: Nature and origins of competence in the everyday world* (pp. 203–235). New York: Cambridge University Press.

Epstein, S. (1981). The unity principle versus the reality and pleasure principles, or the tale of the scorpion and the frog. In M. D. Lynch, A. A. Norem-Hebeisen, & K. J. Gergen (Eds.), *Self-concept: Advances in theory and research* (pp. 27–38). Cambridge, MA: Ballinger.

Ericsson, K. A. (1985). Memory skill. *Canadian Journal of Psychology, 39*, 188–231.

Erikson, E. H., Erikson, J. M., & Kivnick, H. (1986). *Vital involvement in old age: The experience of old age in our time*. London: Norton.

Featherman, D. L. (1983). The life-span perspective in social science research. In P. B. Baltes & O. G. Brim, Jr. (Eds.), *Life-span development and behavior* (Vol. 5, pp. 1–59). New York: Academic Press.

Featherman, D. L. (1986). Biography, society, and history: Individual development as a population process. In A. B. Sørensen, F. E. Weinert, & L. R. Sherrod (Eds.), *Human development and the life course: Multidisciplinary perspectives* (pp. 99–149). Hillsdale, NJ: Lawrence Erlbaum.

Felton, B. J. (1987). International cohort variation on happiness: Some hypotheses and exploratory analyses. *International Journal of Aging and Human Development, 25*, 27–42.

Filipp, S.-H., & Klauer, T. (1986). Conceptions of self over the life span: reflections on the dialectics of change. In M. M. Baltes & P. B. Baltes (Eds.), *The psychology of control and aging* (pp. 167–205). Hillsdale, NJ: Lawrence Erlbaum.

Finch, C. E. (1988). Neural endocrine approaches to the resolution of time as a dependent variable in the aging processes of mammals. *Gerontologist, 28*, 29–42.

Fries, J. F. (1983). The compression of morbidity. *Milbank Memorial Fund Quarterly, 61*, 397–419.

Fries, J. F., & Crapo, L. M. (1981). *Vitality and aging*. San Francisco: Freeman & Co.

Greenough, W. T. (1986). What's special about development? Thoughts on the bases of experience-sensitive synaptic plasticity. In W. T. Greenough & J. M. Juraska (Eds.), *Developmental Neuropsychology* (pp. 387–407). Orlando, FL: Academic Press.

Greenwald, A. G. (1980). The totalitarian ego: Fabrication and revision of personal history. *American Psychologist, 35,* 603–618.

Guthke, J. (1972). *Zur Diagnostik der intellektuellen Lernfähigkeit.* Berlin: Deutscher Verlag der Wissenschaften.

Guthke, J. (1982). The learning test concept: An alternative to the traditional static intelligence test. *German Journal of Psychology, 6,* 306–324.

Gutmann, D. (1987). *Reclaimed powers: Toward a new psychology of men and women in later life.* New York: Basic Books.

Harris, L. (1975). *The myth and reality of aging in America.* Washington, DC: National Council on the Aging.

Havighurst, R. J. (1963). Successful aging. In R. H. Williams, C. Tibbits, & W. Donahue (Eds.), *Processes of aging* (Vol. 1, pp. 299–320). New York: Atherton Press.

Heckhausen, J., Dixon, R. A., & Baltes, P. B. (1989). Gains and losses in development throughout adulthood as perceived by different adult age groups. *Developmental Psychology, 25,* 109–121.

Henry, J. P. (1988). The archetypes of power and intimacy. In J. E. Birren & V. L. Bengtson (Eds.), *Emergent theories of aging* (pp. 269–298). New York: Springer.

Holliday, S. G., & Chandler, M. J. (1986). Wisdom: Explorations in adult competence. In J. A. Meacham (Ed.), *Contributions to human development* (Vol. 17, pp. 1–96). Basel: Karger.

Horn, J. L. (1970). Organization of data on life-span development of human abilities. In L. R. Goulet & P. B. Baltes (Eds.), *Life-span developmental psychology: Research and theory* (pp. 423–466). New York: Academic Press.

Hoyer, W. J. (1985). Aging and the development of expert cognition. In T. M. Schlechter & M. P. Toglia (Eds.), *New directions in cognitive science* (pp. 69–87). Norwood, NJ: Ablex.

Hunt, E. (1978). Mechanics of verbal ability. *Psychological Review, 85,* 109–130.

Kahn, R.L., & Antonucci, T. C. (1980). Convoys over the life course: Attachment, roles, and social support. In P. B. Baltes & O. G. Brim, Jr. (Eds.), *Life-span development and behavior* (Vol. 3, pp. 253–286). New York: Academic Press.

Kliegl, R. (1989). *Formation of expert knowledge in a mnemonic skill: Twelve case studies of young and old adults.* Unpublished manuscript, Max Planck Institute for Human Development and Education, Berlin, Federal Republic of Germany.

Kliegl, R., & Baltes, P. B. (1987). Theory-guided analysis of development and aging mechanisms through testing-the-limits and research on expertise. In C. Schooler & K. W. Schaie (Eds.), *Cognitive functioning and social structure over the life course* (pp. 95–119). Norwood, NJ: Ablex.

Kliegl, R., Smith, J., & Baltes, P. B. (1989). Testing-the-limits and the study of adult age differences in cognitive plasticity of a mnemonic skill. *Developmental Psychology, 25,* 247–256.

Labouvie-Vief, G. (1981). Proactive and reactive aspects of constructivism: Growth and aging in life-span perspective. In R. M. Lerner & N. A. Busch-Rossnagel (Eds.), *Individuals as producers of their development* (pp. 197–230). New York: Academic Press.

Labouvie-Vief, G. (1985). Intelligence and cognition. In J. E. Birren & K. W. Schaie (Eds.), *Handbook of the psychology of aging* (2nd ed., pp. 500–530). New York: Van Nostrand Reinhold.

Labouvie-Vief, G. (Ed.). (1986). *Developmental dimensions of adult adaptation: Perspectives on mind, self, and emotion*. Unpublished manuscript, Wayne State University, Department of Psychology, Detroit.

Lachman, M. E. (1986). Personal control in later life: Stability, change, and cognitive correlates. In M. M. Baltes & P. B. Baltes (Eds.), *The psychology of control and aging* (pp. 207–236). Hillsdale, NJ: Lawrence Erlbaum.

Langer, E. (1989). *Mindfulness*. Reading, MA: Addison-Wesley.

Lawton, M. P. (1982). Environments and living arrangements. In R. H. Binstock, W.-S. Chow, & J. H. Schulz (Eds.), *International perspectives on aging* (pp. 159–192). New York: United Nations Fund for Population Activities.

Lawton, M. P. (1988). Behavior-relevant ecological factors. In K. W. Schaie & C. Schooler (Eds.), *Social structures and aging: Psychological processes* (pp. 57–78). Hillsdale, NJ: Lawrence Erlbaum.

Lehr, U. (1987). *Zur Situation der älterwerdenden Frau*. Munich: C. H. Beck.

Lehr, U., & Thomae, H. (Eds.). (1987). *Formen seelischen Alterns*. Stuttgart: Enke.

Lerner, R. M. (1984). *On the nature of human plasticity*. New York: Cambridge University Press.

Lindenberger, U. (1990). *The effects of professional expertise and cognitive aging on skilled memory performance*. Unpublished doctoral dissertation, Free University of Berlin.

Maddox, G. L. (1987). Aging differently. *Gerontologist, 27,* 557–564.

Mandl, H., & Spada, H. (Eds.). (1988). *Wissenspsychologie*. Munich and Weinheim: Psychologie Verlags Union.

Markus, H., & Nurius, P. (1986). Possible selves. *American Psychologist, 41,* 954–969.

Markus, H., & Wurf, E. (1987). The dynamic self-concept: A social psychological perspective. *Annual Review of Psychology, 38,* 299–337.

Meacham, J. A. (1982). Wisdom and the context of knowledge: Knowing that one doesn't know. In D. Kuhn & J. A. Meacham (Eds.), *On the development of developmental psychology* (pp. 111–134). Basel: Karger.

Mosher-Ashley, P. M. (1986–1987). Procedural and methodological parameters in behavioral-gerontological research: A review. *International Journal of Aging and Human Development, 24,* 189–229.

Neisser, U. (1988). Five kinds of self-knowledge. *Philosophical Psychology, 1,* 35–59.

Neugarten, B. L. (Ed.). (1968). *Middle age and aging: A reader in social psychology*. Chicago: University of Chicago Press.

Neugarten, B. L. (1987). Kansas City studies of adult life. In G. L. Maddox (Ed.), *The encyclopedia of aging* (pp. 372–373). New York: Springer.

Palmore, E. (1979). Predictors of successful aging. *Gerontologist, 19,* 427–431.

Parmelee, P. A., & Lawton, M. P. (1990). The design of special environments for the aged. In J. E. Birren & K. W. Schaie (Eds.), *Handbook of the psychology of aging* (3rd ed., pp. 464–488). New York: Van Nostrand Reinhold.

Perlmutter, M. (Ed.). (in press). *Late-life potential*. Washington, DC: Gerontological Society of Ameria.

Plomin, R., & Thompson, L. (1986). Life-span developmental behavioral genetics. In P. B. Baltes, D. L. Featherman, & R. M. Lerner (Eds.), *Life-span development and behavior* (Vol. 8, pp. 1–31). Hillsdale, NJ: Lawrence Erlbaum.

Riley, M. W. (1983, December). *Aging and society: Notes on the development of new understandings*. The Leon and Josephine Winkelman Lecture, School of Social Work, University of Michigan.

Riley, M. W. (1985). Age strata in social systems. In R. H. Binstock & E. Shanas (Eds.), *Handbook of aging and the social sciences* (Vol. 3, pp. 369–411). New York: Van Nostrand Reinhold.

Roether, D. (1983). Entwicklungspsychologische Beiträge zum lebenslangen Lernkonzept. *Zeitschrift für Gerontologie, 16*, 234–240.

Roether, D. (1986). *Lernfähigkeit im Erwachsenenalter: Ein Beitrag zur klinischen Entwicklungspsychologie*. Leipzig: Hirzel.

Rowe J. W., & Kahn, R. L. (1987). Human aging: Usual and successful. *Science, 237*, 143–149.

Rybash, J. M., Hoyer, W. J., & Roodin, P. A. (1986). *Adult cognition and aging: Developmental changes in processing, knowing, and thinking*. Elmsford, NY: Pergamon Press.

Ryff, C. D. (1982). Successful aging: A developmental approach, *Gerontologist, 22*, 209–214.

Ryff, C. D. (1984). Personality development from the inside: The subjective experience of change in adulthood and aging. In P. B. Baltes & O. G. Brim, Jr. (Eds.), *Life-span development and behavior* (Vol. 6, pp. 243–279). New York: Academic Press.

Salthouse, T. A. (1984). Effects of age and skill in typing. *Journal of Experimental Psychology: General, 113*, 345–371.

Salthouse, T. A. (1985). *A theory of cognitive aging*. Amsterdam: North-Holland.

Schaie, K. W. (1979). The primary mental abilities in adulthood: An exploration in the development of psychometric intelligence. In P. B. Baltes & O. G. Brim, Jr. (Eds.), *Life-span development and behavior* (Vol. 3, pp. 67–115). New York: Academic Press.

Schaie, K. W. (Ed.). (1983). *Longitudinal studies of adult psychological development*. New York: Guilford Press.

Schaie, K. W., & Willis, S. L. (1986). Can adult intellectual decline be reversed? *Developmental Psychology, 22*, 223–232.

Schmidt, L. R. (1971). Testing the limits im Leistungsverhalten: Möglichkeiten und Grenzen. In E. Duhm (Ed.), *Praxis der klinischen Psychologie* (Vol. 2, pp. 9–29). Göttingen: Hogrefe.

Schwartz, A. N. (1974). Staff development and morale building in nursing homes. *Gerontologist, 14*, 50–53.

Schwarzer, R., Lange, B., & Jerusalem, M. (1982). Selbstkonzeptentwicklung nach einem Bezugsgruppenwechsel. *Zeitschrift für Entwicklungspsychologie und Pädagogische Psychologie, 14*, 125–140.

Shock, N. W. (1977). System integration. In C. E. Finch & L. Hayflick (Eds.), *Handbook of the biology of aging* (pp. 639–665). New York: Van Nostrand Reinhold.

Shock, N. W., Greulich, R. C., Costa, P. T., Andres, R., Lakatta, E. G., Arenberg, D., & Tobin, J. D. (1984). *Normal human aging: The Baltimore Longitudinal Study on Aging* (Report No. 84-2450). Washington, DC: NIH Publications.

Singer, W. (1987). Activity-dependent self-organization of synaptic connections as a substrate of learning. In J.-P. Changeux & M. Konishi (Eds.), *The neural and molecular bases of learning* (pp. 301–336). New York: John Wiley & Sons.

Smith, J., & Baltes, P. B. (1990). Wisdom-related knowledge: Age/cohort differences in response to life-planning problems. *Development Psychology, 26*, 494–505.

Smith, J., Dixon, R. A., & Baltes, P. B. (1989). Expertise in life planning: A new research approach to investigating aspects of wisdom. In M. L. Commons, J. D. Sinnott, F. A. Richards, & C. Armon (Eds.), *Adult development: Vol. 1. Comparisons and applications of developmental models* (pp. 307–331). New York: Praeger.

Smith, M. B. (1978). Perspectives on selfhood. *American Psychologist, 33,* 1053–1063.

Sowarka, D. (1989). Weisheit und weise Personen: Common-Sense-Konzepte älterer Menschen. *Zeitschrift für Entwicklungspsychologie und Pädagogische Psychologie, 21,* 87–109.

Staudinger, U. M. (1989). *The study of life review: An approach to the investigation of intellectual development across the life span* (Studien und Berichte des Max-Planck-Instituts für Bildungsforschung, No. 47). Stuttgart: Klett Verlag.

Staudinger, U. M., Cornelius, S. W., & Baltes, P. B. (1989). The aging of intelligence: Potential and limits. *Annals of the Academy of Political and Social Sciences, 503,* 43–59.

Sternberg, R. J. (Ed.). (in press). *Wisdom: Its nature, origins, and development.* New York: Cambridge University Press.

Stones, M. J., & Kozma, A. (1985). Physical performance. In N. Charness (Ed.), *Aging and human performance* (pp. 261–291). New York: John Wiley & Sons.

Suls, J. N., & Mullen, B. (1982). From the cradle to the grave: Comparison and self-evaluation across the life span. In J. N. Suls (Ed.), *Psychological perspectives on the self* (Vol. 1, pp. 97–128). Hillsdale, NJ: Lawrence Erlbaum.

Thomae, H. (1979). The concept of development and life-span developmental psychology. In P. B. Baltes & O. G. Brim, Jr. (Eds.), *Life-span development and behavior* (Vol. 2, pp. 282–312). New York: Academic Press.

Thomae, H. (1987). Alternsformen: Wege zu ihrer methodischen und begrifflichen Erfassung. In U. Lehr & H. Thomae (Eds.), *Formen seelischen Alterns* (pp. 173–195). Stuttgart: Enke.

Thompson, L. A., & Kliegl, R. (1989). *Adult age differences in connecting thoughts during elaborative encoding.* Manuscript submitted for publication.

Veroff, J., Douvan, E., & Kulka, R. A. (1981). *The inner American: A self-portrait from 1957 to 1976.* New York: Basic Books.

Weinert, F. E. (1986). Developmental variations of memory performance and memory-related knowledge across the life-span. In A. B. Sørensen, F. E. Weinert, & L. R. Sherrod (Eds.), *Human development and the life course: Multidisciplinary perspectives* (pp. 535–554). Hillsdale, NJ: Lawrence Erlbaum.

Whitbourne, S. K. (1985). *The aging body.* New York: Springer.

Williams, R. H., & Wirths, C. G. (1965). *Lives through the years: Styles of life and successful aging.* New York: Atherton Press.

Willis, S. L. (1987). Cognitive training and everyday competence. In K. W. Schaie (Ed.), *Annual Review of Gerontology and Geriatrics* (Vol. 7, pp. 159–188). New York: Springer.

Wills, T. A. (1981). Downward comparison principles in social psychology. *Psychological Bulletin, 90,* 245–271.

Wisocki, P. (1984). Behavior modification in the elderly. In M. Hersen, R. M. Eisler, & P. Miller (Eds.), *Progress in behavioral modification* (Vol. 16, pp. 121–157). New York: Academic Press.

Wood, J. V. (1989). Theory and research concerning social comparisons of personal attributes. *Psychological Bulletin, 106,* 231–248.

2 Medical perspectives upon successful aging

JAMES F. FRIES

Introduction: The minimum morbidity model and the compression of morbidity

Successful aging, viewed from a medical or public health viewpoint, consists of optimizing life expectancy while at the same time minimizing physical, psychological, and social morbidity, overwhelmingly concentrated in the final years of life. Thus, the achievement of successful aging requires that the onset of infirmity, on average, increase more rapidly than average life expectancy, compressing morbidity into a shorter period (e.g., Fries, 1980, 1983, 1987a, 1987b; Fries & Crapo, 1981). Successful aging implies and requires morbidity compression.

The national illness burden in developed nations has shifted over recent decades from acute to chronic illness and from younger to older individuals (e.g., Fries & Crapo, 1981). Increasingly, the problems of chronic illness mix with and finally give way to problems of senescence. Our future population will contain more old individuals as successive birth cohorts continually increase in size and because, until recently, life expectancy from age 65 has also been increasing. Projections made from these trends have led some to postulate a gloomy future of increasing dependency, worsening health, and spiraling health care costs. The ability of society to pay ever-increasing costs for ever-more vegetative existence has been called into question.

However, there is the much more hopeful paradigm of the compression of morbidity elaborated here and elsewhere (e.g., Fries, 1988). Rather than assuming that disease is a fixed part of life and the life span indefinitely extensible, the compression of morbidity thesis states that the species' life span is finite and the onset of chronic disease is relatively easily delayed. Thus, the period from onset of chronic infirmity to death may be shortened, with benefit, to both individuals and society.

The basic syllogism of the compression of morbidity is that because the age of first chronic infirmity can be postponed but the life span itself is genetically fixed, the period of infirmity can be shortened. In more complete formulation, the theorem holds that (a) if morbidity may be defined as that period from the onset of the first irreversible chronic disease or aging marker until death, (b) if the date of occurrence of that marker can be postponed until later in life, and (c) if the rate of such postponement can be greater than the rate of increase in adult life expectancy, then (d) morbidity for the average person can be compressed into a shorter period of time.

This model is a dynamic one, with changes envisioned in both average life expectancy and average time of first infirmity. Critical to prediction of future morbidity are the relative rates of change in these two markers, each projected to increase. A central issue, therefore, is whether it is easier to prevent death or to prevent sickness.

In the first three quarters of the twentieth century, there seems little doubt that morbidity for the average person increased (e.g., Fries & Crapo, 1981; Gruenberg, 1977; Schneider & Brody, 1983). Health advances over this period in the United States, for example, were characterized by sharp reductions in infant mortality and major increases in average life expectancy from birth, from 47 years at the turn of the century to 75 years today. Over this period, there was decline and virtual elimination of most of the acute infectious causes of death prominent early in the century and concomitant major increases in chronic and morbid diseases such as atherosclerosis, cancer, and osteoarthritis.

Nevertheless, by the late 1970s indications began to appear that these historic trends might be ready for equally historic changes. Thus, with decreases in infant mortality and other deaths in early life, essentially intact cohorts began to achieve senior status. For example, nearly 90% of white females are expected to live to the age of 70 or more. This suggested that the exchange of chronic diseases for acute, a driving force toward increasing morbidity, was nearly complete and that morbidity could not continue to increase by this mechanism. Second, for the first time there was a decrease in chronic illness. Atherosclerosis mortality, responsible for nearly half of all deaths, began to decrease remarkably in the United States in about 1970, at an average decline of about 3% a year (e.g., Stern, 1979). Finally, to a clinician such as myself, there was a manifest change in senior health problems, with the frailty resulting from senescence increasingly dominant over specific medical disability. At autopsy, seniors were found frequently free of obvious pathological "causes" of death. These observations suggested that life expectancy increases might soon begin to slow. A variety of demographic projections suggested that the optimal human average life expectancy might closely approximate 85 years (e.g., Fries, 1980). With life expectancy for females already beginning to crowd 80 years, this again suggested slower future increases in average life expectancy.

The compression of morbidity hypothesis was advanced in 1979 without specification of its exact timing but with the suggestion that we might expect to see morbidity compression over the next 50 years. The thesis contained a number of implicit predictions. Life expectancy increases would slow, and this phenomenon would first be noted in females. The male–female gap in life expectancy (which had increased during the 1970s in the United States to 7.9 years) should decrease. Interventions based on primary prevention (such as smoking cessation, exercise, and cholesterol reduction) should have greater effects on decreasing morbidity than decreasing death rates. Changes in habits (such as decreasing smoking) should result in decreased health care need rather than, as feared by some, increasing costs by increasing the length of life. And, examination of the patterns responsible for decreases in chronic disease should reveal that changes in age-specific incidence have been more important than changes in survival after initial diagnosis.

Evidence accruing over the past 9 years is strongly supportive of the hypothesis, demonstrates that the compression of morbidity is occurring in the United States at the present time, and indicates strategies for further compression.

Recent evidence for the hypothesis

Physical plasticity in seniors

Studies from all areas of gerontology have demonstrated increased variability between individuals with increasing age. Intervention studies consistently show that physical reserves in individuals over the age of 70 can be increased (e.g., Larson & Bruce, 1986). An extensive literature documents the training effects of aerobic exercise; decreases in resting pulse rate, decreases in blood pressure, and increases in maximum cardiac output occur at all ages (e.g., Bortz, 1982; Bruce, 1984; Paffenbarger, Hyde, Wing, & Hsieh, 1986). Lane and colleagues (1986, 1987) studied the development of musculoskeletal disability by year of age in a cross-sectional study comparing nearly 500 runners and a similar number of carefully matched community controls aged 54–76. Functional ability showed virtually no decline with age in the active group, and preliminary longitudinal data confirm these findings. The rate of development of disability was nearly 10 times greater in the control population than in the aerobically active one. Similarly, bone density was increased by 40% in both males and postmenopausal women who run compared with matched controls; the medical target here is 650,000 yearly osteoporotic fractures (e.g., Brody, 1985). Reaction time is improved by aerobic activity and by racquet sports (Spirduso, 1980). The ability to improve in physical and emotional function parameters ranging from depression to mobility has been repeatedly demonstrated. Improvement in serum cholesterol, systolic blood pressure, and many other aging markers is readily achieved by appropriate interventions (e.g., Fries & Crapo, 1981). The social science literature, discussed abundantly elsewhere, similarly demonstrates both increased variability with age and the ability of well-conceived interventions to improve status in the 70s and 80s (e.g., Baltes, 1987; Berkman & Syme, 1979; Fries & Crapo, 1981; Plemons, Willis, & Baltes, 1978).

Associations between habits and health

The strong associations between life-style and health are increasingly a matter of public knowledge. Beginning with the demonstration of a link between smoking behavior and lung cancer and the early observations of the Framingham study, risk factor models have been developed that express these relationships (e.g., Surgeon General, 1983; Farquhar, 1987). Risk factor models are successful in explaining the majority of the variance with specific medical end points such as coronary artery disease. Commonly recognized risk factors include cigarette smoking, excess alcohol consumption, inadequate exercise, increased dietary saturated fat, failure to use automobile seat belts, excessive salt intake, inadequate fiber intake, and obesity. With most risk factors the mechanisms linking habits and health are sufficiently understood so as to establish causality. Risk factor models imply the ability to modify the rate of accumulation of chronic pathology and thus the ability to alter disease incidence rates (e.g., Bairey, 1986).

Risk factor models for vascular disease and for most solid cancers are well established, and risk factors have been identified to some degree for osteoarthritis, diabetes, emphysema, cirrhosis, ulcers, gallbladder disease, varicose veins, and a great many other problems, probably representing 75% or more of mortality and morbidity. To these could be added the social risk factors of pollution, education level, and socioeconomic status.

A substantial remainder, perhaps 20% or 25%, of human disease is probably not risk factor related and will not be affected by strategies described in this paper; such conditions, including Alzheimer's disease, rheumatoid arthritis, multiple sclerosis, and Parkinson's disease, may prove amenable to biomedical solutions.

Changing national habit patterns

A massive "experiment of nature" is under way in the United States and, to a lesser extent, in other developed nations. Risk factors are consistently being reduced (e.g., Surgeon General, 1983; Goldman & Cook, 1984). Cigarette smoking, defined in terms of per capita tobacco consumption, has declined by over 40%, and the rate of change is accelerating. Saturated fat intake has similarly declined by more than one third, there has been a slight decrease in alcohol consumption, seat belt use is increasingly prevalent, there has been a decrease in the national average serum cholesterol, and at least 30 million Americans regularly practice aerobic exercise. If risk factor models are even approximately accurate, these changes are currently reducing age-specific incidence rates for heart disease, stroke, and important cancers.

Decreasing age-specific incidence of chronic disease

The age-specific incidence of mortality from vascular disease has been steadily declining in the United States; these data are firm and generally accepted. Age-specific incidence rates, however, are much harder to measure, and data often are not adequate. In the numerically most important areas, however – heart disease, lung cancer, and seat belt use – data are now convincing.

Pell and Fayerweather (1985) found a steady decline in age-specific incidence rates of myocardial infarction among male employees of the E. I. du Pont de Nemours & Company over a 24-year period; a total decline of 28.2% was observed. As predicted by the compression of morbidity model, the declines were most striking at younger ages. Males averaging 30 years of age showed incidence rates declining by 50%; those at age 40, 39.4%; those at age 50, 25.9% and those at age 60, 22.3%. The slope for declining incidence was significantly steeper than the slope of the relatively small declines in survival after the initial event measured by 24-hour and 30-day case fatality rates ($p > .001$).

U.S. hospital discharge survey data show steadily declining hospitalization rates for myocardial infarction. The Kaiser-Permanente study in northern California (e.g., Friedman, 1979) confirmed decreased incidence rates over time for acute myocardial infarction. The Minnesota Heart Survey (Gillum et al., 1983) reported a significant decline in hospitalization rates for acute myocardial infarction between 1970 and 1980. Analysis of short-term hospital stays in U.S. hospitals over time (National Center for Health Statistics 1965, 1968, 1974, 1978) suggests that the average age of hospitalization for cardiovascular disease increased more rapidly over a 13-year period (average increase of 4 years) than did life expectancy (2 years) over the same period.

Changes in lung cancer incidence rates are easier to estimate, because cure is unusual and survival times have not been changing (e.g., Bailar & Smith, 1986). Thus, incidence rates must almost exactly parallel mortality rates. Moreover, as with cardiovascular disease, models predicting risk of developing lung cancer are related to exposure factors (such as pack-years of cigarette exposure), and a reduction of exposure (fewer pack-years at a given age) logically requires postponement of incidence (e.g., Surgeon General, 1983).

Recently, in full agreement with the compression of morbidity model, Horm and Kessler (1986) have documented the first declining rates of lung cancer mortality in men in the United States; the overall decline began in 1982. Moreover, mortality has been decreasing for men under 45 since at least 1973 and for men between 45 and 54 years of age since 1978. As with the heart disease data, declines occur first and are most pronounced at younger ages.

Automobile seat belt use has been steadily increasing in the United States, partly because of public education and partly because of increasingly strict laws. Positive effects, recently examined by Williams and Lund (1986), include substantial reductions in both mortality and injury, with serious injury being approximately 10 times as prevalent as death. Effects on morbidity, therefore, are more pronounced than effects on mortality.

Randomized controlled trials of primary prevention

Randomized controlled trials (RCT) constitute the most rigorous technique known for testing of medical hypotheses. A number of very large primary prevention RCTs have been performed, and these experiments document unequivocally that these interventions affected sickness far more than death.

The Multiple Risk Factor Intervention Trial (MRFIT) study (1982, 1986) was a 7-year 12,000-subject RCT of the effects of reduction of smoking, reduction of hypertension, and reduction of serum cholesterol through diet. Unfortunately, all-cause mortality actually increased in the treatment group! (There was a statistically nonsignificant 7% decrease in coronary death rates.) On the other hand, dramatic decreases in morbidity were observed; morbidity was decreased an average of 23%, statistically significant at the $p < .001$ level. There were two more deaths in the treated group than in the control group, but there were 171 fewer subjects with angina pectoris, 35 fewer with intermittent claudication, 15 fewer with heart failure, and 29 fewer with peripheral occlusive disease. In total, there were 268 fewer morbid events in the prevention group. This represents experimental demonstration of the ability to compress morbidity in the most important single area, cardiovascular disease. Because mortality was not changed, one would *not* expect a compensating increase in other forms of morbidity not measured.

These data are fully consistent from study to study. The Lipid Research Clinic Coronary Primary Prevention Trial (1984), a massive placebo-controlled randomized study of over 4,000 individuals, examined the effect of lowering total serum cholesterol by use of cholestyramine. Coronary deaths were decreased by 20%, statistically significant at the .05 level. All-cause mortality, however, was reduced only 3%, an insignificant amount. As in the MRFIT study, all-cause morbidity was reduced by 20%, statistically significant at the .001 level. In absolute terms, deaths were decreased by 3 and morbid events by 176.

The Veterans' Administration Cooperative Study Group on Anti-hypertensive Agents (1970) gave similar results. Treatment was found statistically effective in preventing congestive heart failure and stroke (morbidity), but no significant reduction of coronary heart disease deaths or total deaths was found. The most recently released large trials show the same pattern. The Helsinki Heart Study (Frick et al., 1987) used Gem-fibrosil to reduce cholesterol in the treatment group. Total deaths were equal in the two groups; coronary heart disease was decreased in the treatment group. The Physicians' Aspirin Study (Physicians' Health Study Research Group, 1988) involved 60,000 American Physicians randomized to placebo or aspirin, one tablet taken every other day. There was a major decrease in heart attacks, wildly trumpeted in the press. Total deaths, however, were exactly the same, 44 and 44 in the treatment and control groups respectively. Thus, it has been unequivocally documented that experimental preventive measures in the largest and most important disease area, heart disease, decrease morbidity rates more than mortality rates, resulting in compression of morbidity.

It is interesting to speculate about the reasons behind the paradox of constant total death rates despite decreases in coronary artery deaths in these studies. The fact of death is easy to ascertain, whereas attribution of cause is more difficult; hence it is possible that some hidden misclassification bias occurred. This would be a trivial explanation. Because a 20% decrease in coronary deaths should result in only perhaps a 5% decrease in total deaths, statistical power may not have been adequate for detection of an effect. Nevertheless, for all of the stories to have had similar "bad luck" seems unlikely.

More likely, these studies have affected coronary artery disease death rates, but death from competing causes has occurred at a rate exceeding that expected. Two explanations can be offered. First, the competing risk of senescent loss of reserve function, not usually estimated, could be operative. Second, interaction terms between different causes of death could also be responsible. If proximity to genetic senescence in the individual simultaneously effects susceptibility to several diseases, then the various hazards are not independent of each other and removal of risk factors for one merely makes it likely that the cause of death will be changed, not its occurrence. Because national decreases in chronic disease death rates have been occurring, there should have been some net gain in mortality in these studies unless the intervention itself was sometimes fatal, but these statistical considerations may have rendered a small change undetectable. That the explanation cannot be solely toxicity of the drugs studied is made clear by the consistent results in studies employing only diet or exercise (Oliver, 1988). Of substantial interest is the fact that study subjects have often been unusually well educated and health aware and thus their overall death rates are lower than that of the general population. It is in such groups, already with excellent life expectancy, that difficulty in extending the length of life should be greatest.

Medical care in the last year of life

Some 18% of lifetime medical costs occur in the last year of life. In many studies, notably those of N. P. Roos and Shapiro (1981) and Fuchs (1984), these effects are noted to be further concentrated into the last 1 or 2 months of life. Recognition of this phenomenon is critical for projection of future health care needs. Although these large terminal costs undoubtedly include many futile and expensive expenditures that could be targeted for cost-cutting measures, a more profound point is at issue. Medical expenses are closely tied to time of death and more loosely tied to time from birth. For any given year of age, two subpopulations of persons are present: one consisting of those who will die within the year and one consisting of those who will not. The first subgroup is very expensive to care for; the second is very inexpensive. For each successive year of age, the relative proportions of these two subpopulations change so that there is a greater percentage of those who will die within the year and a smaller percentage who will live through the year. This phenomenon entirely accounts for increased health care costs per year of age above age 65 (Fuchs, 1984). The critical error in most economic prophecies of health care costs for the aged has been assuming lower age-specific mortality rates while, at the same time, assuming constant age-specific health care costs. If death is postponed, the costs of death must be postponed also.

Interestingly, the data of N. P. Roos, Montgomery, L. L. Roos, and Shapiro (1987) demonstrate that hospitalization costs in the months prior to death are essentially constant for all age-groups.

Changing demographic predictions

Current U.S. demographic predictions, including the 1987 predictions from the Social Security Administration, continue to project straight lines with the slopes of the 1970s into the future (e.g., Faber, 1982; Actuarial Study No. 99, 1987). In contrast to the compression of morbidity hypothesis, they thus predict steadily continuing gains in life expectancy over the next century and a gradual widening of the male–female gap in average life expectancy at all ages. Recent national mortality data suggest that this is very unlikely to be the case; indeed, the 1982 predictions are already off by nearly a year in terms of the male–female gap and by seven tenths of a year in terms of female life expectancy!

In fact, the male–female gap in life expectancy from birth has narrowed in the 1980s from a high of 7.9 to 7.0 (e.g., *Metropolitan Life Insurance Statistical Bulletin*, 1988; Public Health Service, 1986). Male life expectancy has rather closely followed projections. However, female life expectancy from birth, projected to be 79.0 in 1986 was instead 78.3, and female life expectancy from age 65 projected at 19.3 was in fact 18.6. Female life expectancy from birth has continued to rise, although more slowly in the 1980s. Most significantly, however, female life expectancy from age 65 did not increase from 1979 to 1986. It is premature to suggest that there will be no further increases in female life expectancy from age 65; indeed, my own projections suggest that an upper limit of approximately 20 years might be eventually possible. But, it seems highly likely that we will never again see the rates of growth in life expectancy at advanced ages that were seen during the years of major decline in chronic vascular disease in the 1970s. It also seems likely that the current "low range" U.S. social security projections, meant to bracket all reasonably likely scenarios, may themselves be too high. Thus, we may look forward to more surviving couples and shorter periods of female dependency than currently estimated, with important social benefit.

The male–female gap is likely to continue to decrease for some time, because the most easily prevented causes of death (accidents, vascular disease, and lung cancer) are still substantially more prevalent in males.

International data are broadly supportive of these trends. For example, Japan has the best longevity record of any country, largely because atherosclerosis is almost nonexistent in that country. Life-expectancy increases for females over 65 have begun to slow in Japan, although less dramatically than in the United States, and the male–female gap in life expectancy from birth in Japan is only 5.7 years.

On the immortalists

Our projections, repeated after an additional decade of data, continue to indicate a mean maximal age of death (maximum average life expectancy) of about 85 years (Fries, in press). (The standard deviation of the age of death, however, is now estimated at 7 years [Fries, 1988] rather than 4 years, as originally calculated [Fries, 1980]). There are those who obviously are threatened by such calculations of the theoretical limits to life.

The theme of the Fountain of Youth recurs in the literature of many nations (Fries and Crapo, 1981) and the quest for immortality has had its advocates in many eras. It is not surprising that our era is no different, or that those individuals drawn to this quest would sometimes seek careers in demography or gerontology or in life-extension institutes, or that they would work diligently to reject evidence of the finitude of life.

The immortalists of today have varied nostrums and notions. Gerovital seems on the decline, but a boomlet for child starvation persists. Both vitamin C in massive doses and lifelong jogging have their advocates. Demographers of this school are currently touting cohort theories (some mysterious betterment in early-life experiences will cause future cohorts to greatly outlive current limits) or life-style theories (simultaneous life-style control and disease elimination may greatly improve life span).

Not to worry that the first of these current demographic theories is inconsistent with historical trends, which have shown rather constant life expectancies from advanced ages for successive cohorts, nor that the second is inconsistent with the experimental studies cited earlier, with regional and international data (e.g., atherosclerosis is essentially absent in Japan, yet Japan has only marginally increased life expectancy; Utah has very low smoking and drinking rates yet unremarkable life expectancy), and with common sense. (Out of 4 billion humans who have lived and died, surely some thousands or millions must have had ideal health habits and been fortunate enough to avoid disease, yet none has achieved remarkable longevity.) After all, these are matters of faith.

The immortalist is further identified by a need to "protest too much" against intimations of mortality. If one argument is shown to fail, try another. If the central argument against the compression of morbidity is that female life expectancy over age 65 was increasing in the 1970s (Manton, 1982), then the plateauing in the 1980s should be similarly argued as proof contrary, by an objective scholar. If a claim that mortality is not compressing (Myers & Manton, 1984a) is proved false (Fries, 1984), that should perhaps weaken the fervor. But no, the arguments merely become more obscure, new and less testable theories are advanced, and the assumptions are left unstated (Myers & Manton, 1984b).

The number of aged individuals, both in absolute terms and as a percentage of the total, will continue to grow impressively in developed nations for the next 40 years as a consequence of increased birth cohorts and decreased early-life mortality. Concern about the social problems that will accompany the increased numbers of elderly is warranted and necessary. But this problem arises because of birth rates to a far greater degree than because of death rates, and its solutions will come in greatest degree through reduction in the average morbidity experienced by individuals.

The medical model versus the minimum morbidity model

The medical demographics of successful aging are a dynamic between two principal points, the average age at first chronic infirmity and the average age at death. If the first increases faster than the second, there is compression of morbidity; if the reverse happens, there is extension of morbidity. The medical model, in essence, ignores the point at which illness begins and focuses attention on treating (or palliating) disease that has been clinically recognized, with a goal of increasing life expectancy by such measures. Such after-the-fact approaches inevitably increase morbidity because life extension with chronic illness is obtained at the cost of a loss in life quality. A second problem is that after-the-fact medical care is expensive and will become increasingly so. In economic terms, the cost of care at the margin increases. Additional gains require higher technology and a higher price tag and provide decreasing amounts of marginal gain. Tradition and many strong national forces continue to insist upon almost-complete dedication to this model.

The compression of morbidity model presents a strategy to minimize morbidity. By moving the age at onset of first chronic infirmity upward, years of healthy life are gained. Morover, the behavioral and preventive initiatives required are relatively low in technological content and are likely to be less expensive. Available data on trends in morbidity and in the quality of life are sadly deficient; at present they do not allow direct measurement of the compression of morbidity. Development of such data is essential to the study of these central issues of public health; indeed, because the most important questions can be addressed only by longitudinal study, it is critical that we immediately begin to include appropriate measures of morbidity and of the quality of life in such studies.

Policy implications and conclusions

The future for the national morbidity thus largely depends upon a self-fulfilling prophecy. If we continue as health professionals to neglect preventive and social science issues, morbidity will likely increase. If we continue to emphasize high technology and serial replacement of tiring body parts, costs will increase. There is an option for a healthier future, but our long-term response to the choice is not yet recorded.

Is the contemporary academic medical center appropriate to current national health needs? Are medical-student and premedical curricula adequate to develop needed skills and knowledge? Do social incentives reward healthy behaviors, or do they take from the premiums of the healthy to pay for the illnesses of those with unhealthy life-styles? Is current medical practice too oriented toward performance of technical procedures and not enough toward human interaction? Are research resource allocations between the several fields appropriately balanced? Is the strength of the arguments to allow less intensive care of the terminally ill increasing? Should individuals be granted greater autonomy in determining for themselves what is to be done to their bodies toward the end of their lives? Are we collecting data on the right end points? Are there methods by which the social sciences and the physical sciences can live in harmony within a health establishment dedicated to reducing the national illness burden? These questions require serious attention.

NOTE

This manuscript was prepared for presentation to the Conference on Estimating the Upper Limit to Human Life Expectancy, Berkeley, California, April 29–30, 1988 (National Institute of Aging), as well as to the 1987 workshop in Ringberg sponsored by the European Network on Longitudinal Studies on Individual Development; it is published here in slightly different form. This work was supported in part by a grant to The American Rheumatism Association Medical Information System (ARAMIS) from the National Institutes of Health (AM21393).

REFERENCES

Actuarial Study No. 99. (1987). Social Security Administration Publication No. 11-11546. Washington, DC: U.S. Public Health Service.
Bailar, J. C., & Smith, E. M. (1986). Progress against cancer? *New England Journal of Medicine, 314,* 1226–1232.

Bairey, C. N. (1986). Exercise and coronary artery disease. *Western Journal of Medicine, 144,* 205–211.

Baltes, P. B. (1987). Theoretical propositions of life-span developmental psychology: On the dynamics between growth and decline. *Developmental Psychology, 23,* 611–626.

Berkman, L. F., & Syme, S. L. (1979). Social networks, host resistance, and mortality: A nine-year follow-up study of Alameda County residents. *American Journal of Epidemiology, 109,* 186–204.

Bortz, W. M. (1982). Disuse and aging. *Journal of the American Medical Association, 248,* 1203–1208.

Brody, J. A. (1985). Prospect for an aging population. *Nature, 315,* 63–66.

Bruce, R. A. (1984). Exercise, functional aerobic capacity, and aging: Another viewpoint. *Sports and Exercise, 16,* 8–13.

Faber, J. F. (1982). *Life tables for the United States, 1900–2050.* Actuarial Study No. 87 (Social Security Administration Publication No. 11-11534). Washington, DC: U.S. Department of Health and Human Services.

Farquhar, J. (1987). *The American way need not be hazardous to your health.* Reading MA: Addison-Wesley.

Frick, M. H., Elo, O., Haapa, K., Heinonen, O. P., Heinsalmi, P., Helo, P., Huttunen, J. K., Kaitaniemi, P., Koskinen, P., Manninen, V., Maenpaa, H., Malkonen, M., Manttari, M., Norola, S., Pasternack, A., Pikkarainen, J., Romo, M., Sjoblom, T., & Nikkila, E. A. (1987). Helsinki Heart Study: Primary-prevention trial with gemfibrozil in middle-aged men with dyslipidemia. *New England Journal of Medicine, 317,* 1237–1245.

Friedman, G. D. (1979). Decline in hospitalization for coronary heart disease and stroke: The Kaiser-Permanente experience in northern California, 1971–1977. In R. J. Havlik & M. Feinleib (Eds.), *Proceedings of the Conference on the Decline in Coronary Heart Disease Mortality* (Publication No. 79-1610, pp. 116–118). Washington, DC: National Institutes of Health.

Fries, J. F. (1980). Aging, natural death, and the compression of morbidity. *New England Journal of Medicine, 303,* 130–136.

Fries, J. F. (1983). The compression of morbidity. *Milbank Memorial Fund Quarterly, 61,* 397–419.

Fries, J. F. (1984). The compression of morbidity: Miscellaneous comments about a theme. *Gerontologist, 24,* 354–359.

Fries, J. F. (1987a). An introduction to the compression of morbidity. *Gerontologica Perspecta, 1,* 5–8.

Fries, J. F. (1987b). Reduction of the national morbidity. *Gerontologica Perspecta, 1,* 54–65.

Fries, J. F. (1988). Aging, illness, and health policy: Implications of the compression of morbidity. *Perspectives in Biology and Medicine, 31,* 407–427.

Fries, J. F. (in press). The compression of morbidity: Near or far? *Milbank Memorial Fund Quarterly.*

Fries, J. F., & Crapo, L. M. (1981). *Vitality and aging.* New York: W. H. Freeman.

Fuchs, V. R. (1984). Though much is taken. *Milbank Memorial Fund Quarterly, 62,* 143–156.

Gillum, R. F., Folson, A., Leupker, R. V., Jacobs, D. R., Jr., Kottke, T. E., Gomez-Marin, O., Prineas, R. J., Taylor, H. L., & Blackburn, H. (1983). Sudden death and acute myocardial infarction in a metropolitan area,

1970–1980: the Minnestoa Heart Survey. *New England Journal of Medicine, 309,* 1353–1358.

Goldman, L., & Cook, E. F. (1984). The decline in ischemic heart disease mortality rates: An analysis of the comparative effects of medical interventions and changes in lifestyle. *Annals of Internal Medicine, 101,* 825–836.

Gruenberg, E. M. (1977). The failure of success. *Milbank Memorial Fund Quarterly, 55,* 3–24.

Horm, J. W., & Kessler, L. G. (1986). Falling rates of lung cancer in men in the United States. *Lancet, 1,* 425–426.

Lane, N. E., Bloch, D. A., Jones, H. H., Marshall, W. H., Wood, P. D., & Fries, J. F. (1986). Long-distance running, bone density, and osteoarthritis. *Journal of the American Medical Association, 255,* 1147–1151.

Lane, N. E., Bloch, D. A., Wood, P. D., & Fries J. F. (1987). Aging, long-distance running and the development of musculoskeletal disability: A controlled study. *American Journal of Medicine, 82,* 772–780.

Larson, E. B., & Bruce, R. A. (1986). Exercise and aging. *Annals of Internal Medicine, 105,* 783–785.

Lipid Research Clinic Coronary Primary Prevention Trial results. I. Reduction of incidence of coronary heart disease. (1984). *Journal of the American Medical Association, 251,* 351–364.

Manton, K. G. (1982). Changing concepts of morbidity and mortality in the elderly population. *Milbank Memorial Fund Quarterly, 60,* 183–244.

Metropolitan Life Insurance Statistical Bulletin 68 (1988). Pp. 18–23.

Multiple Risk Factor Intervention Trial Research Group (1982). Multiple Risk Factor Intervention Trial. *Journal of the American Medical Association, 248,* 1465–1477.

Multiple Risk Factor Intervention Trial Research Group (1986). Coronary heart disease death, non-fatal acute myocardial infarction and other clinical outcomes in the Multiple Risk Factor Intervention Trial. *American Journal of Cardiology, 58,* 1–13.

Myers, G. C., & Manton, K. G. (1984a). Compression of morbidity: Myth or reality. *Gerontologist, 24,* 346–353.

Myers, G. C., & Manton, K. G. (1984b). Recent changes in the U.S. age at death distribution: Further obeeservations. *Gerontologist, 24,* 572–575.

National Center for Health Statistics (1965, 1968, 1974, 1978). *Inpatient utilization of short-stay hospitals by diagnosis: United States* (Series 13, Nos. 6, 12, 26, 46). Washington, DC: Author.

Oliver, M. F. (1988). Reducing cholesterol does not reduce mortality. *Journal of the American College of Cardiology, 12,* 814–817.

Paffenbarger, R. S., Hyde, R. T., Wing, A. L., & Hsieh, C. C. (1986). Physical activity, all-cause mortality, and longevity of college alumni. *New England Journal of Medicine, 314,* 605–613.

Pell, S., & Fayerweather, W. E. (1985). Trends in the incidence of myocardial infarction and in associated mortality and morbidity in a large employed population, 1957–1983. *New England Journal of Medicine, 312,* 1005–1011.

Physicians' Health Study Research Group, Steering Committee of (1988). Preliminary report: Findings from the aspirin component of the Ongoing Physicians' Health Study. *New England Journal of Medicine, 318,* 262–264.

Plemons, J. K., Willis, S. L., & Baltes, P. B. (1978). Modifiability of fluid intelligence in aging: A short-term longitudinal training approach. *Journal of Gerontology, 33,* 224–231.

Public Health Service, Department of Health and Human Services (1986). *Health, United States, 1986* (Publication No. [PHS] 87-123211). Washington, DC: Author.

Roos, N. P., Montgomery, P., Roos, L. L., & Shapiro, E. (1987). Health care utilization in the years prior to death. *Milbank Memorial Fund Quarterly, 65,* 231–254.

Roos, N. P., & Shapiro, E. (1981). The Manitoba Longitudinal Study on aging: Preliminary findings on health care utilization by the elderly. *Medical Care, 19,* 644–657.

Schneider, E. L., & Brody, J. A. (1983). Aging, natural death, and the compression of morbidity: Another view. *New England Journal of Medicine, 309,* 854–856.

Spirduso, W. W. (1980). Physical fitness, aging, and psychomotor speed: A review. *Journal of Gerontology, 35,* 850–865.

Stern, M. P. (1979). The recent decline in ischemic heart disease mortality. *Annals of Internal Medicine, 91,* 630–640.

Surgeon General, Report of the (1983). *The health consequences of smoking: Cardiovascular diseases* (pp. 344–347). Washington, DC: Public Health Service.

Veterans' Administration Cooperative Study Group on Anti-hypertensive Agents. (1970). Effects of treatment on morbidity in hypertension. *Journal of the American Medical Association, 213,* 1143–1152.

Williams, A. F., & Lund, A. K. (1986). Seat belt use laws and occupant crash protection in the United States. *American Journal of Public Health, 76,* 1438–1442.

3 Successful aging in a post-retired society

DAVID L. FEATHERMAN, JACQUI SMITH, AND
JAMES G. PETERSON

Successful aging: A transactional view from the social sciences

Viewed from the perspective of the social sciences, successful aging is a quality of the transaction between the changing person and changing society over the entire life span but especially during a person's later years. As a sociological construct, successful aging is not an attribute of the person. Strictly speaking, it is neither an individual-difference variable such as cognitive wisdom nor the relative prevalence of vitality over morbidity in the later years of life. These orientations are wholly legitimate intellectually. They offer highly valuable insights, from the point of view of the person as a psychological or biological entity, within a given environment. Although both constructs may reflect influences from the social and physical ecology of the person, wisdom and vitality tend to be studied as person-centered states or trait variables and in terms of the determinants of individual differences in them, including variations by sociocultural and demographic categories. However, the static or dynamic nature of the embedding sociocultural system typically is not an explicit part of the *definition* of what constitutes successful aging in these formulations. That is, the nature of society and its dynamic properties are cast as influences on successful aging and not as part of its very essential manifestation and definition.

By contrast, the sociological orientation to successful aging can take at least two forms. The first begins from the perspective of the social collectivity, rather than the person, and asks how the aging of a person or persons might lead, optimally, toward the betterment of society, that is, toward improving the quality of life for the population in general or perpetuating the social system beyond the lifetime of the oldest cohorts. This is an interactional or contextual view, and not necessarily transactional. In such a view, maximizing the life-years or the physiological vitality of each older person may not follow necessarily from the idea of successful aging. For example, the philosopher-ethicist Norman Daniels (1988), among others, has proposed that rationing of expensive acute-care technologies may be just and may maximize justice both in the population at large and over a cohort's lifetime.

A second contextual view of successful aging, from the starting point of the societal collectivity, recognizes that societies and civilizations, too, can assume various properties of vitality and aging. They and their many levels of component institutions – for example, the economy, education and culture, family and polity – can be characterized as growing or declining, as resilient to challenges and open to change or vulnerable, and so forth. One of the newest fields in American sociology, organizational ecology (Hannan & Freeman, 1986; Hawley, 1968), is developing principles concerning the life and death and the adaptational vigor of various organizational forms in response to or anticipation of change in their environment. In addition, it is possible to speak of population aging, the culmination of what demographers have called the demographic transition of the 19th and 20th centuries, and of its impact on the quality of institutional life and vigor of a society. Within this perspective, successful aging is a construct applied to the society itself – the successfully aging society. In this instance, it is feasible to consider what successful aging of the person is, within the conditions and constraints of the successfully aging society. This, too, is a relational definition and not transactional.

For example, while wisdom may be an important prototype for the study of successful aging of the contemporary elderly person, it most definitely is so from the point of view of enhancing or optimizing the positive bases for self-esteem and for positive social evaluation of a given person's worth (what sociologists call social honor or prestige). Yet wisdom could lose its special significance as a collective "virtue" (in the sense used by Erik Erikson, 1950), apart from its impact on self-esteem, if the social or collective utility of the elderly were to change under the pressures of collective interests.

Consider the following hypothetical case. There is persisting refusal of many American women to bear children, under prevailing suboptimal conditions for women in the economy, unstable marital life, and the economic vulnerability of single-parent households (Sweet & Bumpass, 1987). Add restrictive and highly selective immigration policies that give preference to low-fertility or postfertility individuals. These conditions that add to the "graying" of the society, plus uncertainties about the public funding of the retired "baby-boomers," could encourage a change in public attitudes and opinions about the "prestige" value of wisdom and leisure for the elderly. The elderly may be needed to make society function, in an everyday sense, and not in just some abstract or intellectualized way. And therefore successful aging, as an honorific state to be attained, could be instanced by attributes other than cognitive wisdom. We may tend to conflate wisdom with successful aging because human civilizations rarely if ever have contained so many old people or needed them very critically (see Nydegger, 1983).

We need not accept this speculative assertion to understand the contextual, mainly sociological, perspective on successful aging. Yet neither of the foregoing examples was truly transactional, a view in which the nature of the person and the fabric of society each contribute a necessary but not sufficient part of a dynamic interplay. In the *transactional view*, successful aging is defined at the point of intersection between the developing person and the changing societal context. (See Samaroff & Chandler, 1975, for an elaboration of transactional models, especially in child developmental research.) Within this third social science perspective, *successful aging is a social psychological construct*, belonging uniquely neither to the person nor to the society and not emphasizing either starting point (person vs. society) over the other.

Thus, as a first approximate definition, *successful aging is a social psychological, processual construct that reflects the always-emerging, socially esteemed ways of adapting to and reshaping the prevailing, culturally recognized conditions of mind, body, and community for the elderly of a society.* Notice that this definition focuses on a process, namely, adaptation, rather than on an explicit outcome as a criterion for success, for example, happiness, health. The rationale for a processual, rather than a state or outcome, criterion rests on the dynamic, transactional perspective on aging and on human development in general (Featherman & Lerner, 1985).[1]

In this paper, we adopt and elaborate this social psychological approach. We wish to develop several propositions about successful aging of persons within a hypothetical state, a "post-retired society," a state characterized by dynamic, uncertain change for persons over the life course and for evolving social institutions.[2] We also want to describe the course of our empirical research that, perforce, is longitudinal not only in the sense of tracking the developmental histories of persons into and through old age but also in the sociological sense of characterizing the course of evolving institutional changes that impel, impede, and deflect the ontogenies of contemporary adults in advanced, modern societies. In the perspective of the social scientist, these sociological and historical forces are the efficient causes (albeit not exclusive ones) of both individual development and the modalities of individual differences in adult development during the later years.

Successful aging as adaptive competence

We begin by providing a generic social psychological definition of success-ful aging across the human life span. It is generic in the sense that this definition could stand no matter what type of society we consider, even though the expression of successful aging, its manifestation in everyday life, surely is infused by the qualities and especially the level of dynamics within each society and its historical period.

Successful aging is but one expression of a generic transactional process, namely, adaptive competence. In turn, and now just in terms of the person, *adaptive competence is a generalized capacity to respond with resilience to challenges arising from one's body, mind, and environment* (see Rowe & Kahn, 1987). Thus, successful aging draws upon reactive and proactive capacities to respond with resilience, adaptively, to those challenges that are unique to later life. Challenges can be biological, mental, self-conceptual, interpersonal, socioeconomic or due to other sources of change in the status quo. The forms, sequences, and meanings of these challenges for the person are provided, in variety, by social structures of interpersonal discourse and relationships, within community life and culture symbolism.

This equation of successful aging, as a process construct of active *adaptation* to challenges of a dynamic and differentiated sociocultural ecology of persons and environments, is an explicitly social psychological or transactional definition. It is a process term and not a trait or state. The process phrase "adaptation to a dynamic ecology" draws attention to important attributes of individual behavior that are captured, historically, by the concept of human intelligence. For example, for the philosopher John Dewey (Ratner, 1939) and the psychologist Robert Sternberg (1985), human intelligence involves a mindful, reflective, and actively reflexive relationship between self and environment. Human intelligence is activated by discrepancies between expectations and realities, or by challenges to the status quo and to habituated behavior. Recent "revision-ist" efforts within psychology to redirect the study of human intelligence (Berg & Sternberg, 1985; Cantor & Kihlstrom, 1985; Sternberg, 1985) refer to adaptational processes in broadly encompassing terms, including, for example, accommodating reactions to limiting conditions, active man-ipulation of constraints and opportunities within a setting, and purposive exits from unfavorable environments for more optimal ones. Thus, in aging successfully, the person may engage in any variety of these types of adaptational processes and draw upon both intrapersonal and ex-trapersonal resources in responding to challenge.

We stress, following P. B. Baltes and M. M. Baltes (this volume) that *successful aging, qua adaptive competence, can be defined as involving an expansion of developmental reserves* (P. B. Baltes, 1987). The latter, in turn, increases the range of functioning of a given person, relative to the opportunities and constraints within a specific social ecological niche and relative to cohort standards of statistically "usual" biobehavioral aging (Rowe & Kahn, 1987).

By referring to successful aging of the person as adaptive *competence*, our perspective acknowledges and emphasizes the apparently latent, perhaps biological, tendencies within our species to actively seek stimulation, to create novel experience, and to be proactive and not just reactive (White, 1959). Competence involves a lifelong capacity for motivated self-expansion and expression that is grounded in collective cultural experience (Dewey, 1910; Mead, 1934; Vygotsky, 1962; Wells & Stryker, 1988) but that also seeks for uniqueness within it, the "competent self" (Meyer, 1986; Ryff, 1984; M. B. Smith, 1968). Finally, competence also refers to behavioral effectiveness of the transactions between self and environment, to "positive" adaptations that maximize gains over losses in functioning (Bloom, 1977; Rowe & Kahn, 1987; White, 1959; Wine & Smye, 1981). That environment is inherently social and sets bounds upon the acceptable definition of *effectiveness* within communal standards that are derived through processes of social comparison (Foote & Cottrell, 1955; Inkeles, 1966). Thus, under the concept of adaptive competence, the transactional definition of successful aging brings together a broad conception of intelligent human response to challenges and an emphasis on the mind's capacity for purposive initiation, self-expression, and self-expansion. Intelligent reflexiveness directs the course of affirmative adaptation to changing societal institutions and cultural meanings. It seeks to optimize developmental outcomes within a given or expected biocultural milieu (i.e., developmental gains over losses; P. B. Baltes, 1987). This point is important, for the transactional view seeks to understand the "what" and "how" of adaptive competence for a given person, sociocultural group, or societal population in terms of their grounding within a particular biocultural milieu and within the scope of the actual and expected pace of change in historical, bioevolutionary contexts (Featherman & Lerner, 1985). Therefore, successful aging can take on many phenotypical expressions in historical time and sociocultural space, even if the generic transactional process of adaptive competence remains fundamentally stable.

Aside from the historical, sociocultural, and individual variability in its manifestation, adaptive competence is multidimensional: (1) emotional, in the sense of coping strategies and skills in response to stressors (Garmezy & Masten, 1986); (2) cognitive, in manifestations of problem-solving heuristics (Simon, 1975); and (3) behavioral, in effective performance and social competence (Cornelius & Caspi, 1987; Wine & Smye, 1981). Although recognizing this multidimensionality (really, multi-processuality), this chapter limits its focus to certain cognitive facets of successful aging qua adaptive competence. This simplification is simply a strategic choice and reflects the fact that our unfolding empirical research began with the cognitive components.

In our cognitive research we view *adaptive competence as the ability to draw upon an extensive knowledge system about one's functioning in the world and as an expertise with respect to problem-solving heuristics.*[3] This usage is similar to Gladwin's (1967, p. 32) definition of competence, as reported by M. Brewster Smith (1968, pp. 274–275):

> Competence ... develops along three major axes, all closely interrelated. First is the ability to learn or to use a variety of alternative pathways or behavioral responses in order to reach a given goal.... Second, the competent individual comprehends and is able to use a variety of social systems within the society, moving within these systems and utilizing the resources they offer. Third, competence depends upon effective reality testing. Reality testing involves not merely the lack of psychopathological impairment to perception but also a positive, broad, and sophisticated understanding of the world, ... an ecological unit encompassing within a single interacting system the individual and as much of his social environment as is relevant.

By emphasizing more than expertise based upon rich knowledge systems (e.g., problem-solving heuristics), a holistic approach to understanding successful aging qua adaptive competence seeks a more comprehensive formulation than just the cognitive. In the social psychological perspective developed herein, a person's adaptive competence includes aspects of social competence as well as cognitive expertise, as implied also by Gladwin's seminal definition of competence. Nevertheless, in the following sections on successful aging, the discussion of adaptive competence is highly focused on only a few of the many component dimensions that we ultimately hope to identify.

From well-structured to ill-structured challenges: Ontogeny and developmental tasks

If the successfully aging older person is adaptively competent, what is he or she competent at doing? Is the adaptive competence of the elderly to be judged against the same life tasks and by the same standards as for their children or grandchildren? Seemingly not, of course, but then by what do we reference, for any life period and its incumbents, what *successful* means or what *competence* is? Here, the concept of *developmental task* (Havighurst, 1956; Oerter, 1986) is of some use.

Developmental tasks

Developmental tasks are sequences of tasks over the life course whose satisfactory performance not only is important for the person's sense of competence and esteem in the community but also serves as preparation for the future. Havighurst included three components in his original conception of developmental tasks: first, the levels of biological, physical, and psychological maturation of the person that permit performance of presented tasks; second, the various task demands imposed by community and culture upon persons of different ages and maturational levels; and third, individuals' own aspirations, values, and life goals throughout life. Havighurst's was a bicultural, contextual definition that included not only reflections of a person's "readiness" to assume roles in society but also the structuring and sequencing of such roles through the life course as part of communal life.

Some researchers, building upon Havighurst's framework, have suggested that developmental tasks can be identified, at least indirectly, through survey research techniques. The evidence may take the form of consensus in individuals' beliefs about psychological and behavioral gains and losses with aging (Heckhausen & P. B. Baltes, 1990) or of convergent attitudes about the salience and sanctioning of age-norms for behavior within a community (Neugarten & Datan, 1973; Passuth, Maines, & Neugarten, 1985). Riley's (1985a) age-stratification model of society incorporates such thinking. She views society as composed of age-graded sets of social positions and roles into which cohorts of individuals are recruited sequentially, based upon their maturational readiness, education through socialization about age-graded norms, and intercohort negotiations about timing of succession.

Do age-graded developmental tasks have an explicit reality and representation in the minds of persons (as "schemata" and "scripts" used for life planning; see, e.g., Schank & Abelson, 1977)? Or, by contrast, are opinion and attitude surveys about age-graded norms for behavior merely eliciting general cultural information and beliefs that have little influence on actual behavior (Hogan & Astone, 1986; Marini, 1984)? These are unsettled questions. However, as an abstraction for analyzing sequences of roles and role requirements over the life course and for assessing adequacy of role performances, the concept is useful in developmental research.

From the individual's point of view, developmental tasks draw upon the level of adaptive competence (Oerter, 1986). That is, satisfactory performance at any developmental task draws upon a person's cognitive, emotional, and behavioral skills, like coping (Haan, 1977; Lazarus, 1966), and higher order executive processes that link skill levels with resources in the environment for effective performance (Waters & Sroufe, 1983). The executive processes that lead to effective activity involve planning and problem-solving heuristics of different kinds (Cantor, Norem, Niedenthal, Langston, & Brower, 1987), presumably in response to the type of task and its difficulty. A later section develops this idea, hypothesizing that these heuristics for mobilizing skills at tasks may have an ontogenetic history that is tied to experiences in different social structures, for example, work settings and career lines.

The construct, developmental task, also has an important sociological side that sets conditions on the expression of a person's adaptive competence through life. By implication, these sociological facets also set conditions on successful aging qua the satisfactory performance of the developmental tasks of later life. The sociological side has to do with the qualitative features of the presented developmental tasks, for example, complexity, uncertainty of task definition, predictability of its timing in the life course, or its prevalence. Some analysts of "life events" qualifying as developmental tasks show that the developmental consequences of such events on persons vary systematically by such qualitative characteristics (Brim & Ryff, 1980; McLanahan & Sørensen, 1985).

Unfortunately, life-span developmental research has not yet produced a systematic identification and scientific consensus about the changing characteristics (both objective and as subjectively perceived) of developmental tasks. Developmentalists have yet to undertake a detailed task analysis that decomposes and recomposes tasks into different levels of globality (Fisher, 1980; Oerter, 1986). This work, therefore, is only a first step in analyzing the developmental tasks over differentiated life courses by gender, race, economic stratum, and so forth.

Lacking this solid empirical base from longitudinal life-span research, developmentalists construct varying lists of the developmental tasks of later adulthood and old age, often drawing inspiration from Eriksonian theory (Atchley, 1983; Marshall, 1980). Making a successful transition into retirement, assembling a "convoy" of others for social support, carrying out a successful life review, maintaining functional independence, and controlling the circumstances of one's own death are a few of the many developmental tasks sometimes listed for old age. Other analysts have not constructed lists per se but instead have engaged speculatively or empirically with hermeneutic techniques in qualitative task analysis (P. B. Baltes, Dittmann-Kohli, & Dixon, 1984; Dittmann-Kohli & Kramer, 1985; Kitchener & King, 1981; Labouvie-Vief, 1980).

These qualitative appraisals of fundamental differences between the tasks of earlier and later adult life lead to one inferential hypothesis:

namely, *throughout the life course, the developmental tasks become less well-structured and more ill-structured* (Dittmann-Kohli, 1984; K. S. Kitchener & King, 1981; Wood, 1983). Put more accurately, the working proposition is that the balance of qualitative features across the many developmental tasks, at any point in life, shifts from predominantly well-structured to ill-structured as the life course unfolds. It is unclear at what age or after what critical event ill-structured tasks outnumber well-structured tasks; so, too, is any indication of the regularity or irregularity in the rates of change over the life span. Is it that ill-structured problems simply increase, or do well-structured tasks just become much less common in later life? We do not know and would be loath to speculate at this level of detail without a longitudinal task analysis (currently unavailable).[4]

Well-structured and ill-structured tasks

What is the distinction between well-structured and ill-structured life problems or developmental tasks from a sociological perspective?[5] Analysts within the cognitive and decisional sciences (Churchman, 1971; Neisser, 1976; Simon, 1978) have disagreed over the uniquely identifying characteristics of ill-structured tasks. However, Wood (1983) has offered a formal system to differentiate degrees of "structured-ness" in tasks or problems, using statistical decision theory (Lindgren, 1976). The scientist could use such criteria in an effort to characterize the objective features; they also could be part of the referential system that problem solvers employ as they seek to discern the type of problem they face (Hayes, 1987). Wood's system focuses on four constituent elements by which problems can be characterized and placed on a continuum from well- to ill-structured:

- the states of nature – that is, initial and goal states – that comprise the "problem space"
- the set of acts open to the decision maker in finding a pathway from initial states to goal states
- the set of outcomes, including constraints, of the decision maker's actions along the pathway
- the utility or value to the decision maker of attaining various states and goals

Stated succinctly, according to Wood's system, a problem is ill-structured if any of the four elements is either *unknown* or *not knowable* with at least a range of probabilistic certainty. Differences among well- to moderately well-structured problems reflect the deterministic (most well-structured) or kind of probabilistic (moderate- to low-structured) nature of the four elements. Given at least some known probabilities for all four elements, however, the decision maker can arrive at a single solution. By contrast, the unknowability associated with at least one of the four essential elements in an ill-structured problem denies the possibility of a single, arguably correct solution (Wood, 1983, pp. 252–254).

In a less formalistic and more qualitative framework, the contrast between well-structured and ill-structured problems can be expressed, for heuristic purposes, as the difference between a "puzzle" and a "dilemma" (Kitchener, 1983). In a puzzle, like a chess game, the first best and often only solution is sought. One does not question the assumptions on which the game is based. Indeed, in well-structured problems, the solution is guaranteed if one but persists in applying standard rules or techniques. In the world of childhood, adolescence, and perhaps early adulthood as well, the developmental tasks associated with well-articulated, circumscribed roles within the family, the school, the playground, and even perhaps the early career of supervised work tend to be more well-structured. That is, the relative degree of structure is toward the *well-structured* end of the continuum. More like puzzles, these developmental tasks are *relatively* more likely to be seen as having definite solutions (Yussen, 1985; Resnick, 1987). The developmental tasks making up the social worlds of the early life course may tend toward the more well-structured end of the continuum, in part, because they emanate from within rather formally organized institutional settings, with comparatively clearer definitions of, and perhaps even relatively more consensus about, circumscribed roles and rule-based expectations for appropriate behavior. (Later in the paper we challenge this broad generalization about the early life course when applied to contemporary cohorts of young adults and some significant fraction of children.)

By contrast, the life period of old age for contemporary cohorts of the elderly tends to be lived out in less formally organized settings, where the positional statuses are comparatively fuzzier and lack consensual value and where the roles are more informal and tenuous (Rosow, 1985; Dittmann-Kohli, 1984). Developmental tasks identified by some gerontologists, like having a productive retirement or controlling the circumstances and conditions of one's death, are not well-structured puzzles with limited solutions. Instead, they are dilemmas, or dialectical problems with contradictory ends and purposes, relative solutions, and ambiguous end points that often change in form and salience as they are pursued (Churchman, 1971; Wood, 1983). These developmental tasks are less well-structured and more ill-structured, possessing one highly distinguishing characteristic: The bane of the ill-structured task is that one rarely knows when a solution has been achieved.

If the life world of the elderly is composed of many more ill-structured dilemmas than well-structured problems (and we do not know empirically), then successful aging may be based on quite different developmental reserves than the adaptive competence of the young. For instance, the cognitive competencies required for the solution of the well-structured tasks of the schoolchild may constitute an "academic intelligence" that is different in the forms and content of knowledge and thinking from the "practical intelligence" of the middle-aged executive or the retired housewife caring for her invalid mother (Resnick, 1987; Scribner & Cole, 1973; Yussen, 1985). The developmental tasks of youth and old age may call for very different problem-solving heuristics, as in the cognition of deciphering what kind of problem one faces and of determining optimal solution strategies and conditions under which the problem can be considered solved (Wood, 1983; Kluwe, 1986; Friedman, Scholnick, & Cocking, 1987). Some cognitive developmentalists suggest that styles of thinking and knowing for some adults begin to shift after midlife from "problem solving" to "problem finding" (Rybash, Hoyer, & Roodin, 1986). Interestingly, cognitive scientists who study ill-structured or ill-defined problem-solving skills conclude that a key asset in success at these tasks is creative problem finding (Hayes, 1987). Creative problem finding often includes divergent thinking, using one's own accumulated knowledge and values as starting points to explore through successive approximations alternative definitions of what the ill-defined problem "really" is and how it might be approached and resolved. Whether the gains in problem-finding skills in middle and later adulthood arise from some endogenous cognitive development or from the proliferation of ill-structured tasks, whose mastery hinges on the acquisition of additional skills (beyond those sufficient for well-defined, well-structured tasks), is an unanswered question.

If the changing balance of ill-structured and well-structured life problems and tasks does call for qualitatively different cognitive reserves for adaptive competence over the life span, then the life-span shift in the prevalence of well- and ill-structured tasks within society disadvantages the elderly. Perhaps this is why the attribute of "wisdom" is regarded by some developmentalists as a psychological facet of successful aging. That is, cognitive wisdom provides some elderly who have acquired it with especially appropriate reserves for adapting well to the ill-structured dilemmas that prevail in later life. Wisdom may not provide any distinctive adaptational advantage in the competitive, achievement- and speed-oriented world of technical efficiency that characterizes the institutional life and organizational roles of youth and middle-aged adults (Labouvie-Vief, 1982). Logically, however, wisdom could be expected to enable more of the elderly to adapt to or reshape ill-structured problematics in ways that the rational, logical, and technical efficiencies of the young may be less suited to accomplish (J. Smith & P. B. Baltes, 1990).

In short, *if successful aging is to be defined as adaptive competence, then it must also be defined so that the performance standard of success reflects an elaborated capacity to surmount the ill-structured dilemmas (as well as the well-structured puzzles) that are the essence of the social organization and associated developmental tasks of old age.* Herein lies a substantial challenge. If adaptive competence in youth is developed, in the main, with reference to prevalent well-structured tasks, then how is adaptive competence extended or transferred into successful aging once the balance of well- versus ill-structured problematics in life shifts from problem-solving puzzle-like tasks to dilemmas? Is there a discontinuity or disjunction, based on the social organization of the life course, between the basis of adaptive competence in youth and the adaptive competence qua successful aging in later adulthood? And if so, what are the societally structured pathways to successful aging that might circumvent the more typical disjunction?

These questions lead us to consider a more precise definition of adaptive competence that reflects the unique developmental tasks of later adulthood and old age. This conceptual approach and the ongoing research that explores its validity will be transactional or social psychological, for they will cast the condition, successful aging, as a dialectical outcome of changing characteristics of the societally structured life course (specifically, the shifting balance of well- and ill-structured tasks) and of changing cognitive requirements for problem-solving heuristics that underlie adaptive success as the individual moves into later life.[6]

Adaptive competence for successful aging: The mind at work

Our research group is pursuing the following developmental hypothesis regarding adaptive competence in life-span perspective: Adaptive competence for successful aging may be developed from experiences and skills acquired in some specifically structured occupations and career lines during the adult years. By implication, other occupations and career lines, those without the putatively requisite social psychological relationships of structured environment and cognitive response, do not promote the acquisition of adaptive competence vis-à-vis the unique developmental tasks of post-retired life. We have chosen two career lines in engineering as prototypical cases to examine this possibility in preliminary empirical studies. The most general hypothesis is that different "frames of mind" are developed during the successful pursuit of these career lines. Further, the distinctive frames of mind are differentially suited, as effective problem-solving heuristics and epistemic orientations (worldviews), to the increasing prevalence of ill-structured dilemmas in the post-retired years.

Given that we are studying the mind at work, our more specific working definition of adaptive competence is both cognitive and reflects a focus on job and career characteristics. Thus, *adaptive competence is an expert knowledge system about one's functioning in the world (of work) and about the nature of tasks that must be performed effectively* (in order to progress in a job sequence or to change fields; e.g., Scribner, 1986; Sternberg & Wagner, 1986). Such a knowledge system, we suggest, would involve an awareness of one's basic abilities, interests, and motives, as well as of strategies for maintaining and using these abilities in situations of environmental challenge, constraint, and opportunity. The knowledge base would include, for example, "schemas" and "scripts" (Schank & Abelson, 1977) about structured job sequences, the "problem space" (Newell & Simon, 1972) of tasks and jobs within a firm, and knowledge of the rapid technological changes in one's field and of impending obsolescence in one's skills. Behavior that reflects high-level knowledge in these areas often is the basis for peer-acknowledged expertise and peer-conferred expert status within one's field.

In terms of the cognitive science construct *expertise, adaptive competence* is defined as exceptional factual and procedural knowledge about (1) the tasks to be performed on the job, (2) the sequences of jobs and criteria by which career movements (up, down, lateral, out) occur, and (3) the mental and behavioral strategies for building, maintaining, and restoring expert status within such jobs and career lines over the working life. This knowledge is likely to be expressed in terms of a general intellectual and epistemic orientation to dealing with work and career-related matters. Adaptive competence can be characterized as an expertise composed of cognitive, metacognitive, and epistemic components (K. S. Kitchener, 1983; Featherman, 1987).

How does the expert knowledge associated with adaptive competence relate to the specialized technical knowledge that workers and professionals have acquired, and presumably continue to accumulate, during their careers? To some extent, they are interdependent, as can be seen from our definition of the knowledge system associated with adaptive competence. It is possible, however, to imagine instances where individuals might have a high-level technical expertise in a field and yet be relatively naive concerning more general aspects of career and self-management. Similarly, other individuals might well have a clear understanding of career management yet be deficient in technical expertise. We expect that to be recognized as an "expert" in one's field (at least by midcareer) an individual should be high on technical expertise and possess high-level knowledge concerning career management. When *both* these criteria are met, an individual might also be considered to be high in adaptive competence (within the developmental tasks of middle adulthood).

It is likely that the balance between technical knowledge and career management knowledge will change in the course of a career. Early in a career, for example, "expert" status may well be attributed primarily on the basis of high-level technical knowledge and performance. Late in a career, the focus for expert status attribution may shift to high-level knowledge in career management issues, possibly in combination with previous expressions of technical brilliance.

To summarize, in our research program we view the adaptive competence of adults in relation to the developmental tasks of work and career management. It is composed of at least two, probably related, high-level knowledge systems, or expertises: one about the technicalities and practicalities of performing one's job effectively and another about the building, maintaining, elaborating, and restoring of careers in one's field. One important component of both expertises is the epistemological system, or worldview, that organizes both what is known about job and career (i.e., factual and procedural knowledge) and one's knowledge about such knowledge (i.e., metacognitive knowledge). It is these higher level epistemic components of both expertises that direct inquiry, structure one's definition of problems and their solution, and define what is "true" and "false" about effective job performance and career management (K. S. Kitchener & King, 1981; Wood, 1983).

Rational problem-solving and reflective planning orientations to work tasks

In our empirical research, we are interested in two, perhaps extreme, forms of epistemic cognition – two frames of mind – that organize the expertise in relation to work and career management: a rational problem-solving orientation to dealing with environmental challenges and a reflective planning orientation. Table 3.1 summarizes these orientations, as they have been defined in various literatures under differing labels (see Nadler, 1981; Peterson, 1985; Rittel & Webber, 1974; and Schön, 1983; for reviews of the origins of these orientations within engineering, cognitive science, and the organizational social psychology literatures).

We shall elaborate these epistemic orientations subsequently, but in brief, the *rational problem-solving orientation* implies a short-term reactive adaptation to environmental challenges: When a problem arises, the individual quickly seeks to restore the situation to normal (i.e., to how it was previously or how it ought to be). In one sense, this approach promotes an efficient search for one best (or the first effective) solution to a puzzle. Solutions that worked in the past are expected to do so again. This orientation focuses on the problem to be solved rather than on what gives

Table 3.1. *Two work orientations among engineers and planners*

Rational problem solving	Reflective planning
• One best (or optimal) solution	• No best solution; but several solutions can serve one purpose
• Boundaries and constraints are given or easily specified	• Boundaries are fuzzy or not known at all
• The solution can be evaluated (often quantitatively)	• Solutions are often qualitative in nature
• Primarily a solitary and highly autonomous activity	• Requiries both group and highly individual work effort
• Problems are not necessarily considered unique; this implies that there are similar solutions to vastly different problems	• Problems are unique; therefore, solutions are unique
• The solution, if found to be unsatisfactory, can often be incrementally improved and (re)implemented	• "One-shot" approach to implementation; it is difficult to change, for example, an implemented but unsatisfactory urban housing plan
• Often a "fixedness" on the problem itself such that the solution fits only the problem and has no larger purpose or scope	• Purpose driven over a timeline; the purpose of planning is to design or (re)structure a new solution system; this purpose subsumes the goal of simply solving the problem; over time, the planning process (by not fixating on the problem itself) derives a self-improving solution system that seeks to anticipate and adjust to future changes
• Not a timeline process; often the problem has changed by the time a solution (designed to solve that specific problem) is reached	

rise to the problem or on the purposes that are to be served by implementing the solution.

The *reflective planning orientation*, on the other hand, connotes an anticipation of problems and environmental changes before they reach a level that requires action. It also consists of a consideration of many possible ways of restoring order and an evaluation of appropriate action based on a broad or contextual and long-term perspective. In this view, problems are less often seen as puzzles and more often as dilemmas or dialectical issues with conflicting, competing end points that defy a "one best solution" approach. Solutions are seen as conditional and transitory. Because of the inherently fuzzy nature of both what the problem "is" and how to "solve" it, persons taking the reflective planning orientation frequently involve others in all stages of problem solving, whereas those who take the rational problem-solving view often see people as a distraction or nonessential.

Both the rational problem-solving and reflective planning orientations could be manifest at expert levels of functioning in the context of a career. Indeed, in our theoretical framework, we consider that these orientations direct the processes (albeit, different modalities) of building, maintaining, and restoring expert status in a career line (Featherman, 1987; Featherman & Peterson, 1986). However, we speculate that the reflective planning orientation is more likely to transfer across domains, that is, from work to nonwork life. The strategies associated with this orientation are more general and less dependent on specialized knowledge about the problem areas (Featherman, 1987). In this sense, higher levels of adaptive competence may be associated with something like a reflective planning orientation.

Let us be more specific about these two epistemic orientations, using the terminology of cognitive science and the problem-solving and planning literatures. In those literatures, *planning* and *problem-solving* have a variety of meanings and nonstandard usages (see Friedman et al., 1987, and Scholnick & Friedman, 1987, for a critique). *In our view, planning is a generic construct defining a particular approach to tasks and a style (or strategy, heuristic) of thinking that is multidimensional (see Table 3.1) and that involves a search for (a) alternative options, (b) options that are not immediately obvious, and (c) innovative end solutions.* Planning, in this sense, is not coextensive with problem-solving. *Problem-solving, according to our definition, connotes an approach to tasks or a thinking strategy that focuses on finding the most efficient path to one correct solution.* In contrast to a reflective planner, a rational problem solver is not motivated to look for innovative end solutions, goals, or alternative options. A good problem solver, however, may look for innovative means to final solutions; but this innovation is in the service of efficiency. In the cognitive science literature, *planning* has often been used as a label for one problem-solving heuristic (e.g., the Newell & Simon, 1972, genre of means–ends analysis). This is a narrower definition of planning than we have in mind. For example, the Newell–Simon approach tends to characterize planning as an ordered scheme of connections between actions, ideas, or subgoals directed toward a final goal that is accepted or given a priori (Schank & Abelson, 1977).

By contrast, our usage of *planning* within our construct of reflective planning can be likened to and seeks to extend Wilensky's (1983) process called "understanding." Reflective planning, like understanding, often requires the planner to "follow the goals and plans of actors in a situation in order to make inferences.... Rather than actually create a plan, an understander must be able to use knowledge about plans to understand the plan under which someone else is operating" (Wilensky, 1983, p. 9). For example, the reflective planner as consultant to a city planning board would be using such a planning strategy when inferring the purposes to be served by a series of goals that are presented to the consultant; the rational problem solver by contrast might take the goals as given and plan by "satisficing" (Simon, 1956) via means–ends analysis alone.

In summary, rational problem-solving and reflective planning are two different heuristics or styles of thinking in problem-solving situations. For purposes of exposition we have tended to dichotomize these as qualitative frames of mind and to infer that a person will manifest either one or the other orientation. It is much more likely that the two heuristics are related and not independent, as for instance when reflective planning incorporates but goes beyond the principles of rational problem-solving qua means–ends analysis. (This possibility is suggested by research on "critical thinking" and "reflective judgement" as related but empirically separate competencies; e.g., K. S. Kitchener & King, 1981.) Still, one might ask, "Are these two heuristics equally useful or effective for all tasks or in all problem-solving settings?" The cognitive science literature suggests that they may not be (Neisser, 1985; Scholnick, Friedman, & Cocking, 1987; Wood, 1983; but see Simon, 1956). In brief, the literature on balance takes the view that what we term reflective planning may be a more effective heuristic in instances of ill-structured dilemmas, whereas rational problem-solving may be more effective for well-structured tasks.

If this proves to be a valid generalization (our preliminary studies have not confirmed this), then the implications for successful aging and adaptive competence with respect to the developmental tasks of later life become clearer. Namely, adaptive competence for successful aging may be connected to acquired cognitive capacities for reflective planning in connection with the ill-structured dilemmas that, putatively, proliferate in later adulthood and old age.

In addition, we can speculate that successful aging also might be optimal among individuals who can deploy both reflective planning and rational problem solving selectively, while appraising the changing circumstances and kinds of problem settings and tasks that challenge these competencies. The latter research hypothesis is important, for it is likely that with aging we encounter *both* well- and ill-structured tasks, even if the latter proliferate. One's adaptive competence across a greater range of experiences would be enlarged – one's developmental reserves expanded – to the degree that reflective planning deploys both frames of mind selectively. If our empirical research can document this connection, it will satisfy our definition of successful aging, namely, that of an expansion of developmental reserves that enable the person to maintain or increase the range of environmental "niches" in which the person can function well, even under circumstances of change in person and environmental context (see P. B. Baltes, 1987).[7]

Work and the development of frames of mind: A prototypical case

How is all of this related to work life and careers? How and when is the mind at work being prepared to meet the challenges of later adulthood? Within which kinds of work settings, occupations, and career lines during adulthood are the developmental reserves expanded for successful aging after retirement? In our empirical research we address these questions through the use of occupational and career line prototypes within engineering. Engineering may be a good prototype for the study of adaptive competence in general and of successful aging in particular for several reasons. For one reason, engineering involves a set of occupations in which the mind is challenged to keep pace with technological changes and to solve novel problems; the mind at work is at work. Some psychologists (Scribner, 1986; Sternberg, 1985) have argued that the cognitive impact of work may be greatest when the required mental processes must be novel, nonentrenched, or nonautomatic (not automatized or habituated). This is consistent with sociological, descriptive research (Kohn & Schooler, 1983; Schooler, 1987) showing a correlation between the complexity and nonroutinization of work and measures of intellectual flexibility and complexity.

A second reason why engineering seems to provide a good prototype is that the limits of performance, based on various adaptive competencies, often are challenged by the nature of the labor market for engineers, the volatility of competition in the product markets in which engineers work, and the rapid change in the technological knowledge base that is required for effective performance in such settings. Thus, the study of how engineers develop, maintain, elaborate, and restore their expertise and their adaptive competence may provide a "window" into the more general study of how adults, and especially the elderly, adapt to the many challenges of uncertain change (Featherman, 1987).

Our preliminary studies (Peterson, 1985; Featherman & Peterson, 1986) have suggested that the specific types of job tasks and career lines in engineering may be important sources of individual variation in intellectual functioning, specifically, in problem-solving strategies deployed on the job, in the career, and, perhaps, in later life adaptational heuristics. The male engineers we have analyzed all completed a bachelor's or equivalent degree in engineering. From detailed work and job histories on these men (median age is 54 years), we have identified two career lines that branch from a common educational background: a line of jobs in engineering that extends through midlife into the later career; and a line beginning in engineering but shifting, about midcareer, into planning and design jobs and management (Figure 3.1).

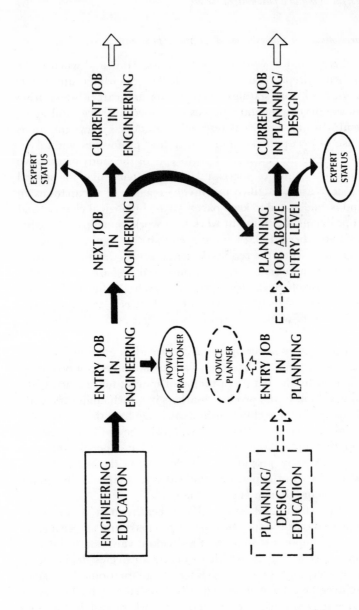

Figure 3.1. Two career lines in engineering.

Peterson (1985) has observed that nearly all jobs in the first career line involve problem-solving tasks (i.e., resolving problems, testing, evaluating, troubleshooting, simulating, analyzing). In the second career line, which branches from the first, men typically report and describe doing tasks that are qualified by different terms; we call these planning tasks (i.e., developing plans, designing, determining, creating).

What is important is that men in these two career lines and sets of common work tasks typically manifested qualitatively distinguishable problem-solving heuristics. Specifically, on instruments that elicit *rational problem-solving* and *reflective planning* orientations toward tasks on the job, engineers more typically engage in rational problem-solving, and planners adopt reflective planning as the approach that makes them "most effective at my work" (Peterson, 1985). The differences were greatest among the more mature, most "expert" in their fields. ("Experts" had won national and international acclaim and awards; "novices," by contrast, were certified practitioner engineers of similar age and career duration but without such distinction.) Apparently, these different epistemic orientations, these distinguishable problem-solving heuristics or modes of critical thinking, are related to the social organization of work, career structure, and task sets. Which orientation is assumed and becomes dominant (at least in the context of work) seems not to be a reflection of quantitative, analytical intelligence, because experts in both fields were highly competent in that dimension. Instead, what seems to be suggested is that qualitatively different epistemologies emerge – regarding the kinds of problems there were to be solved and the kinds of solutions one contemplates – among men of common educational origins but with different job, task, and career histories.

Thus, our preliminary studies support the inference that different bases for adaptive competence may become manifest during the work career, perhaps because of occupational socialization. (Our preliminary studies have not as yet ruled out the possibility that these different career lines select and retain men with initial tendencies toward one or the other of the epistemic orientations.) Clearly, high adaptive competence within the work of engineering careers can be achieved by either or both of these problem-solving heuristics. That is, expert status in one's career and effectiveness at daily tasks seem to follow from expertise at either one or the other of these orientations; but expertise at reflective planning is more likely to be required for expert status in planning careers, and vice versa.

However, what is the connection between high adaptive competence at work tasks and career management during adult life and the requisite adaptive competencies for successful aging after retirement? Are career experts, with their acquired competencies, all likely to age successfully?

Our empirical research leads us to think that men who have attained the status of expert in their fields may be more likely to age successfully than those who have not attained this status. In that sense, there is some basis for saying that being adaptively competent at some of the developmental tasks of adulthood may lead to being adaptively competent in old age. On the other hand, our theory of adaptive competence and emerging research also suggest a different outcome. Namely, not all career experts will age successfully, and those that do or do not can be predicted from the sociological and social psychological characteristics of their adult work careers. Put another way, some adaptive competencies for career expertise may facilitate successful aging after retirement, whereas other adulthood competencies rooted developmentally in different work and career lines may not. Let us examine these possibilities.

Do career experts age more successfully than career novices?

In our empirical research on careers in engineering, we examine the possibility that those who have achieved peer-acknowledged status as experts in their fields possess a high level of career management knowledge, that is, career management expertise. Among nonexperts ("novices") of equivalent age, such factual and procedural knowledge is less well formulated and deployed. Further, we are testing the proposition that expertise in career management, especially in these prototypical engineering careers, provides a developmental reserve for adapting to the life management tasks associated with retirement preparations and with the developmental tasks of post-retired life that is less available to nonexperts. In short, we expect to show that engineers who retire as experts are able to age more successfully than those who retire as novices and to connect this difference to their respective knowledge systems about career management.

Our preliminary studies about career management expertise are focused on three elements of procedural and factual knowledge about building, elaborating, maintaining, and restoring expert status in highly challenging careers, like engineering, where the mind is nearly always at work. The three elements of the knowledge system (Table 3.2) refer to career management processes: specialization, optimization, and compensation.[8]

Specialization is the process of gaining basic factual and procedural knowledge and the cognitive metaprocessing systems that enable the worker to master customary tasks or problems that are confronted on the job. Optimization subsumes specialization. As a process it refers to the cumulation of (sub)specializations and additional specializations beyond

Table 3.2. *Elements of career management expertise*

Specialization	Process of mastering the factual, procedural, and metaprocessing knowledge systems basic to a domain of activity (here, engineering) and planning
Optimization	Strategy of adding to and coordinating cumulating (sub)specialties, involving metacognitive or metaprocessing executive strategies; permits the construction of a global expertise from component expertises
Compensation	Processes of adaptive competence that are directed toward restoring (rather than adding to) and coordinating existing specializations; often used to restore global expertise that is failing or becoming obsolescent

the basic. It also involves processes that sequence and give priority to the acquisition of these various dimensions of specialization. Optimization is based on extensive metacognitive heuristics and other metaprocessing executive strategies of problem solving. Finally, compensation is a special form of optimization in which the executive system of metacognitions is directed toward both restoring and coordinating existing specializations, rather than adding to them. Compensation, we find empirically, can take the form of conservation or of substitution. In conservation, the optimization strategy shifts attention, energy, and other resources into a smaller subset of subspecialties in order to maintain the best available balance between gains and losses of expert status and job performance expertise. In substitution, compensation results from changing the composition of job-related specialization, without necessarily reducing the scope of the subspecialties that make up one's base of expert status. Substitution may involve respecialization, or career "retooling," with the objective of restoring expert status on the basis of newly acquired expertise that compensates, perhaps, for obsolescence in former domains.

In our empirical work, we use engineers' knowledge and use of specialization, optimization, and compensation to define, in functional terms, what phase a work career is in – a building phase, a maintenance phase, a restoration phase, or a loss management (terminal decline) phase (Figure 3.2). That is, it is the accumulation of career management expertise, based on the three processes, that enables engineers to become peer-acknowledged experts. It is this expert knowledge that is used to restore expert status when the foundations of that status are challenged by

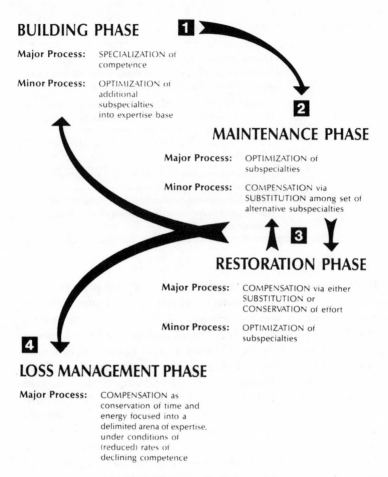

BUILDING PHASE

Major Process: SPECIALIZATION of competence

Minor Process: OPTIMIZATION of additional subspecialties into expertise base

MAINTENANCE PHASE

Major Process: OPTIMIZATION of subspecialties

Minor Process: COMPENSATION via SUBSTITUTION among set of alternative subspecialties

RESTORATION PHASE

Major Process: COMPENSATION via either SUBSTITUTION or CONSERVATION of effort

Minor Process: OPTIMIZATION of subspecialties

LOSS MANAGEMENT PHASE

Major Process: COMPENSATION as conservation of time and energy focused into a delimited arena of expertise, under conditions of (reduced) rates of declining competence

Figure 3.2. Conceptual schema of the phases of expertise in a career and related hierarchical processes of expertise management in each phase.

changing definitions and requirements for expertise in the field. Likewise, when confronted by evidence of inexorable obsolescence of mental skills and technical knowledge that are demanded for peak engineering performance, it is this expert knowledge system about career management that enables workers to slow the pace of loss.

And here we link our research on career experts with that of P. B. Baltes and M. M. Baltes on "expert" life management performances of the very old (P. B. Baltes & M. M. Baltes, this volume). Baltes and Baltes have offered evidence that successful aging by the very old may rest upon the effective use of "selective optimization with compensation." That is, faced with challenges of impending limitation of functioning in mind or body or with limitation of range of self-management and agency by a restrictive social ecology, the most effective elderly engage in compensatory actions. Compensation often takes the form of reducing the range of claimed responsibility or aspiration for agency, so that the end result is making the best of what is possible; it is a specialization of functioning in order to achieve an optimal outcome under limiting conditions. Selective optimization with compensation may be most apparent when the limits of (declining) performance capacity are being tested (P. B. Baltes & M. M. Baltes, this volume).

If the theory of selective optimization with compensation is an apt characterization of one modality of successful aging, then our experts at career management may be more likely to age successfully than are their novice counterparts. During the course of adult work careers, acquisition of expertise in specialization, optimization, and compensation provides the building blocks for expert status over the working life. Workers in career lines that customarily test the limits of performance, as we think can be shown for the prototype careers in engineering, and who attain and maintain the status of expert acquire this expert knowledge system, perforce. Workers in nonchallenging careers may not develop these adaptational reserves. The same expertise that fosters and sustains expert status in challenging careers also may provide career experts, but not career novices, with the building blocks for selective optimization with compensation, especially whenever "testing-the-limits" conditions arise beyond retirement and in very old age. This expertise also may support other forms of successful aging, qua life career management (Staudinger, 1989), insofar as expert career management skills are honed on increasingly ill-structured career problems beyond midlife, such as coping with issues like "plateauing."

Thus, developmental reserves for adaptive competence at career management tasks also may serve the purposes of successful aging. This is most likely to occur for workers who are career experts and who have attained and maintained this status within career lines that routinely test the limits of performance capacity with challenges from uncertain change and ill-structured tasks.

Do all career experts age successfully?

It is unlikely that all career experts will age successfully, even if they have worked in highly challenging career lines and have acquired expertise in specialization, optimization, and compensation in adapting to the viscissitudes of career management in these settings. There are two reasons why expertise in career management may not be transferable to successful aging. First, most expertises are domain specific and do not transfer from domain to domain (Chi, Feltovich, & Glaser, 1982; Salthouse, 1987a, 1987b); having an expert knowledge system and using it effectively in a career does not guarantee being an "expert in life management" after retirement. Second, the developmental tasks of post-retirement are not equivalent to those of midlife, including career management within the world of work and socially organized career pathways. To reintroduce the terminology of well- and ill-structured tasks, adaptive competence at career management involves expertise developed with reference to well-structured and moderately ill-structured work and career tasks (Featherman, 1987; Yussen, 1985).

Still, we are testing the hypothesis that transfer of expertise from the domain of career management to the domain of post-retired life management is possible for some expert engineers. Our hypothesis is that career experts who have acquired a reflective planning orientation will age more successfully than career experts who use a rational problem-solving approach to tasks. This expectation is based on the wider experience of reflective planners with job tasks that are relatively more ill-structured than well-structured and on the tendency of reflective planners to be adaptive, creative experts. Such experts are more efficient in finding new problems and in expanding old problems and in knowing who to ask to solve such problems. By contrast, rational problem solvers have more experience at engineeering tasks with well-structured boundaries. They are highly efficient in finding best solutions themselves; they are routinized or convergent experts.

If the life world of post-retirement does contain developmental tasks that become increasingly less well-structured and more ill-structured, then a basis for transfer of expertise from work careers to life management careers is found. And in this late-life setting, it is the expert reflective planners who may be relatively better equipped to age successfully, because of prior experience and expertise in highly effective problem solving of ill-structured tasks.

Are reflective planning and wisdom related forms of adaptive competence?

Our research program has not yet produced data on the relationship, if any, between reflective planning and wisdom. However, the argument that they are related forms of adaptive competence is provided some credibility from inferences and extensions we draw from the Berlin wisdom project (P. B. Baltes & J. Smith, 1990; Dittmann-Kohli, 1984; J. Smith & P. B. Baltes, 1990; Staudinger, 1989). In the Berlin

Table 3.3. *Similarity of wisdom and the reflective planning orientation*

P. B. Baltes and J. Smith (1990) use the following assessment criteria for *wisdom*. Wisdom is viewed as an expert knowledge system in the domain of fundamental life pragmatics consisting of

- *Rich factual knowledge*: General and specific knowledge about the conditions of life and its variations
- *Rich procedural knowledge*: General and specific knowledge about strategies of judgment and advice concerning matters of life
- *Life-span contextualism*: Knowledge about the contexts of life and their temporal (developmental) relationships
- *Relativism*: Knowledge about differences in values, goals, and priorities
- *Uncertainty*: Knowledge about the relative indeterminacy and unpredictability of life and ways to manage

Similarly, Featherman and Peterson (1986), (following Nadler, 1981; and Rittel & Webber, 1974) define the *reflective planning orientation* as follows:

- Expertise (including factual, procedural, and epistemic knowledge) about approaches to and the process of creating or restructuring a solution system
- Purposive, volitional, and requiring the abandonment of the assumption of static problems and problem solutions
- Belief in the uniqueness of every problem (its plan and solution)
- View of problem solving as a time-based, historical process; recognition of the relativity of solutions
- Acknowledgment of the social, interpersonal, and societal relevance of technical problems
- Application of both divergent (i.e., novelty search) and convergent thinking
- Awareness of uncertainty and the fallibility of the one-best-solution approach

research, wisdom is viewed as expert knowledge about the important and fundamental matters of life, their interpretation and management. Five criteria of wisdom have been specified. A prerequisite for expertise in the domain of fundamental life pragmatics is a rich factual and procedural knowledge base. The Berlin group also nominated several meta-level (or interpretative) knowledge dimensions, namely, life-span contextualism, relativism, and an understanding of life's uncertainties. A functional consequence of this expert knowledge is exceptional insight into life's conditions and problems, "good" judgment, and the capacity to give "good" advice. Wisdom, in this sense, includes being able to make reflective judgments (Table 3.3).

Like cognitive wisdom in the Berlin research, reflective planning, as practiced by our expert engineers, also is an expertise. It is a cumulative knowledge system about creating or restructuring a solution system, under conditions of high uncertainty. It is a process driven by purposes that lie behind the actual problem to be solved. It reflects relativity and uncertainty and is socially rooted in values and human purposes. By contrast, the rational problem-solving orientation does not share many attributes with wisdom, either as a knowledge system or as a cognitive process.

These apparent similarities between the conceptual definitions of wisdom and planning and the differences between wisdom and problem solving have prompted our thinking about the developmental relationship among these constructs. We have hypothesized that the midcareer shifts in job tasks we observe among many engineers – from traditional problem-solving jobs and tasks into jobs that involve primarily planning and design responsibilities – may be associated with a corresponding shift in problem-solving heuristics – from rational problem solving to reflective planning. This occupational resocialization explanation would be consistent with research showing a developmental shift toward "reflective judgement," as is observed during and after graduate education in some disciplines (K. S. Kitchener & Wood, 1987). Or, the shift in orientation could reflect fundamental cognitive developmental changes in the affected men. Postformal operational shifts in cognitive functioning have been reported for older adults (Hoyer, 1985; Labouvie-Vief, 1980). Finally, are the men who undertake new careers in planning jobs and assume a new epistemology for problem solving compensating for failing or obsolescent technical competencies? That is, are they engaging in an early form of selective optimization with compensation (P. B. Baltes & M. M. Baltes, this volume)?

We cannot, as yet, verify these proposals about the developmental origins of reflective planning and its apparent relationship to cognitive wisdom. We have hypothesized that our expert engineers with a reflective planning orientation will score higher on the Berlin measures of cognitive wisdom than will the experts who take a rational problem-solving approach. If that relationship is supported in our research, it will provide one inferential link between reflective planning and successful aging. Reflective planning, like cognitive wisdom, may draw upon the same cognitive reserves for successful aging, given the special characteristics of developmental tasks in late life. Both may be composed of the same underlying capacities (e.g., reflective judgment, critical thinking, tolerance of uncertainty, and other related dimensions of mind and personality). Alternatively, both may be reflections of the more latent construct, adaptive competence, as expressed during later adulthood and old age.

Only further research will illuminate these possibilities. However, the entire line of research is directed toward finding possible life-span processes that provide some adults with developmental reserves of adaptive competence both during the adult years and in later life. Despite the possible discontinuity between the relatively well-structured developmental tasks of childhood, youth, and early adulthood, on the one hand, and the more ill-structured features of later life, on the other, we pursue the view that successful aging is a life-span phenomenon. In our conceptual framework, successful aging is more likely among persons whose work, family, and community roles have instilled deep knowledge and who have successfully managed their careers during adulthood; in addition, it is more likely in those who also have had more extensive experience with ill-structured tasks and who approach problem solving with a reflective planning orientation. We believe it is such persons who have learned to plan and who plan to learn (Michael, 1973) over the entire adult life course. Such persons seem highly adaptive and adaptively competent, especially in a life period of increasingly uncertain change in mind, body, self, and environment.

The post-retired society and the role of planning in its successful aging

The transactional view states that successful aging is not a characteristic of persons. Rather, it is a descriptive term for the dialectical relationship between the adaptive competence of the person and the developmental tasks of a dynamic society. The emphasis is on potentialities for change in both person and society and on the dynamic steady states of adaptation, both between persons and their communities and between these communities and their wider societal setting.

In the first portion of this chapter we defined successful aging from the point of view of the person, in transactional terms, as adaptive competence. The focus was on developmental reserves for resilience in the face of increasingly uncertain change arising from ill-structured developmental tasks. The view was ontogenetic, or developmental. In this last section we take a different view, from the perspective of the embedding social systems of institutions and demographic structures and their dynamics. This is the reciprocal view of the transaction that constitutes successful aging. It is evolutionary or historical rather than ontogenetic.

To repeat a point made earlier, the "content" of successful aging, apart from its generic adaptational quality, is always historical or situational. That is, what successful aging "is," is conditioned by the fabric of society and by the historical moment; its content is time-dependent, time-bound. (By extension, it takes on many forms even within a historical epoch, varying possibly by gender, race, class, and so on.) Therefore, in attempting to provide a view of successful aging for the present and immediate future, how can we characterize at least American society and its dynamics as they pertain to the adaptational challenges during adult development? The reply to this question is necessarily speculative, perhaps even imprudent and premature; the disciplined historical analysis required to substantiate any answer has yet to be done. Nevertheless, the intellectual task is not unimportant if one wishes to be faithful to the transactional view. Thus, what follows is but a synoptic, first, and tentative approximation for purposes of illustration and discussion. The construct of post-retired society will be a frame of reference.

The post-retired society

By *post-retired society* we refer to an abstraction about American society; it is a heuristic construction rather than an empirically derived phenomenon. We do not suggest that there is a general "type" of society that is or becomes post-retired. Nevertheless, we have in mind several constituent characteristics of American society that, together, are our frame of reference for successful aging in that context.

First, this is a society becoming demographically older by virtue of fertility limitation and extension of longevity; it is an aging, or "graying," society, lacking massive immigration of high-fertility individuals and families. There is little doubt that contemporary American society, like most industrialized ones in the West, manifests this characteristic.

Second, shifts in the age composition of an aging society produce a secondary effect, namely, an increase in the prevalence and visibility of ill-structured life dilemmas associated with the presence of more elderly. The evolution of a larger, healthier, and better educated post-retirement age stratum, through the succession of cohorts, increases the diffusion of general awareness of the developmental issues and dilemmas associated with the post-retired years and aging. Politically active, vocal interest groups of elderly, with effective leadership in the Congress, lobby for their welfare and an end to age discrimination. For example, ending mandatory retirement, expanding social security, fostering independent living, guaranteeing long-term health care, and even the issue of life extension versus the right to die enter national policy discourse.

However, the key outcome of the demographic shifts is not just greater exposure to and awareness of the problems of the elderly and of being "old." Some of the problems of the elderly and their possible solutions are discussed in dialectical terms, as if the welfare of the burgeoning elderly population and that of the young were not only interrelated but also in possible opposition (Braungart & Braungart, 1986; Preston, 1984). They are discussed as "age policy" or life-cycle dilemmas (i.e., "generational equity") involving uncertain rules of justification for rationing scarce, life-sustaining, and welfare-promoting resources (Daniels, 1988). The dilemmas may have no final solutions in societies with slow-growth economies, "stable" population structures, and a pluralistic polity. For example, "aging" policies set in terms of vertical equity across contemporary age categories (really birth cohorts with different histories of benefits and needs) and even welfare policies that involve "means testing" do not necessarily provide horizontal equity, "justice over the life span," for any given cohort (Daniels, 1988). In any case, the graying of the population seems to have increased the range and volume of ill-structured problems (originating from the developmental tasks of the elderly) on the agenda of national policy and in the minds and personal lives of many citizens irrespective of their ages.

A third defining element of the post-retired society construct also increases the ill-structured dilemmas facing the population: The adult life course itself is becoming less well-structured, even during the earlier years. This evolving, historical change is connected to the demographic aging of American society, albeit indirectly, through the historical forces affecting the declining rates of nuptuality and fertility (see Sweet & Bumpass, 1987, for fuller treatments). In brief, the historical forces are the trailing edge of industrialization and an American demographic transition that is focused most sharply in the life courses of adult women: greater economic opportunities in a service economy for well-educated, never-married women to lead independent lives, and the ascendency of cultural values embracing self-selection of life goals and the pursuit of personal interest (Lesthaeghe, 1983; Sørensen & McLanahan, 1987). American women remain enrolled in colleges and universities at rates that currently exceed those of the males in their cohorts; by the end of this century the rates of male and female participation in the labor force may reach parity; and about 30% of contemporary American women may never marry, and 30% of American-born women are likely to remain childless. These facts and projections may be related to the gradual and steady rise in the divorce rate since the American Civil War.

For example, some analysts (England & Farkas, 1986; Sweet & Bumpass, 1987) regard the fundamental changes in the character of family life as reflecting a new calculus of economic gains and losses in the minds of women and men. For women, the economic advantages of remaining single and pursuing a full-time career may tend to outweigh those of marriage and parenthood, especially considering the personal costs of pursuing a "dual career" of domestic and paid labor, the lower wages paid to married women, and the probable high costs of eventually becoming a single mother (Fuchs, 1986; Garfinkel & McLanahan, 1987). For men, the gains from marriage may be diminishing, to the degree that the historic availability of a spouse-homemaker-mother role complex declines in response to career pursuits, economic independence, and voluntary childlessness by their potential spouses.

These interpretations aside, the consequences of the observed trends in work and family life for young and middle-aged adults seem clear: The once-normative, age-graded impetus to form families is eroded and eroding. The problematics of "loving and working" for contemporary American adults is far less well-structured than it must have been during the 1950s, when social scientists used the term *family life cycle* to capture the highly prevalent, age-regular pattern of marrying, bearing, and rearing children into their own adulthood (see Vinovskis, 1988, for a review of this research).

There is also limited evidence to support the speculation that the once rather well-structured features of the early and middle adult life course, in this case the adult work career, may be giving way to ill-structured features. The aging of the labor force may be altering the social mobility chances of successive cohorts and is changing the predictability of advancements within career lines (Hout, 1988). For example, professional career lines are being shortened ("plateauing"), especially in bureaucratic, internal labor markets in which the demographic density of middle-aged and older workers has increased. Many middle- and upper-level managers are without next career steps; they are without explicit organizational timetables that, in recent times, had provided predictability of job and salary advancements and were used as reference points for gauging one's effectiveness and professional esteem (Lawrence, 1987; *Wall Street Journal*, April 10, 1987, Section 2). The lesser predictability is not only a matter of reorganization of professional career lines, for longitudinal analysis of the stability and instability of annual income for all American families shows a surprising amount of interannual vacillation (Duncan, 1988).

These constructions of the dynamics of a post-retired society suggest that the predominance of ill-structured over well-structured features of developmental tasks may emerge at earlier ages or life periods for contemporary cohorts of adults than for their predecessors. If this speculative conclusion is correct, what are its implications for the *society's* successful aging, that is, for society's effective functioning and longevity? One way to restate this question is in terms of societal problem solving and of the styles of thinking that underlie social planning and policy formulation in a society faced with a greater volume and range of ill-structured dilemmas. To put the suggested answer in the form of a question: Is it possible that the adoption of a reflective planning orientation as a societal problem-solving heuristic increases the adaptive competence of a post-retired society, just as a similar strategy by individuals increases their successful aging?[9]

Toward a planning society

Commentaries about planning and problem solving in widely different arenas of American life – education, industrial management, and public administration – suggest that an affirmative answer to the question posed at the end of the last section has some support. Writing within the liberal educational philosophy of John Dewey (Ratner, 1939) and Robert Hutchins (1968), Resnick (1987) suggests that the schools should prepare persons to be "*adaptive learners*, so that they can perform effectively when situations are unpredictable and tasks demand change" (1987, p. 18; my italics). This goal for modern education is required, she states, because of discontinuities between the modes of learning required and the challenges encountered in the contemporary adult worlds of work and community life, on the one hand, and in today's schools, on the other. In the terminology of this paper, Resnick sees the well-structured school and its curriculum as failing to provide adaptive competence for the ill-structured settings of modern adult life. She recommends that the schools reorganize their curricula to provide epistemic training in how to organize knowledge, parse problems, self-monitor learning, and handle related problem-solving tasks that "drive" effective education through life (see also Yussen, 1985; cf. Glaser, 1984). This proposal for the teaching of adaptive competence skills calls for the application of reflective planning to modern education. Resnick's appraisal and recommendations seem at variance with other advice from American educators for the teaching of specific cultural knowledge (Hirsch, 1987).

Similarly, industrial engineers and management analysts increasingly argue that conventional decision making within American industry may be ill-suited to the requirements for competitiveness within a rapidly changing world marketplace, (Cohen & Zysman, 1988; Nadler, 1986; Nadler, Perrone, Seabold, & Yussen, 1984; Thurow, 1987). Many such studies call for redesigning the "planning" of process technology and the management of production by supplanting the "satisficing" approach of rational problem solving (in our terms) by reflective planning or "conceptual planning" (Nadler, 1986; see also Quinn, 1988; and Schön, 1983). For example, Michael (1973) discusses "future responsive societal learning" and "long-range societal planning" as managerial orientations that go beyond the social engineering approach to industrial problem solving and planning. (The social engineering approach is a top-down, rational problem-solving approach.) In this framework, the planning process should promote novel, multiple uses of technology as markets change; promote continuous feedback about failures in achieving goals (quality control); and involve expertise at the bottom as well as at the top of the bureaucratic hierarchy. Thus, a planning orientation, akin to reflective planning, may provide greater adaptive competence for American industry and economic success within the new realities of the world economy.[10]

Finally, some political scientists and historians who study American public policy formulation and decision making make the case for new thinking about lessons from history. For example, Neustadt and May (1986) use case histories from American politics and government to show the errors of taking events in the past and prior policy decisions as strictly applicable to the present and future. The ways in which policymakers think about the past and use historical examples are reflected in the fate of nations. Mechanistic, deterministic views appear to be less adaptive than reflective, purposively rational planning. In the latter style of thinking about time, the many possible consequences of acts – their policy implications – as well as history are considered.

These examples underscore the view that the adaptive resilience of a society hinges upon its problem-solving heuristics for life-span education, world economic competitiveness, and transnational political action. The aging of contemporary Western societies puts additional pressure on policy planning and decision making. The contemporary world situation may well require a society to depend on reflective planning approaches to ensure its resiliency and viability.

The constituting reference points of the post-retired society have suggestive implications for the successful aging of American society as well as for the individuals within it. Whether the specific implications hold in other societies with similar configurations of these characteristics is unclear, but the general didactic point remains: *Successful aging of individuals is related to the functioning and maintenance of communal life as the human ecology changes over time, that is, to the successful aging of society through its adaptive competence.* Let us close with a summary comment on this transactional view of successful aging.

Successful aging is individuals' learning to plan and society's planning to learn

The theme of this paper is that successful aging of individuals may differ across history and societies. But one relationship abides, namely, the link between the form of successful aging and the constraints on the functioning of the communities and societies within which these individuals reside. The heuristic construct of a post-retired society was used to illustrate this link for contemporary America. We have suggested a generic definition of successful aging, adaptive competence, and have provided several manifestations of it within a post-retired society.

One manifestation in particular was singled out, a problem-solving heuristic called reflective planning. We have argued that reflective planning enlarges adaptive competence in historical circumstances and for developmental tasks in the life course when ill-structured dilemmas are more prevalent than well-structured puzzles. Thus, for individuals, successful aging may be increased by "learning to plan." This thesis was explored conceptually using data from ongoing longitudinal research on successful individual aging. We predicted that cognitive and behavioral reserves for adaptive competence in later life may be acquired, selectively, from work and career management experiences during adult life. In a more speculative vein, we have suggested that the same problem-solving heuristic may be involved in successful adaptations to the challenges of a post-retired society, in which the ill-structured dilemmas of uncertain change abound. Indeed, it was the increasing prevalence of ill-structured life tasks and dilemmas, both through the later life course and in the evolving history of modern American society, that led us to suggest the adaptive "fit" of the reflective planning orientation. Thus, for social institutions and their key managers and decision makers, successful societal adaptation may be increased by "planning to learn," or planning that is more fully reflective.

A longer life of post-retired leisure provides the opportunity for reflective planning and a rationale for learning to plan (Riley, 1985b). The increase in the rate and the uncertain outcomes of complex changes in society and in the geopolitical system may force individuals and institutions to plan to learn in future-oriented, life-span frameworks. This argument about successful aging is transactional, for it infers that what constitutes successful aging is unknowable from characteristics of the person, of the life course, or of an epoch of a society's history taken apart from each other. Successful aging is a construct that lies at the boundary of personal biography, society, and history. If in contemporary post-retired American society successful aging is linked to some degree to individual differences in reflective planning and expertise in career management, this is a transitory relationship. In a transactional, social psychological perspective, the same statement applies to wisdom and other facets of successful aging.

For example, why is wisdom, and not some other attribute of behavior or mind, the honorific characteristic of later life (the cardinal "virtue," in an Eriksonian sense)? Does the "choice" of wisdom reflect the evolutionary history of old age as a life period and its societal function (or lack thereof)? Is this choice related to the availability (or relative absence) of roles and organized positions within society whose incumbents can be called "productive" or can attain high status and otherwise derive personal esteem? In the demographic evolution of a longer term of post-retired life in the postindustrial West, and with the likely prevalence of wider biological and psychosocial variations within this age stratum, will the signal importance of wisdom subside or be superseded by other positive attributions? Will the social and political reconstruction of the developmental tasks and available "productive" roles for this evolving life period be influenced by what wisdom is or by the search and "discovery" of other positive attributes and functions of being long-lived? And if the reorganized social world of old age increases the prevalence of well-structured roles and status-conferring positions within formal institutions, will it be the rational problem solvers or the reflective planners who age more successfully or who are deemed to be more wise?

Successful aging is a transactional construct. To understand it, we need longitudinal research that is longitudinal in both a biographical and a historical dimension. The research should be about the aging of persons as well as about the dynamics of society. It should dwell upon the adaptive competence of person and society as each is affected by the other: Successful aging is individuals' learning to plan and society's planning to learn.

NOTES

Research and writing of this paper were supported by grants from the John D. and Catherine T. MacArthur Research Program on Successful Aging and the National Institute on Aging. We thank Christine Caldwell and Nadine Marks for their assistance in research. W. Andrew Achenbaum, Margret and Paul Baltes, O. Gilbert Brim, Jr., Norman Garmezy, and Gerald Nadler kindly commented on related manuscripts; their collegiality and the helpful advice of anonymous reviewers of the ESF draft are gratefully acknowledged.

1 This approach is consistent with the view of Rowe and Kahn (1987) that successful aging involves resilience, that is, a restorative and expansive potentiality in the face of challenges to the person, as well as vitality, that is, a state of unusual physical, mental, or behavioral functioning relative to one's age peers.

2 In a subsequent section we define *post-retired society* as a heuristic construct that has at least three characteristics: (1) a demographically aged population, (2) discussion of welfare policies as life-cycle dilemmas that derive from a demographically aging society (i.e., generational equity), and (3) an increased perception that developmental tasks, from childhood throughout old age, are less solvable, or more "ill-structured."

3 Current thinking about expertise, at least within the experimental traditions of cognitive psychology, is summarized by Glaser (1984), and its manifestations in adulthood are detailed by Salthouse (1987a, 1987b). Our cognitive approach to competence also is consistent with Cantor and Kihlstrom's (1985) conception of personality and "intelligent" behavior in real-world settings.

4 At the current time, there is a paucity of empirical information on which to base this working hypothesis. However, Brandtstädter and Baltes-Götz (this volume) report that middle-aged and older adults *perceive* the impact of uncontrollable, exogenous factors on personal development to increase. Others (P. B. Baltes, 1973; Brim & Ryff, 1980; Seligman & Elder, 1986) have suggested that uncontrollable events and life changes, as *objectively defined*, cumulate across the life span. The working hypothesis is also consistent with commentaries and unsystematic task analyses by educational psychologists who argue that the objective learning tasks and school and home settings through which children and adolescents learn and acquire problem-solving skills are considerably more formalized, closed ended, rule bound, and group oriented than in the subsequent worlds of work and community life (Resnick, 1987; Scribner & Cole, 1973; Yussen, 1985). The status of this hypothesis cannot be settled without further data, including both objective task analysis and studies of how tasks are perceived and understood by the person facing them. In addition, such studies must take note of the sociological conditions that surround the problem solver. For example, one may wish to argue that the young child faces more objectively indeterminate life outcomes and perceives tasks to be more undefined (by lack of prior experience) than does the child's parent. Although these assumptions may prove correct , it also may be true that the sociocultural and interpersonal context of the child more readily provides the "correct" answers and imposes preferred directions to problems and life tasks for the child than for the parent. Thus, neither analysis of the intrinsic characteristics of tasks nor analysis of individuals' perceptions of tasks is sufficient. As we argue subsequently, the sociological setting of developmental tasks and of solution finding is less well organized by contemporary culture, and the tasks of later life are set within fewer formalized institutional contexts than those in the first decades of life (Rosow, 1985). That this alleged state of affairs can change (and, indeed, seems to be under way at least in American society) is suggested in the subsequent discussion of the post-retired society.

5 The terminology used here follows from Churchman (1971). Others have contrasted these two classes of tasks as "well-defined" versus "ill-defined" (Hayes, 1987). We prefer *ill-structured* as a term to emphasize that organizational timetables, peer reference groups, and other instances of objective social structure set conditions on the ways that everyday problems and developmental tasks are defined and solutions are sought (e.g., Kohli, 1986; Kluwe, 1986; Meyer, 1986). For example, the developmental tasks faced by the school-aged child in a middle-class neighborhood are far more well-structured than those of age peers who may have to fight their way to the classroom in the urban ghetto. This example also illustrates that any hypothesis about the life-span prevalence of well- and ill-structured tasks necessarily refers to rather gross tendencies; variations according to gender, social class, race, and other social categories may constitute significant departures from the prevalent mode for the population or age stratum.

6 Professor Andrew Achenbaum has suggested to us that ill-structured dilemmas may proliferate (if they do in fact) with aging because "by their very nature late-life challenges are *intrinsically* more formidable or intriguing to an older person who has become experienced in seeing issues in a broader context or in making connections among several realms of life as they approach the finitude of their existence." Perhaps cumulative personal experience and the dialectics of unresolved life conflicts promote such a schema of thinking and knowing, he has suggested (personal communication, 1988). We accept this as one life-span explanation for the putative shift in the prevalence of ill- over well-structured life tasks. Yet we eschew any explanation that takes a wholly person-centered developmental view. That is, our working hypothesis is that the organizational context of later life tends, on average, to offer fewer guidelines, imperatives, and structurally provided facilitators (but perhaps more inhibitors) to achieve the developmental tasks of later life. For example, Margret Baltes and colleagues (e.g., Baltes & Reisenzein, 1986) point out that older persons residing in nursing homes, a small fraction of the elderly to be sure, may engage in a variety of ironic "dependence-casting" interactions with professional staff in order to gain some control over social contacts and a modicum of independence over the circumstances of one's final months of life within a well-structured institutional setting. This is an example of an ill-structured dilemma set within a seemingly well-structured setting (Marshall, 1980). The example reminds us that a structural analysis of developmental tasks (i.e., how well-structured or well-defined a task is) calls for a sophisticated theory of action (Brandtstädter, 1984; Giddens, 1984; Wells & Stryker, 1988). This action theory must consider the intrinsic nature of the task but in relationship to the embedded sets of intrapersonal and organizational definitions of the situation. Importantly, structural analysis of action recognizes the degree of accessibility of resources — including the clarity of purpose or goal — within the organizational setting, which either impedes or aids the fulfillment of purposive action (mastering the developmental task). The latter will include aspects of empowerment or interpersonal influence in both subjectively perceived and objectively enacted dimensions, as in the Baltes research. Such complexity in task analysis makes the judgment of what is ill-structured or well-structured a difficult task in itself.

7 Research in progress explores the hypothesis that rational problem solving precedes the development of reflective planning. To explore this possibility we are examining the relationship of expertise in and use of these styles of thinking and knowing to developmental levels of reflective judgment (K. S. Kitchener & King, 1981; K. S. Kitchener & R. F. Kitchener, 1981).

8 See P. B. Baltes and M. M. Baltes (this volume) for a related set of constructs. We suggest that these three constructs have a life-span applicability for the expression of competence across behavioral domains.

9 We do not intend to engage in reification by referring to societal problem solving. The reference is elliptical, for it applies to the heuristics used by public officials and by managers, administrators, professionals, and other decision makers in public sector institutions.

10 This idea has some empirical basis in the research by Quinn (1988) on managers of American business enterprises. Quinn shows that when managers go "beyond rational management," or in our terms, beyond rational problem solving, both they and their firms tend to thrive. Specifically, Quinn's findings

suggest that a combination of rational problem solving and reflective planning is the optimal operating style of the more effective managers in the most flourishing and resilient firms.

REFERENCES

Atchley, R. C. (1983). *Aging: Continuity and change.* Belmont, CA: Walsworth.

Baltes, M. M., & Reisenzein, R. (1986). The social world in long-term care institutions: Psychosocial control toward dependency? In M. M. Baltes & P. B. Baltes (Eds.), *The psychology of control and aging* (pp. 315–344). Hillsdale, NJ: Lawrence Erlbaum.

Baltes, P. B. (1973). Life-span models of psychological aging: A white elephant? *Gerontologist, 13,* 475–512.

Baltes, P. B. (1987). Theoretical propositions of life-span developmental psychology. *Developmental Psychology, 23,* 611–626.

Baltes, P. B., Dittmann-Kohli, F., & Dixon, R. A. (1984). New perspectives on the development of intelligence in adulthood: Toward a dual-process conception and a model of selective optimization with compensation. In P. B. Baltes & O. G. Brim, Jr. (Eds.), *Life-span development and behavior* (Vol. 6, pp. 34–78). New York: Academic Press.

Baltes, P. B., & Smith, J. (1990). Toward a psychology of wisdom and its ontogenesis. In R. J. Sternberg (Ed.), *Wisdom: Its nature, origins, and development* (pp. 87–120). New York: Cambridge University Press.

Berg, C. A., & Sternberg, R. J. (1985). A triarchic theory of intellectual development during adulthood. *Developmental Review, 5,* 334–370.

Bloom, B. L. (1977). *Community mental health.* Monterey, CA: Brooks/Cole.

Brandtstädter, J. (1984). Personal and social control over development: Some implications of an action perspective in life-span developmental psychology. In P. B. Baltes & O. G. Brim (Eds.), *Life-span development and behavior* (Vol. 6, pp. 2–33). New York: Academic Press.

Braungart, R. G., & Braungart, M. M. (1986). Life-course and generational politics. In R. Turner & J. Short (Eds.), *Annual review of sociology* (Vol. 12, pp. 205–231). Palo Alto, CA: Annual Review.

Brim, O. G., Jr., & Ryff, C. D. (1980). On the properties of life events. In P. B. Baltes & O. G. Brim, Jr. (Eds.), *Life-span development and behavior* (Vol. 3, pp. 368–388). New York: Academic Press.

Cantor, N., & Kihlstrom, J. F. (1985). Social intelligence: The cognitive basis of personality. In P. Shaver (Ed.), *Self, situations and social behavior* (pp. 15–33). Beverly Hills, CA: Sage.

Cantor, N., Norem, J. K., Niedenthal, P. M., Langston, C. A., & Brower, A. M. (1987). Life tasks, self-concept ideas, and cognitive strategies in a life transition. *Journal of Personality and Social Psychology, 53,* 1178–1191.

Chi, M. T. H., Feltovich, P. J., & Glaser, R. (1982). Categorization and representation of physics problems by experts and novices. *Cognitive Science, 5,* 121–152.

Churchman, C. W. (1971). *The design of inquiring systems: Basic concepts of systems and organization.* New York: Basic Books.

Cohen, S. S., & Zysman, J. (1988). Manufacturing innovation and American industrial competitiveness. *Science, 239,* 1110–1115.

Cornelius, S. W., & Caspi, A. (1987). Everyday problem solving in adulthood and old age. *Psychology and Aging, 2,* 144–153.

Daniels, N. (1988). *Am I my parents' keeper: An essay on justice between the young and old.* New York: Oxford University Press.

Dewey, J. (1910). *How we think.* New York: D. C. Health.

Dittmann-Kohli, F. (1984). Weisheit als mögliches Ergebnis der Intelligenzentwicklung im Erwachsenenalter. *Sprache und Kognition, 2,* 112–132.

Dittmann-Kohli, F., & Kramer, D. (1985 July). *Task analysis in cognitive aging research: Comparison of tradition and real life approaches.* Paper presented at the eighth biennial meeting of the International Society for the Study of Behavioral Development, Tours, France.

Duncan, G. (1988). The volatility of family income over the life course. In P. B. Baltes, D. L. Featherman, & R. M. Lerner (Eds.), *Life-span development and behavior* (Vol. 9, pp. 318–358). Hillsdale, NJ: Lawrence Erlbaum.

England, P., & Farkas, G. (1986). *Households, employment and gender.* New York: Aldine.

Erikson, E. H. (1950). *Childhood and society.* New York: Norton.

Featherman, D. L. (1987, July). *Work, adaptive competence, and successful aging: A theory of adult cognitive development.* Lecture given at the World Congress of the International Society for the Study of Behavioral Development, Tokyo, Japan.

Featherman, D. L., & Lerner, R. M. (1985). Ontogenesis and sociogenesis: Problematics for theory and research about development and socialization across the lifespan. *American Sociological Review, 50,* 659–676.

Featherman, D. L., & Peterson, J. G. (1986, November). *Adaptive competence in work careers: Socialization for successful aging.* Poster presented at the annual meeting of the Gerontological Society of America, Chicago, IL.

Fisher, K. W. (1980). A theory of cognition development: The control and construction of hierarchies of skills. *Psychological Review, 87,* 477–531.

Foote, N. N., & Cottrell, L., Jr. (1955). *Identity and interpersonal competence: A new direction in family research.* Chicago: University of Chicago Press.

Friedman, S. L., Scholnick, E. K., & Cocking, R. R. (1987). *Blueprints for thinking: The role of planning in cognitive development.* Cambridge: Cambridge University Press.

Fuchs, V. R. (1986). Sex differences in economic well-being. *Science, 232,* 459–464.

Garfinkel, I., & McLanahan, S. (1987). *Single mothers and their children: A new American dilemma.* Washington, DC: Urban Institute.

Garmezy, N., & Masten, A. S. (1986). Stress, competence and resilience: Common frontiers for therapist and psychopathologist. *Behavior Therapy, 17,* 500–521.

Giddens, A. (1984). *The constitution of society: Outline of the theory of structuration.* Los Angeles and Berkeley, CA: University of California Press.

Gladwin, T. (1967). Social competence and clinical practice. *Psychiatry, 30,* 30–43.

Glaser, R. (1984). Education and thinking. *American Psychologist, 39*(1), 93–104.

Haan, N. (1977). *Coping and defending: Processes of self-environment regulation.* New York: Academic Press.

Hannan, M. T., & Freeman, J. (1986). The ecology of organizations: Structural inertia and organizational change. In S. Lindenberg, J. S. Coleman, & S.

Nowak (Eds.), *Approaches to social theory* (pp. 151–172). New York: Russell Sage Foundation.

Havighurst, R. J. (1956). Research on the developmental task concept. *School Review: A Journal of Secondary Education, 64,* 215–223.

Hawley, A. (1968). Human ecology. In D. L. Sills (Ed.), *International encyclopedia of the social sciences.* New York: Macmillan.

Hayes, J. (1987). *The complete problem solver.* Hillsdale, NJ: Lawrence Erlbaum.

Heckhausen, J., & Baltes, P. B. (1990). *Perceived controllability of expected psychological change.* Manuscript submitted for publication.

Hirsch, E. D., Jr. (1987). *Cultural literacy.* New York: Houghton Mifflin.

Hogan, D. P., & Astone, N. M. (1986). The transition to adulthood. *Annual Review of Sociology, 12,* 109–130.

Hout, M. (1988). More universalism, less structural mobility: The American occupational structure in the 1980's. *American Journal of Sociology, 93,* 1358–1400.

Hoyer, W. J. (1985). Aging and the development of expert cognition. In T. M. Schlecther & M. P. Toglia (Eds.), *New directions in cognitive science* (pp. 69–87). Norwood, NJ: Ablex.

Hutchins, R. (1968). *The learning society.* New York: Mentor.

Inkeles, A. (1966). Social structure and the socialization of competence. *Harvard Educational Review, 36,* 265–283.

Kitchener, K. S. (1983). Cognition, metacognition and epistemic cognition: A three-level model of cognitive processing. *Human Development, 26,* 222–232.

Kitchener, K. S., & King, P. M. (1981). Reflective judgement: Concepts of justification and their relationship to age and education. *Journal of Applied Developmental Psychology, 2,* 89–116.

Kitchener, K. S., & Kitchener, R. F. (1981). The development of natural rationality: Can formal operations account for it? In J. A. Meacham & N. R. Santelli (Eds.), *Social development in youth: Structure and content* (pp. 160–181). Basel: S. Karger.

Kitchener, K. S., & Wood, P. K. (1987). Development of concepts of justification in German university students. *International Journal of Behavioral Development, 10,* 171–185.

Kluwe, R. H. (1986). Psychological research on problem solving and aging. In A. B. Sørensen, F. Weinert, and L. Sherrod (Eds.), *Human development and the life course: Multidisciplinary perspectives* (pp. 509–534). Hillsdale, NJ: Lawrence Erlbaum.

Kohli, M. (1986). Social organization and subjective construction of the life course. In A. B. Sørensen, F. Weinert, and L. Sherrod (Eds.), *Human development and the life course: Multidisciplinary perspectives* (pp. 271–293). Hillsdale, NJ: Lawrence Erlbaum.

Kohn, M. L., & Schooler, C. (1983). *Work and personality: An inquiry into the impact of social stratification.* Hillsdale, NJ: Ablex.

Labouvie-Vief, G. (1980). Beyond formal operations: Uses and limits of pure logic in life-span development. *Human Development, 23,* 141–161.

Labouvie-Vief, G. (1982). Dynamic development and mature autonomy. *Human Development, 25,* 161–191.

Lawrence, B. S. (1987). An organizational theory of age effects. In S. Bacharach &

N. DiTomaso (Eds.), *Research in the sociology of organizations* (pp. 37–71). Greenwich, CT: JAI Press.

Lazarus, R. S. (1966). *Psychological stress and the aging process*. New York: Academic Press.

Lesthaeghe, R. (1983). A century of demographics and cultural change in Western Europe. *Population and Development Review, 9*, 441–435.

Lindgren, B. W. (1976). *Statistical theory* (3rd ed.). New York: Macmillan.

Marini, M. M. (1984). Age and sequencing norms in the transition to adulthood. *Social Forces, 63*, 229–244.

Marshall, V. W. (1980). *Last chapters: A sociology of aging and dying*. Monterey, CA: Brooks/Cole.

McLanahan, S., & Sørensen, A. B. (1985). Life events and psychological well-being over the life course. In G. H. Elder (Ed.), *Life course dynamics* (pp. 217–238). Ithaca, NY: Cornell University Press.

Mead, G. H. (1934). *Mind, self, and society*. Chicago: University of Chicago Press.

Meyer, J. (1986). The self and the life course: Institutionalization and its effects. In A. B. Sørensen, F. Weinert, & L. Sherrod (Eds.), *Human development and the life course: Multidisciplinary perspectives* (pp. 199–216). Hillsdale, NJ: Lawrence Erlbaum.

Michael, D. N. (1973). *On learning to plan – And planning to learn*. San Francisco: Jossey-Bass.

Nadler, G. (1981). *The planning and design approach*. New York: John Wiley & Sons.

Nadler, G. (1986). The role of design processes in engineering. Lecture presented at installation as IBM Professor of Engineering Management, University of Wisconsin – Madison.

Nadler, G., Perrone, P., Seabold, D., & Yussen, S. (1984). Planning and design in education. Unpublished manuscript, University of Wisconsin – Madison.

Neisser, U. (1976). *Cognition and reality: Principles and implications of cognitive psychology*. San Francisco: W. H. Freeman.

Neisser, U. (1985). Toward an ecologically oriented cognitive science. In T. M. Shlechter & M. P. Toglia (Eds.), *New directions in cognitive science* (pp. 17–32). Norwood, NJ: Ablex.

Neugarten, B. L., & Datan, N. (1973). Sociological perspectives on the life cycle. In P. B. Baltes, & K. W. Schaie (Eds.), *Life-span developmental psychology: Personality and socialization* (pp. 53–69). New York: Academic Press.

Neustadt, R. E., & May, E. R. (1986). *Thinking in time: The uses of history for decision makers*. New York: Free Press.

Newell, A., & Simon, H. A. (1972). *Human problem solving*. Englewood Cliffs, NJ: Prentice-Hall.

Nydegger, C. (1983). Family ties of the aged in cross-cultural perspective. *Gerontologist, 23*, 26–32.

Oerter, R. (1986). Developmental tasks through the life span: A new approach to an old concept. In P. B. Baltes, D. L. Featherman, & R. M. Lerner (Eds.), *Life-span development and behavior* (Vol. 7, pp. 233–269). Hillsdale, NJ: Lawrence Erlbaum.

Passuth, P. M., Maines, D. R., & Neugarten, B. L. (1985). *Age norms and age constraints: A replication*. In preparation.

Peterson, J. G. (1985). *Personal qualities and job characteristics of expert engineers and planners*. Unpublished doctoral dissertation, University of Wisconsin – Madison.

Preston, S. (1984). Children and the elderly: Divergent paths for America's dependent. *Demography, 21*, 435–458.

Quinn, R. E. (1988). *Beyond rational management*. San Francisco: Jossey-Bass.

Ratner, J. (1939). *Intelligence in the modern world: John Dewey's philosophy*. New York: Modern Library.

Resnick, L. B. (1987 December). The 1987 presidential address: Learning in school and out. *Educational Researcher*, pp. 13–20.

Riley, M. W. (1985a). Age strata in social systems. In R. H. Binstock and E. Shanas (Eds.), *Handbook on aging and the social sciences* (pp. 369–414). New York: Van Nostrand Reinhold.

Riley, M. W. (1985b). Women, men, and the lengthening life course. In A. Rossi (Ed.), *Gender and the life course* (pp. 333–348). New York: Aldine.

Rittel, H. W. J., & Webber, M. M. (1974). Dilemmas in a general theory of planning. *Design Methods Group – Design Research Society Journal, 8*, 31–39.

Rosow, I. (1985). Status and role change through the life cycle. In R. Binstock & E. Shanas (Eds.), *Handbook of aging and the social sciences* (2nd ed., pp. 62–93). New York: Van Nostrand Reinhold.

Rowe, J., & Kahn, R. (1987). Human aging: usual and successful. *Science, 237*, 142–149.

Rybash, J. M., Hoyer, W. J., & Roodin, P. A. (1986). *Adult cognition and aging: Developmental changes in processing, knowing and thinking*. New York: Pergamon Press.

Ryff, C. D. (1984). Personality development from the inside: The subjective experiences of change in adulthood and aging. In P. B. Baltes & O. G. Brim, Jr. (Eds.), *Life-span development and behavior* (Vol. 6, pp. 244–279). New York: Academic Press.

Salthouse, T. M. (1987a). Age, experience and compensation. In C. Schooler & K. W. Schaie (Eds.), *Cognitive functioning and social structure over the life course* (pp. 142–157). Norwood, NJ: Ablex.

Salthouse, T. A. (1987b). The role of experience in cognitive aging. In K. W. Schaie (Ed.), *Annual review of gerontology and geriatrics* (Vol. 7, pp. 135–158). New York: Springer.

Samaroff, A. J., & Chandler, M. J. (1975). Reproductive risk and the continuum of caretaking causality. In F. D. Horowitz (Ed.), *Review of child development research* (Vol. 4, pp. 187–244). Chicago: University of Chicago Press.

Schank, R. C., & Abelson, R. P. (1977). *Scripts, plans, goals, and understanding*. Hillsdale, NJ: Lawrence Erlbaum.

Scholnick, E. K., & Friedman, S. L. (1987). The planning construct in the psychological literature. In S. L. Friedman, E. K. Scholnick, & R. R. Cocking (Eds.), *Blueprints for thinking* (pp. 3–38). New York: Cambridge University Press.

Scholnick, E. K., Friedman, S. L., & Cocking, R. R. (1987). Reflections on reflections: What planning is and how it develops. In S. L. Friedman, E. K. Scholnick, & R. R. Cocking (Eds.), *Blueprints for thinking* (pp. 515–534). New York: Cambridge University Press.

Schön, D. A. (1983). *The reflective practitioner*. New York: Basic Books.

Schooler, C. (1987). Cognitive effects of complex environments during the life-span: A review and theory. In C. Schooler & K. W. Schaie (Eds.), *Cognitive functioning and social structure over the life course* (pp. 24–49). Norwood, NJ: Ablex.

Scribner, S. (1986). Thinking in action: Some characteristics of practical thought. In R. J. Sternberg & R. K. Wagner (Eds.), *Practical intelligence* (pp. 13–30). New York: Cambridge University Press.

Scribner, S., & Cole, M. (1973). Cognitive consequences of formal and informal education. *Science, 182,* 553–559.

Seligman, M. E. P., & Elder, G. H., Jr. (1986). Learned helplessness and life-span development. In A. B. Sørensen, F. E. Weinert, & L. Sherrod (Eds.), *Human development in the life course: Multidisciplinary perspectives* (pp. 377–428). Hillsdale, NJ: Lawrence Erlbaum.

Simon, H. A. (1956). Rational choice and the structure of the environment. *Psychological Review, 63,* 129–138.

Simon, H. A. (1975). The functional equivalence of problem solving strategies. *Cognitive Psychology, 7,* 268–288.

Simon, H. A. (1978). Information processing theory of human problem solving. In W. K. Estes (Ed.), *Handbook of learning and cognitive processes* (Vol. 5, pp. 271–296). Hillsdale, NJ: Lawrence Erlbaum.

Smith, J., & Baltes, P. B. (1990). Wisdom-related knowledge: Age/cohort differences in response to life-planning problems. *Developmental Psychology, 26,* 494–505.

Smith, M. B. (1968). Toward a conception of the competent self. In J. A. Clausen (Ed.), *Socialization and society* (pp. 271–320). New York: Little Brown and Company.

Sørensen, A., & McLanahan, S. (1987). Married women's economic dependency: 1940–1980. *American Journal of Sociology, 93,* 659–687.

Staudinger, U. M. (1989). *The study of life review: An approach to the investigation of intellectual development across the life span* (Studien und Berichte des Max-Planck-Instituts für Bildungsforschung, No. 47). Stuttgart: Klett Verlag.

Sternberg, R. (1985). Human intelligence: The model is the message. *Science, 230,* 1111–1118.

Sternberg, R. J., & Wagner, R. K. (1986). *Practical intelligence: Nature and origins of competence in the everyday world.* New York: Cambridge University Press.

Sweet, J. A., & Bumpass, L. L. (1987). *American families and households.* New York: Russell Sage Foundation.

Thurow, L. (1987). A weakness in process technology. *Science, 238,* 1659–1663.

Vinovskis, M. A. (1988). The historian and the life course: Reflection on recent approaches to the study of American family life in the past. In P. B. Baltes, D. L. Featherman, & R. M. Lerner (Eds.), *Lifespan development and behavior* (Vol. 8, pp. 33–59). Hillsdale, NJ: Lawrence Erlbaum.

Vygotsky, L. S. (1962). *Thought and language.* Cambridge: MIT Press.

Waters, E., & Sroufe, L. A. (1983). Social competencies as a developmental construct. *Developmental Review, 3,* 79–97.

Wells, E., & Stryker, S. (1988). Stability and change in self over the life course. In P. B. Baltes, D. L. Featherman, & R. M. Lerner (Eds.), *Life-span development and behavior* (Vol. 8, pp. 192–230). Hillsdale, NJ: Lawrence Erlbaum.

White, R. W. (1959). Motivation reconsidered: The concept of competence. *Psychological Review, 66,* 297–337.

Wilensky, R. (1983). *Planning and understanding.* Reading, MA: Addison-Wesley.

Wine, J. D., & Smye, M. D. (1981). *Social competence*. New York: Guilford.

Wood, P. K. (1983). Inquiring systems and problem structure: Implications for cognitive development. *Human Development, 26,* 249–265.

Yussen, S. R. (1985). The role of metacognition in contemporary theories of cognitive development. In D. Forrest-Pressley & G. Waller (Eds.), *Contemporary research in cognition and metacognition*. Orlando: Academic Press.

4   The optimization of cognitive functioning in old age: Predictions based on cohort-sequential and longitudinal data

K. WARNER SCHAIE

Introduction

Social scientists who are concerned with examining the hypothesis that optimization can occur with advancing age and who direct their efforts to discover the factors that allow some but not all individuals to optimize their abilities to maintain high-quality lives generally would seem to make three implicit assumptions. The first assumption has a negative flavor: Declines from asymptotic levels attained during early adulthood are assumed to occur in old age in both biological and behavioral functioning, whether at the level of observed performance or of reserve capacity. The second assumption, by contrast, is more positive: Individuals are thought to differ widely in their adaptation to experienced losses, and patterns of individual maintenance in decline may be both varied and subject to multiple influences. The third assumption concerns the model chosen for the study of aging pheonmena: Decline with age is often thought to be gradual, continuous, and irreversible in nature. Evidence with respect to these assumptions has long been examined in the area of cognitive functioning, the topic of this chapter.

Whether older adults can maintain levels of adaptation that allow continuation of independent living and the expression of accomplishments in late life is necessarily contingent upon the maintenance of levels of intellectual functioning that have not fallen significantly below the normative levels expected by our society. It is quite true that many individuals throughout much of their life manage to cope at below-average levels of competence. However, it is these very individuals who are at greatest risk of requiring institutional care, when even slight age-related change lowers their competence from a marginal to an unacceptable level. Moreover, maintenance of leadership roles in society and continued productivity in competitive creative or scientific endeavors would seem to demand that the older person so engaged remains at high levels of functioning when compared with younger peers.

Strong evidence exists that a substantial proportion of individual differences in performance on everyday tasks (Willis & Schaie, 1986a) and in the perception of competence in real-life situations (Schaie, Gonda, & Quayhagen, 1982) can be accounted for by performance levels on measures of the primary mental abilities. The occurrence of average declines in mental abilities with advancing age has been reliably established (see Schaie, 1983). But there remains much controversy as to the patterns of individual differences in such decline. Individual differences in performance patterns, moreover, may be particularly profound in persons at high ability levels (Schaie, 1984, 1988b). In addition, previous research (Schaie, 1983, in press) has demonstrated differential cohort trends over time that influence the proportion of individuals of advanced age who remain capable of optimal functioning.

In view of the above considerations, I will argue that optimization in old age in the area of basic intellectual skills does not imply the attainment of new levels of high performance. Rather, I would suggest that the name of the game is indeed preservation of the levels that one has attained at an earlier age. Furthermore, in the face of cumulative environmental insults and biological constraints, optimization of intellectual functioning in old age should be expected to be selective rather than generalized.

In this chapter, I will examine evidence from my longitudinal–sequential studies of adult intelligence that can help determine the most likely predictors of optimal cognitive functioning in late life. As part of the Seattle Longitudinal Study (SLS) of adult cognitive functioning, we have tried to identify a large number of endogenous and exogenous variables that might have either positive or negative effects upon the maintenance of an individual's cognitive functions as he or she ages. The variables included here are those that in previous work have been demonstrated to explain many of the individual differences in intellectual changes with advancing age. The variables to be examined here include the effects of cardiovascular disease, cognitive styles, perceptual speed, associative memory, and several demographic antecedents. Before doing so, however, I will review the nature of the data base upon which my analyses and conclusions rely. In addition, I will examine in some detail evidence that suggests that there are a number of different patterns in which intellectual change in old age occurs. This approach is dictated by the recognition that an optimal adaptive pattern in old age may not necessarily be restricted to the maintenance of prior levels of functioning in all areas. Instead, if we give credence to the position that older individuals engage in selective optimization (e.g., P. B. Baltes & M. M. Baltes, 1980), we would expect a variety of patterns of selective maintenance of skills, which might well depend on alternative antecedent correlates. Finally, I will comment briefly on the implications of cohort trends in abilities for the optimal functioning of older adults.

Description of the data base

The data to be discussed come from the SLS, a multiwave panel study that uses as its population frame the membership of a metropolitan health maintenance organization (see Schaie, 1983). All 3,442 participants at first test were community-dwelling adults who were randomly selected from each 7-year age stratum included in each panel. These data were collected in 1956 ($N = 500$; ages 22–70), 1963 ($N = 997$; ages 22–77), 1970 ($N = 705$; ages 22–84), 1977 ($N = 612$; ages 22–84), and 1984 ($N = 628$; ages 22–84). At each successive data point, as many of the survivors of the previous wave as possible were reexamined. Thus we have 1357 participants for whom 7-year longitudinal data at Time 2 are available for four data sets: 1963 ($N = 303$; ages 29–77), 1970 ($N = 420$; ages 29–84), 1977 ($N = 340$; ages 29–91), and 1984 ($N = 294$; ages 29–91). Fourteen-year longitudinal data at Time 3 are available for 723 participants in three data sets: 1970 ($N = 162$; ages 36–84), 1977 ($N = 337$, ages 36–91), and 1984 ($N = 224$; ages 36–91). Twenty-one year longitudinal data at Time 4 exist for 355 participants in two data sets: 1977 ($N = 130$; ages 43–91) and 1984 ($N = 225$; ages 43–91). Finally, there is one 28-year longitudinal data set in 1984 at Time 5 ($N = 97$; ages 50–91). The age and sex distribution of this sample by 7-year age strata is provided in Table 4.1.

All participants were in good health when tested and were representative of the upper 75% of the socioeconomic stratum. For the total data base, educational levels averaged 13.27 years (range: 4–20 years), and occupational status averaged 6.25 on a 10-point scale, using census classifications ranging from unskilled labor to professional.

Throughout the study, the five primary mental abilities identified by L. L. Thurstone and T. G. Thurstone (1941) to exhibit the greatest variance (see also Schaie, 1985) were assessed. The Test of Behavioral Rigidity (Schaie & Parham, 1975) and a demographic information form were also used. Beginning in 1977, we added some measures of perceptual speed, and in 1984, measures of associative memory. Health history data have been abstracted for subsets of our data base that allow study of the effects of specific disease entities. All subjects were tested in small groups

Table 4.1. *First-time participants in the Seattle Longitudinal Study classified by chronological age and gender*

Mean age	Males	Females	Total
25	157	200	357
32	169	205	374
39	209	239	448
46	216	225	441
53	210	235	445
60	202	224	426
67	219	230	449
74	161	151	312
81	78	83	161
Total	1,621	1,792	3,413

in sessions that for the first three waves lasted about 2 hours, for the fourth wave about 3 hours, and for the fifth wave in two sessions of 2.5 hours each (necessary because multiple markers of the abilities and other additional measures were added). For the purpose of this chapter, our primary focus will be upon the five primary mental abilities: Verbal Meaning, the ability to comprehend words, a measure of recognition vocabulary; Spatial Orientation, the ability to mentally rotate objects in two-dimensional space; Inductive Reasoning, the ability to infer rules from examples that contain regular progressions of information; Number, the ability to manipulate number concepts, as measured by checking simple addition problems; and Word Fluency, a measure of recall vocabulary. Inductive reasoning and spatial orientation involve the solution of novel problems, whereas the other abilities represent more acculturated knowledge. In terms of the second-order ability domains involved, inductive reasoning is a measure of fluid ability, spatial orientation is a measure of visualization ability, and the other abilities are largely crystallized in nature (see Horn, 1970).

Because the emphasis of this volume is upon optimization of functioning in advanced age, we will limit our discussion to that part of our data base that extends from late midlife into old age. That is, we will consider only the 1,793 individuals who were 50 years of age or older when they entered the study. For this subset, longitudinal data are available on 1,179 individuals. Of these, 229 persons participated in cognitive training programs involving strategy training on either the Inductive Reasoning or Spatial Orientation ability (Schaie & Willis, 1986; Willis & Schaie, 1986b, 1988). For ease of comparison, all data have been scaled in *T*-score

Table 4.2. *Seven-year age changes for the primary mental abilities*

	Verbal Meaning	Spatial Orientation	Inductive Reasoning	Number	Word Fluency	Composite
From age 53 to age 60 (N = 417)						
Mean	0.48	0.54	0.20	0.68	1.23	0.62
S.D.	5.32	6.33	4.79	5.27	6.34	3.03
From age 60 to age 67 (N = 359)						
Mean	2.08	2.02	2.09	2.27	1.78	2.06
S.D.	6.36	6.33	4.99	5.46	6.46	3.25
From age 67 to age 74 (N = 284)						
Mean	3.01	2.59	2.42	2.53	2.46	2.59
S.D.	6.92	5.95	5.06	5.84	6.12	3.11
From age 74 to age 81 (N = 129)						
Mean	3.82	2.94	2.06	4.08	3.48	3.27
S.D.	6.96	5.81	4.30	5.34	6.10	3.32

Note: All average changes are decrements expressed in *T*-score points.

form (mean = 50, standard deviation = 10) based on the scores of 2,810 subjects at first test. Thus, in population terms, changes or differences reported here imply an order of magnitude of one tenth of a standard deviation unit for each *T*-score point.

Patterns of decline from late middle age into old age

We will begin our discussion by considering the amount of average decrement from late midlife and by examining the various patterns of decline shown by different individuals. To maintain substantial sample sizes, we will base these data on 7-year longitudinal changes cumulated across the four samples (1956, 1963, 1970, and 1977 entry waves) for which longitudinal data are available (also see Schaie, 1988a, for an analysis of the empirical consequences of this approach).

Patterns of average ability changes

Table 4.2 lists average changes in *T*-score points for the five primary mental abilities as well as for a linear composite (analogous to a global IQ estimate). Average decrements from age 53 to 60 are statistically significant for Number (men only) and Word Fluency as well as for the composite score. Although the magnitude of decrement over this age

Table 4.3. *Twenty-eight-year changes for the primary mental abilities*

	Verbal Meaning	Spatial Orientation	Inductive Reasoning	Number	Word Fluency	Composite
From age 25 to age 53 (N = 15)						
Mean	+3.67	1.87	+0.47	1.93	1.07	0.07
S.D.	4.95	8.14	4.52	6.51	8.29	2.74
From age 32 to age 60 (N = 21)						
Mean	1.14	2.71	2.24	1.86	2.91	2.33
S.D.	2.95	7.20	5.65	4.30	9.89	3.45
From age 39 to age 67 (N = 17)						
Mean	1.06	1.12	2.59	3.29	6.65	3.12
S.D.	4.98	8.01	5.37	5.52	6.29	3.44
From age 46 to age 74 (N = 24)						
Mean	3.96	4.29	5.62	3.04	8.12	5.04
S.D.	9.72	8.38	5.00	4.29	5.52	3.57
From age 53 to age 81 (N = 16)						
Mean	8.75	7.69	8.19	7.69	11.25	8.75
S.D.	5.07	6.05	8.08	5.51	8.39	4.52

Note: All changes are in *T*-score points. Values carrying the plus sign represent increments; all others, decrements. These data are based only on the survivors of the sample first tested in 1956 (in contrast to Table 4.2, which is based on pooled data across all longitudinal samples).

range is virtually trivial, there is substantial variability, suggesting that at least some individuals do show significant decrements over this age range. Beyond age 60, 7-year decrements are statistically significant for all abilities ($p < .001$) and increase up to 4.08 population standard deviations for the 7-year interval from age 74 to 81.

Data are also available for a small subset of 93 persons for whom cumulative change can be examined over a 28-year period. Table 4.3 reports these cumulative changes for 28-year periods, beginning from ages 25–53 and ending at ages 53–81. For the youngest group there is a significant increment for Verbal Meaning ($p < .01$), but no other significant change. From age 32 to 60, it is only the composite measure that shows a statistically significant ($p < .01$) but very small cumulative decrement. Even from age 39 to 67, it is only the Word Fluency and composite measures that show statistically significant decrements ($p < .01$). However, statistically significant cumulative decrements of moderate magnitude are found for all variables except Verbal Meaning from age 46 to 74, and large cumulative decrements prevail for all variables from age 53 to 81.

It should be noted that variability is quite large, both for the 7-year and the cumulative 28-year data. Inspection of frequency distributions of observed *individual* changes therefore indicates that many individuals at all ages show little or no decrement on specific abilities over the periods monitored. Variability is considerably less on the composite measure, supporting the notion that although there may be decline in some ability or abilities for most individuals over age 60, the pattern of such decline is indeed quite variable.

Individual patterns of ability changes

Although continuous data are preferred to describe parametric changes in populations, the use of such data involves the assumption that change at the individual level is also linear and continuous in nature. We should like to question this assumption and argue that individual change occurs in a much more sporadic fashion (we will document this point later on). For the purpose of studying individual differences in ability decline, it may therefore be more useful to study decline as events, recognizing that the reliability of the absolute difference embodied in an individual change score is likely to be limited. Thus, converting our continuous data into discrete events will most likely result, not in what some might consider to be a regrettable information loss, but rather in data that are more suitable for the study of patterns of individual change (also see Schaie, 1989a).

We can best examine the question of what proportion of individuals show which pattern of decline by specifying criteria that allow identification of individuals who show decremental change that exceeds possible measurement error. We do so by creating a 1 standard error of measurement (SEM) confidence band about our participants' base scores (see Dudek, 1979).[1] Those individuals whose 7-year change falls below this interval are considered to have reliably experienced age decrement; all others are considered to have maintained their previous level of performance. This is a rather conservative estimate, with an error rate of .16 in favor of accepting the prevalence of reliable decrement and thus, if anything, it is biased against diagnosing excessive numbers of individuals as stable when they are not. The procedure advocated here does not depend on the reliability and/or distribution of change scores; instead, it simply determines whether or not a Time 2 score could or could not have been another estimate of the Time 1 score, given the specified confidence interval about the Time 1 score.

I will first examine the proportion of individuals who show significant

Table 4.4. *Proportions of individuals showing decline in specific abilities*

Ability	53–60	60–67	67–74	74–81
Verbal Meaning	15.2	24.8	26.8	35.7
Spatial Orientation	21.1	27.0	29.6	32.6
Inductive Reasoning	14.0	26.5	23.6	27.9
Number	17.2	26.2	26.2	31.8
Word Fluency	23.6	28.4	27.5	37.2
Composite	18.9	34.3	43.0	50.4

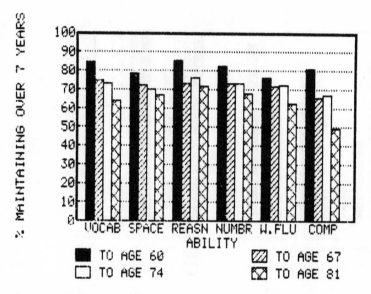

Figure 4.1. Proportion of individuals maintaining or improving performance levels on specific abilities over 7 years.

decline over 7 years on specific abilities as well as on the overall composite score (see Table 4.4). Note that the incidence of significant decrement for specific abilities is quite limited until age 60; until age 74 affects less than a third of our subjects; and even by age 81 is limited to between 30% and 40% of the persons studied. For the composite score, significant decline is somewhat higher and increases by about 10% per decade. For the purpose of this chapter, it seems appropriate to state these findings more positively. As graphed in Figure 4.1, depending upon age-group, from 60% to 85% of all subjects remain stable or improve on specific abilities. And for the composite score, approximately 50% even of the oldest group

Table 4.5. *Proportions of individuals showing decline of abilities*

Number of abilities	53–60	60–67	67–74	74–81
None	41.3	26.7	24.3	15.5
One	35.3	35.1	37.7	37.2
Two	17.0	22.0	21.8	24.8
Three	4.9	10.3	11.3	14.0
Four	1.2	5.0	3.9	6.2
All five	0.5	0.8	1.1	2.3

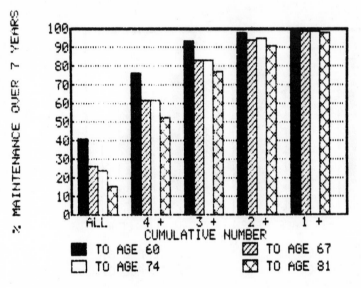

Figure 4.2. Proportion of individuals maintaining or improving performance levels on multiple abilities over 7 years.

did not show evidence of statistically significant decline over the preceding 7 years.

Let us next consider whether cognitive decline is a global or a highly specific event. Table 4.5 lists the proportion of individuals maintaining all of the five abilities monitored over a 7-year period compared with individuals who decline on one or more ability. In fact, very few individuals show global decline. These data are graphed again in Figure 4.2 to show the cumulative proportion of study participants who maintain or improve their level of cognitive functioning in advanced age on one or

Table 4.6. *Proportions of individuals showing different decline patterns over four consecutive 7-year periods*

Ability	Periods of decline				
	None	One	Two	Three	Four
Verbal Meaning	50.5	36.1	11.3	2.1	0.0
	(69.1)	(24.8)	(5.2)	(0.0)	(0.0)
Spatial Orientation	35.1	47.4	16.5	1.0	0.0
	(64.9)	(30.9)	(3.1)	(1.0)	(0.0)
Inductive Reasoning	35.1	56.3	11.6	0.0	0.0
	(58.8)	(39.2)	(2.1)	(0.0)	(0.0)
Number	35.1	47.4	15.5	2.1	0.0
	(61.9)	(32.0)	(6.2)	(0.0)	(0.0)
Word Fluency	27.8	42.3	28.9	1.0	0.0
	(53.6)	(29.9)	(15.5)	(1.0)	(0.0)
Composite	32.0	43.3	18.6	6.2	0.0
	(44.3)	(35.1)	(15.5)	(3.1)	(0.0)

Note: Values in parentheses are adjusted for prior or consecutive periods of reliable increment.

more abilities. It is particularly noteworthy that by age 60, three fourths of our study participants maintained their level of functioning over 7 years on at least four out of the five abilities monitored and that this level of maintenance was true even at age 81 for slightly more than half of the sample.

One may ask, of course, to what extent there is cumulative decrement from one 7-year period to the next. We address that question, again using our small 28-year subset ($N = 93$; mean age = 68.3). Elsewhere we have reported individual profiles of change on this data set, showing that the accumulation of small changes in a linear fashion is quite atypical (Schaie, 1989b). This finding becomes even clearer when we consider cumulative change as multiple change events within individuals. Table 4.6 shows the proportions of our subjects who remained completely stable over a 28-year period or who showed one, two, or three periods of decrement. Note that there was no subject who showed significant decrement over all four 7-year periods (for Inductive Reasoning, no subject showed more than two decrement periods). Data are even more positive when we adjust proportions by not counting as a decrement those instances where the significant decrement is followed by a compensatory significant increment during the next period. These data suggest that individual linear decline is quite atypical and that the population estimates for ability maintenance based on our 7-year data are only minimally inflated by successive decrement events.

What are the processes and mechanisms that govern the selective pattern of optimization apparent from the above data? At this point, we have little to offer at the theoretical level of analysis, except to refer to models of adaptive cognitive aging that have the individual responding to the most urgent presses and needs of the concurrent environment (see Schaie, 1977/78). At the empirical level, however, one might argue that studying individual differences in endogenous and exogenous variables that possibly affect cognitive maintenance will also provide information about the process of optimization. Rather than engage in what I think to be premature theoretical speculations, I will now turn to a description of what we know about the many variables that affect differential cognitive aging.

Variables that mediate maintenance of cognitive functioning

I will now discuss those variables that may be particularly important in mediating the maintenance of high levels of functioning. In our work, we have attended particularly to the presence or absence of cardiovascular disease (e.g., Hertzog, Schaie, & Gribbin, 1978), demographic variables such as education and occupation (Schaie, 1983, 1988, in press), complexity of life-styles (Gribbin, Schaie, & Parham, 1980), the role of perceptual speed (Schaie, 1989c), verbal memory, and the contributions of cognitive styles as expressed through measures of flexibility-rigidity (Schaie, 1983; Willis, 1989). Not all of these variables, of course, have the same conceptual status. For example, it is quite possible that the effects of cardiovascular disease on cognitive maintenance may simply represent the results of life-styles that are unfavorable for both cardiovascular health and maintenance of cognitive function. Likewise, occupational and educational factors may well be the root cause of flexible behaviors and attitudes that favorably affect cognitive maintenance. The complex models that need to be tested to resolve these matters go beyond the scope of a single chapter. I will therefore limit myself to describing the effects or variables that have a direct impact on cognitive maintenance.

I will first consider some of the predictors of high levels of cognitive functioning at various advanced ages for the full data set described earlier. For many of the variables to be considered, however, we will need to refer to the data set employed in our training studies (Schaie & Willis, 1986; Willis & Schaie, 1986b, 1988), for which we have the most detailed data on all of these variables. These studies involved subjects over 64 years of age who received 5 hours of training in cognitive strategies at the ability factor level for either Inductive Reasoning or Spatial Orientation. This data set is particularly valuable because we can examine the effect of possible predictors on both decline and remedial intervention in the elderly.

Base level as predictor of later performance

Because decline in ability is so specific, it is necessary to examine the various abilities separately, in order to test whether base level performance predicts later performance. We use a discriminant function approach to determine whether we can identify variables that distinguish those who maintain their previous performance levels from those who decline. We include the base levels of the five mental abilities as well as the factor scores of Motor–Cognitive Flexibility, Personality–Perceptual (Attitudinal) Flexibility, and Psychomotor Speed from the Test of Behavioral Rigidity (Schaie & Parham, 1975). We also enter gender and cohort membership into this analysis to control for possible confounds due to sample composition. Regression coefficients (beta weights) and multiple correlations (all of which are statistically significant) are reported in Table 4.7. The most striking finding is that at every age level the likelihood of maintaining optimal levels of function appears to be inversely correlated with previous levels. That is, the higher the base level on a given ability, the more likely it is that significant decline will occur; and this inverse relationship appears to be strongest in our oldest age-group. Note, however, that this inverse relationship, in most cases, is strictly a within-variable relationship. Because our decline criteria incorporate the stability coefficients (which are uniformly high), it seems unlikely that these findings can be attributed to statistical regression effects. We have previously examined the validity threat due to statistical regression by means of time-reversal analysis (see Baltes, Nesselroade, Schaie, & Labouvie, 1972; Campbell & Stanley, 1966). In that study we concluded that the observed relationships represent a valid developmental phenomenon and cannot be dismissed as statistical artifacts (Schaie & Willis, 1986).

There are some other base level predictors that contribute to the discriminant functions. High base level on Spatial Orientation appears to be positively related to maintenance on Verbal Meaning, as is high level on Psychomotor Speed. Other base level predictors appear to be quite age-specific. For example, both Motor–Cognitive Flexibility and Attitudinal Flexibility base levels are positively related to several abilities from age 60 to 67 but do not reach significance at other ages. Cohort level has no predictive value, and gender effects are significant only from age 53 to

Table 4.7. *Discriminant functions for the maintenance or decline of the primary mental abilities over 7 years (regression coefficients and multiple correlations)*

Predictors	53–60	60–67	67–74	74–81
Verbal Meaning				
Verbal Meaning	−.347***	−.449***	−.531***	−.508***
Spatial Orientation	.120*	.115*	−.015	.127
Inductive Reasoning	.072	.080	.116	.090
Number	.042	−.034	.136*	.000
Word Fluency	.011	−.064	−.005	.086
Motor–Cognitive				
Flexibility	.071	.191**	.041	.123
Attitudinal Flexibility	.018	.057	−.016	−.055
Psychomotor Speed	.195**	.142*	.121	.119
Sex	−.001	.024	−.045	.005
Cohort	.055	.033	−.007	−.054
Multiple R	.270***	.350***	.395***	.404**
Spatial Orientation				
Verbal Meaning	.039	−.097	.078	−.230*
Spatial Orientation	−.337***	−.401***	−.411***	−.433***
Inductive Reasoning	.065	.105	.101	.152
Number	.067	.018	.017	.018
Word Fluency	−.101	−.138*	−.020	−.066
Motor–Cognitive				
Flexibility	.059	.167**	.043	−.014
Attitudinal Flexibility	−.047	.127*	−.002	.118
Psychomotor Speed	.031	.007	−.128	.177
Sex	−.108*	.007	−.039	.040
Cohort	−.005	.062	.078	−.049
Multiple R	.319***	.350***	.373***	.520***
Inductive Reasoning				
Verbal Meaning	.025	.144	.016	.164
Spatial Orientation	.022	.013	.010	−.027
Inductive Reasoning	−.272***	−.384***	−.525***	−.683***
Number	−.029	.011	−.057	.052
Word Fluency	.058	−.025	−.027	−.037
Motor–Cognitive				
Flexibility	−.007	.032	.113	.100
Attitudinal Flexibility	.021	−.128*	.013	.028
Psychomotor Speed	−.046	.037	.227**	.090
Sex	.022	−.007	−.118*	−.060
Cohort	.025	.034	.097	−.015
Multiple R	.233**	.335***	.435***	.519***

Table 4.7. *(cont.)*

Predictors	53–60	60–67	67–74	74–81
Number				
Verbal Meaning	−.225**	.025	.111	−.020
Spatial Orientation	.002	.086	−.030	−.084
Inductive Reasoning	.111	.054	.173*	.116
Number	−.239***	−.388***	−.394***	−.408***
Word Fluency	.171**	.038	.127	−.027
Motor–Cognitive				
Flexibility	.076	.070	−.011	.156
Attitudinal Flexibility	−.009	−.087	−.026	−.073
Psychomotor Speed	−.059	.028	−.078	.080
Sex	−.029	.045	.008	−.031
Cohort	−.069	−.006	.000	−.035
Multiple R	.318***	.345***	.354***	.378*
Word Fluency				
Verbal Meaning	.052	.052	.035	.269*
Spatial Orientation	.098	−.012	.020	.094
Inductive Reasoning	−.039	.086	−.032	.086
Number	.034	.047	.076	.072
Word Fluency	−.368***	−.329***	−.381***	−.507***
Motor–Cognitive				
Flexibility	.095	−.027	.130	.022
Attitudinal Flexibility	.078	.047	.009	−.188*
Psychomotor Speed	.058	.070	.083	.131
Sex	.069	−.092	−.014	.007
Cohort	−.048	.063	.004	.068
Multiple R	.321***	.334***	.338***	.504***

*$p < .05$. **$p < .01$. ***$p < .001$.

60 for Spatial Orientation and from age 67 to 74 for Inductive Reasoning, in both instances favoring men.

The effects of cardiovascular disease

We have previously studied the effects of cardiovascular disease on mental ability performance and found that those individuals who were at risk from such disease tended, on the average, to decline earlier than did individuals not so affected (see Hertzog, Schaie, & Gribbin, 1978). I would like to report here a recent analysis of the relationship between cardiovascular disease, significant decline over a 14-year period, and significant remediation of decline in a group of 109 subjects (ranging in

Table 4.8 *Incidence of treatment of cardiovascular disease and decline or training gain on inductive reasoning*

	Disease incidents[a]	Disease episodes[b]
Change status		
Total incidence		
Stables	6.89	3.46
Decliners	16.50	6.00
Days in hospital only		
Stables	0.54	0.13
Decliners	6.34	0.85
Gain (decliners only)		
Gain	7.31	3.34
No gain	19.50	7.77

[a]Number of clinic visits and days in hospital.
[b]Number of continuous spells of illness.

age from 62 to 94) who received cognitive training on the Inductive Reasoning ability. Medical histories for these subjects were examined over the 7-year period preceding their pretraining evaluation. All clinic visits and illness episodes (continuous spells of illness) were recorded and coded by disease. The disease experience was then examined for individuals who had declined or remained stable in Inductive Reasoning and for individuals who had experienced or failed to experience significant training gain.

It is of interest to note that no significant relationships could be found between total numbers of disease incidents or episodes and mental ability, suggesting that overall health indices may not be very useful predictors of cognitive behavior. The findings are much more suggestive when we restrict our analysis to the occurrence of cardiovascular disease (including hypertension). These data are shown in Table 4.8. Individuals experiencing significant decline on Inductive Reasoning, on the average, had more than twice the number of cardiovascular-system–related treatment visits ($p < .01$) and about 1 and 1/2 times more cardiovascular illness episodes ($p < .05$) than those who remained stable. Even more dramatic were the incidents of hospitalization for cardiovascular disease, with the decliners averaging approximately 10 times as many hospitalizations as those who remained stable ($p < .01$). Note that because it was necessary for our subjects to be able to perform on paper and pencil tests, we do not include any individuals who experienced strokes severe enough to result in significant sensorimotor impairment.

The relation between cardiovascular disease and significant training gain further supports the finding that this syndrome is of importance in behavioral plasticity in the elderly. When we divide the group who showed significant decline on Inductive Reasoning into those who show and those who fail to show significant gains from cognitive training, we find that those who gain have experienced, on the average, less than half the number of clinic visits or illness episodes than those who do not gain ($p < .01$). Moreover, those who gain from training experienced their first cardiovascular system disease diagnosis approximately 2 years later than those who failed to show significant training gain.

Some important demographic status variables

Although many demographic status variables are not informative in predicting the occurrence of maintenance or decline of cognitive functioning, they do remain important in advanced age as contributors to the prediction of absolute levels of functioning (Schaie, in press). We therefore examined the effects of gender, education, and occupational level (scaled as a continous variable from unskilled to professional) for the four 7-year longitudinal samples with end points at ages 60, 67, 74, and 81 (see Table 4.9). Because the three status variables are correlated with each other, we present standardized regression weights for each (partialing out the effects of the two others) rather than the raw correlations with the ability measures.

Throughout, gender is related to Spatial Orientation favoring men and to Word Fluency favoring women (because of the smaller sample size, the regression weights are not statistically significant for the oldest group, but they are in the expected direction). The number of years of education is positively related throughout to Verbal Meaning, Inductive Reasoning, and Word Fluency. For the two oldest groups, there is also a positive relationship with Number. Occupational level relates positively to Inductive Reasoning and Number. Note, however, that this relationship disappears for the oldest group, where few individuals remain engaged in active occupational pursuits.

The role of perceptual speed and verbal memory

Just as ability decline seems to occur in an individualized, rather than a uniform and universal, fashion, so do the otherwise well documented declines in speed of performance. We have recently documented that although decline with age in perceptual speed assumes linear form for populations, such decline is more likely to occur in a stair-step fashion for

Table 4.9. *Regression weights for gender, education, and occupation showing the effects on level of functioning of the primary mental abilities at 7-year longitudinal end points*

Predictors	53–60	60–67	67–74	74–81
Gender				
Verbal Meaning	.063	.115*	.056	.072
Spatial Orientation	−.252***	−.203***	−.192**	−.152
Inductive Reasoning	.100*	.124*	.074	.073
Number	−.038	.051	−.035	−.026
Word Fluency	.158**	.176**	.140*	.172
Years of education				
Verbal Meaning	.458***	.333***	.507***	.261*
Spatial Orientation	−.010	.164*	−.038	.094
Inductive Reasoning	.309***	.235***	.355***	.252*
Number	.036	.084	.251**	.228
Word Fluency	.272***	.142*	.223**	.292*
Occupational level				
Verbal Meaning	.063	.091	.010	.088
Spatial Orientation	.072	−.057	.010	−.018
Inductive Reasoning	.180**	.151*	.221*	.069
Number	.154*	.153*	.199*	.087
Word Fluency	.048	.147*	.131	−.104

*$p < .05$. **$p < .01$. ***$p < .001$.

individuals. We have also shown that much of the age-related longitudinal change in other ability variables may be attributable to concurrent change in perceptual speed (see Schaie, 1989c). It follows, therfore, that the base level and the change in perceptual speed might well be important predictors of ability decline. Because we have thus far collected perceptual speed data only for one 7-year period, we combined base level data for 542 individuals who were in the 53 years or older groups. The measures of perceptual speed used in this study are the Finding A's and Incomplete Pictures tests from the ETS *Kit of Factor-Referred Cognitive Tests* (Ekstrom, French, Harman, & Derman, 1976). In our analyses, we use the linear combination of the two markers as the optimal estimate of perceptual speed.

In order to appraise the predictive ability of these data for individuals, we once again use our SEM-defined criteria to examine the joint occurrence of decline events in perceptual speed and ability functioning over 7 years (Figure 4.3). When we do so, we find, for all abilities except Spatial

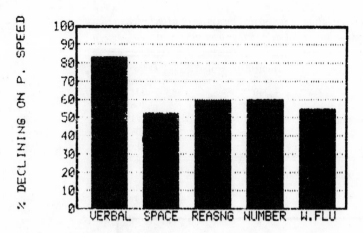

Figure 4.3. Joint occurrence of decline in perceptual speed and in other primary mental abilities.

Orientation, a lower occurrence of ability decline in those individuals whose perceptual speed has not declined. However, the base level of perceptual speed attains a significant relation with ability maintenance only for Inductive Reasoning. As would be expected, there is a high correlation between base level perceptual speed and end point ability functioning. Cross-lagged correlation analysis (Kenny, 1975), however, identified significantly greater cross-lags from speed to ability only for Word Fluency ($p < .05$). On the other hand, significantly greater cross-lags were identified from Spatial Orientation and Inductive Reasoning to perceptual speed.

Although we do not as yet have longitudinal data on verbal memory, we can examine the relationship between concurrent associative memory performance (immediate and 1-hour-delayed recall of a word list) measured at one point in time (1984) and the 7-year longitudinal change in the abilities. These data are available for a small set of people ($N = 111$; mean age = 72). The observed relationships suggest small but significant negative correlations between ability maintenance and memory functioning. This phenomenon is somewhat more general across abilities for delayed recall than for immediate recall (see Table 4.10).

Consequences of cohort differences in ability performance

Although we have noted that cohort level does not contribute to the prediction of individual differences in maintenance of function, there are still consequences of changes in population by cohort that are relevant to our

Table 4.10. *Correlation of concurrent measures of associative memory with magnitude of ability change over seven years*

Abilities	Immediate recall	Delayed recall
Verbal Meaning	−.248**	−.303**
Spatial Orientation	−.355***	−.366***
Inductive Reasoning	−.109	−.224*
Number	−.149	−.204*
Word Fluency	−.078	−.117

*$p < .05$. **$p < .01$. ***$p < .001$.

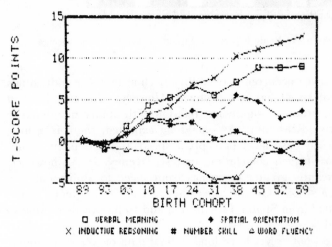

Figure 4.4. Cumulative cohort gradients for the primary mental abilities of Verbal Meaning, Spatial Orientation, Inductive Reasoning, Number, and Word Fluency for cohorts with mean birth years from 1889 to 1959.

discussion. Whether or not older individuals are perceived as functioning optimally will, of course, depend not only on intra-individual change but also on the levels of functioning of younger, comparison groups at any particular point in time. Both positive and negative ability changes across cohorts will therefore affect the extent to which older individuals will be perceived to be at a relative disadvantage. Our own work and that of others has consistently shown the prevalence of cohort differences in abilities throughout this century (see P. B. Baltes, Cornelius, & Nesselroade, 1979; Flynn, 1984; Parker, 1986; Schaie, 1983, in press). Figure 4.4 shows cohort gradients for the abilities discussed in this presentation.

These gradients were obtained by averaging differences between each successive pair of cohorts at all ages for which data are available for the same age levels (typically four age levels). Differences between successive cohorts as expressed in *T*-score points (.1 standard deviation) were cumulated from the oldest cohort, with mean birth year of 1989, up to the most recently measured cohort, with mean birth year of 1959.

It will be noted immediately that the cohort gradients differ markedly across abilities in both slope and shape. Inductive Reasoning comes closest to showing a linear positive cohort progression. Even here there are departures from linearity, with relatively steep increments up to the 1931 cohort and far slower and decelerating increments thereafter. Nevertheless, the cumulative increment across the currently available population is well in excess of a population standard deviation. The next most substantial pattern of positive increment across successive cohorts is shown by Verbal Meaning. After an initial modest dip, this ability rises until the 1924 birth cohort. After another modest dip, there is a further rise to an asymptote attained by the 1945, 1952 and 1959 cohorts. Spatial Orientation also shows a basically positive cohort progression, but with a much flatter and variable profile. This ability reaches an initial asymptote for the cohorts from 1910 to 1931. A further rise to a new peak occurs in 1938, which is followed by a drop to the earlier asymptote in 1952, but with recovery to the higher level by the most recent cohort.

A very different pattern is shown for Number. Here, a peak is reached by the 1910 cohort at a level that is maintained through the 1924 cohort. Thereafter, an almost linear negative slope is found that continues through the most recent cohort, which is below the 1889 base. Word Fluency, moreover, actually shows a negative cohort gradient up to the 1938 cohort, with recovery to the level of the base cohort by the most recent cohort studied.

It should also be noted that the increment of cohort differences has slowed markedly over the past two decades. Cumulative magnitudes of cohort differences between those now in midlife and those in early old age are no greater than the amount of training gains demonstrated for older adults who had not experienced age-related decline (Schaie & Willis, 1986; Willis & Schaie, 1986b). It seems reasonable then to assume that much of the cohort-related aspect of the older person's intellectual disadvantage when compared with younger peers may well be amenable to compensation by suitable educational interventions.

Because of the recent leveling off of some cohort changes and the curvilinear nature of cohort changes for some abilities, we must project substantial reduction in future observed cross-sectional ability differences between young and old adults. Indeed, for an ability such as numerical skill, we can look forward to a period when older adults will be advantaged when compared with younger persons. In addition to the positive inferences drawn from these data, there are also some negative ones. First, we need to note that the effects of positive cohort shifts are no longer apparent once the eighties are reached for any ability other than recognition vocabulary (see Schaie, in press). Apparently, age-related changes do take their toll for most of us in very old age, and environmental interventions at this time are perhaps not very effective in prolonging full functioning into very advanced old age. Second, the asymptote reached by recent cohorts in educational attainment, given the substantial correlations of the abilities with education, may suggest that the positive shifts in potential experienced in early old age by successive cohorts over the past several decades may come to a halt by the end of this century.

Summary and conclusions

In this presentation, we have tried to summarize some new analyses of data from the longitudinal–sequential studies of cognitive functions contained in the SLS archives. We began by examining the extent of ability maintenance in old age and concluded that although decline in cognitive functioning occurs for many individuals as the sixties are reached, such decline is differential in nature. Virtually none of the individuals contained in our data set showed universal decline on all abilities monitored, even by the eighties. We conclude then that optimization of cognitive functioning in old age may well involve selective maintenance of some abilities but not others. Moreover, such optimization is highly individual. The dynamic process that governs the mechanisms leading to the optimization of specific ability dimensions still remains to be discovered.

We next examined a number of variables that may be useful in predicting individual patterns of maintenance and decline. Evidence points to cardiovascular disease as a possible mediator in the maintenance of abilities and as a possible determinant of successful remediation of ability decline in advanced age. Demographic characteristics that may be related to optimal maintenance of intellectual functioning into old age certainly include education, but occupational level was also seen as important, at least up to that stage when most older individuals leave the world of work. High levels of motor–cognitive and attitudinal flexibility appear to be conducive to maintenance of function in early old age. Contrary to the hope that age might be kinder to those of high ability, once decline does occur, it is most likely to reach significant magnitudes in those of high ability. Perhaps this is only fair, because in spite of modest losses, those who start at a high level will still retain preeminence among their peers. Although there is an excess of expected ability decline among those who also decline in perceptual speed, there is evidence that prior level of speed is only modestly predictive of ability maintenance and that maintenance of ability levels may actually be more predictive of maintenance of perceptual speed. Current verbal memory level was found to be related to magnitude of ability change.

In our final section, we briefly examined cohort changes in ability and argued that the curvilinear patterns and slowing of positive cohort changes would be likely to lessen the competitive disadvantage experienced by average older adults when compared with younger peers, at least for the remainder of this century.

Although all of these data provide us with some clues as to the variables that should be studied to understand the vast individual differences in the maintenance of optimal functioning in old age, much more work is needed to integrate this material and expand it to include additional personality and life-style variables. Such work may eventually permit us to provide reasonably accurate predictions of the hazard of individual change in functioning with increasing age, as well as to predict more accurately the diverse patterns of optimizing cognitive performance that have been identified.

NOTES

This chapter was written while the author was a visiting scholar at the Institute of Human Development at the University of California, Berkeley. Preparation of the paper was supported by research grant AG04770 from the National Institute on Aging. The cooperation of members and staff of the Group Health Cooperative of Puget Sound is gratefully acknowledged. Thanks are due to Ranjana Dutta, Ann Gruber-Baldini, and Ann O'Hanlon for assistance in the data reduction. As always, I am indebted to Sherry L. Willis, my wife and colleague, for many insightful suggestions and comments.

1 The SEM used for our classification purposes has the form of $\sigma_{1I} (1 - r_{12}{}^2)^{1/2}$. It should probably more precisely be identified as the standard error of prediction. This error estimate is slightly larger than the conventional SEM, which represents the standard deviation of observed scores if the true score is held constant. Dudek (1979, p. 336) has argued that "if one desires to set confidence intervals for obtained scores (say on a retest), then the appropriate standard error interval is σ_{1I}, and using the [conventional] standard error of measurement in such a situation could lead to a serious underestimation of the interval." The size of this interval is dependent on the homogeneity or heterogeneity of the sample as well as the stability coefficient over the time interval for which change in individuals is to be identified. We deal with this matter by

using as stable as possible parameters for our SEM estimates, basing the Time 1 standard deviation and the stability coefficients upon all subjects for whom 7-year longitudinal data are available ($N = 1,793$).

REFERENCES

Baltes, P. B., & Baltes, M. M. (1980). Plasticity and variability in psychological aging: Methodological and theoretical issues. In G. Gursky (Ed.), *Determining the effects of aging on the central nervous system* (pp. 41–66). Berlin: Schering.

Baltes, P. B., Cornelius, S. W., & Nesselroade, J. R. (1979). Cohort effects in developmental psychology. In J. R. Nesselroade & P. B. Baltes (Eds.), *Longitudinal research in the study of behavior and development* (pp. 61–87). New York: Academic Press.

Balter, P. B., Nesselroade, J. R., Schaie, K. W., & Labouvie, E. W. (1972). On the dilemma of regression effects in examining ability level – related differentials in ontogenetic patterns of adult intelligence. *Developmental Psychology, 6,* 79–84.

Campbell, D. T., & Stanley, J. C. (1966). *Experimental and quasi-experimental designs for research.* Chicago: Rand-McNally.

Dudek, F. J. (1979). The continuing misinterpretation of the standard error of measurement. *Psychological Bulletin, 86,* 335–337.

Ekstrom, R. B., French, J. W., Harman, H., & Derman, D. (1976). *Kit of factor-referenced cognitive tests* (rev. ed.). Princeton, NJ: Educational Testing Service.

Flynn, J. R. (1984). The mean IQ of Americans: Massive gains, 1932 to 1978. *Psychological Bulletin, 95,* 29–51.

Gribbin, K., Schaie, K. W., & Parham, I. A. (1980). Complexity of life style and maintenance of intellectual abilities. *Journal of Social Issues, 36,* 47–61.

Hertzog, C., Schaie, K. W., & Gribbin, K. (1978). Cardiovascular disease and changes in intellectual functioning from middle to old age. *Journal of Gerontology, 33,* 872–883.

Horn, J. L. (1970). Organization of data on life-span development of human abilities. In L. R. Goulet & P. B. Baltes (Eds.), *Life-span developmental psychology: Research and theory* (pp. 424–466). New York: Academic Press.

Kenny, D. A. (1975). Cross-lagged panel correlation. *Psychological Bulletin, 82,* 887–903.

Parker, K. C. H. (1986). Changes with age, year-of-birth cohort, age by year-of-birth cohort interaction, and standardization of the Wechsler Adult Intelligence Tests. *Human Development, 29,* 209–222.

Schaie, K. W. (1977/78). Toward a stage theory of adult cognitive development. *Journal of Aging and Human Development, 8,* 129–138.

Schaie, K. W. (1983). The Seattle Longitudinal Study: A twenty-one year exploration of psychometric intelligence in adulthood. In K. W. Schaie (Ed.), *Longitudinal studies of adult psychological development* (pp. 64–135). New York: Guilford Press.

Schaie, K. W. (1984). Midlife influences upon intellectual functioning in old age. *International Journal of Behavioral Development, 7,* 463–478.

Schaie, K. W. (1985). *Manual for the Schaie-Thurstone Test of Mental Abilities (STAMAT).* Palo Alto, CA: Consulting Psychologists Press.

Schaie, K. W. (1988a). Internal validity threats in studies of adult cognitive development. In M. L. Howe & C. J. Brainard (Eds.), *Cognitive development in adulthood: Progress in cognitive development research* (pp. 241–272). New York: Springer-Verlag.

Schaie, K. W. (1988b). Variability in cognitive function in the elderly: Implications for social participation. In A. Woodhead, M. Bender, & R. Leonard (Eds.), *Phenotypic variation in populations: Relevance to risk management* (pp. 191–211). New York: Plenum.

Schaie, K. W. (1989a). The hazards of cognitive aging. *Gerontologist, 29,* 484–493.

Schaie, K. W. (1989b). Individual differences in rate of cognitive change in adulthood. In V. L. Bengtson & K. W. Schaie (Eds.), *The course of later life: Research and reflections* (pp. 63–83). New York: Springer Publishing Co.

Schaie, K. W. (1989c). Perceptual speed in adulthood: Cross-sectional and longitudinal studies. *Psychology and Aging, 4,* 443–453.

Schaie, K. W. (in press). Late life potential and cohort differences in mental abilities. In M. Perlmutter (Ed.), *Late life potential.* Washington, DC: Gerontological Society of America.

Schaie, K. W., Gonda, J. N., & Quayhagen, M. (1982). Die Beziehung zwischen intellektueller Leistung und erlebter Alltagskompetenz bei Erwachsenen in verschiedenen Altersabschnitten [The relationship of intellectual performance and perceived every-day competence in adults of various ages]. In H. Loewe, U. Lehr, & J. E. Birren (Eds.), *Psychologische Probleme des Erwachsenenalters* (pp. 43–67). Berlin: VEB Deutscher Verlag der Wissenschaften.

Schaie, K. W., & Parham, I. A. (1975). *Manual for the Test of Behavioral Rigidity.* Palo Alto, CA: Consulting Psychologists Press.

Schaie, K. W., & Willis, S. L. (1986). Can intellectual decline in the elderly be reversed? *Developmental Psychology, 22,* 223–232.

Thurstone, L. L., & Thurstone, T. G. (1941). *Factorial studies of intelligence.* Chicago: University of Chicago Press.

Willis, S. L. (1989). Cognitive training in later adulthood: Remediation vs. new learning. In L. Poon, D. Rubin, & B. Wilson (Eds.), *Everyday cognition in adults and late life* (pp. 545–569). New York: Cambridge University Press.

Willis, S. L., & Schaie, K. W. (1986a). Practical intelligence in later adulthood. In R. J. Sternberg & R. K. Wagner (Eds.), *Practical intelligence: Origins of competence in the everyday world* (pp. 236–268). New York: Cambridge University Press.

Willis, S. L., & Schaie, K. W. (1986b) Training the elderly on the ability factors of spatial orientation and inductive reasoning. *Psychology and Aging, 1,* 239–247.

Willis, S. L., & Schaie, K. W. (1988). Gender differences in spatial ability in old age: Longitudinal and intervention findings. *Sex Roles, 18,* 189–203.

5 The optimization of episodic remembering in old age

LARS BÄCKMAN, TIMO MÄNTYLÄ, AND
AGNETA HERLITZ

Introduction

The purpose of this chapter is to survey the literature on aging and memory with special reference to the factors that promote the optimization of episodic remembering in old age. The overall objective of this enterprise is to identify and organize the variables that may contribute to our understanding of how and when older adults exhibit good memory performance. The review focuses on memory tasks that are episodic and explicit in nature, thus requiring conscious recollection of episodes encoded in a particular temporal–spatial context (e.g., lists of words encountered in the laboratory). Although microgenetic longitudinal studies in the form of research on memory training have received increasing attention from investigators during recent years, the bulk of empirical inquiry pertaining to the issue of memory optimization in old age is cross-sectional. This bias is reflected in the present review.

The concept of optimization is complex. It may be analyzed from a variety of perspectives and with different criteria. Taking the perspective that optimization is a concept that is related to the maximal performance level for a given individual in a given task, it follows that we have to know the absolute ceiling of performance for that individual in that task in order to make any definite statements about optimization. As far as the psychology of memory is concerned, determining an individual's performance ceiling in a given task is difficult. Although an individual may have reached the asymptotic level after, say, 3,000 trials, it is an open question what might happen after, say, 50,000 trials. In addition, although it may be sensible to equate optimization with maximization for some individuals in some task situations, there are situations in which this assumption is questionable. From a general psychological perspective, maximizing memory performance (by investing a substantial amount of time and effort) may be suboptimal in the sense that other domains of functioning may suffer (Bäckman & Dixon, 1989). This is especially true for individuals, such as older adults, who have deficits in the basic processing resources that govern memory functioning (Baltes, 1987). Also, if the criterion for what is optimal memory performance is defined in relation to an individual's well-being and life satisfaction, then what is optimal may be something completely different from what is maximal. An illustrative, albeit extreme, example of the importance of forgetting for optimal living is provided by Luria (1965/1968) in his description of the Russian mnemonist Shereshevskii. This person possessed extraordinary memory skills, performing at the maximum in most standard memory tasks. However, according to Luria, Shereshevskii's memories were so elaborate and detailed that they interfered with his everyday life, leading to difficulties in concentration, sleeplessness, and personality disturbances. Surely, forgetting may serve adaptive purposes also for individuals with normal memory skills (e.g., to forget traumatic failures in love, work, social interactions).

Acknowledging the relativism of the concept of optimization, we have chosen to adopt a definition of optimization that covers (1) those situations in which older adults maximize their performance (relative to other situations) and (2) performance increments demonstrated within the same type of task following intervention. Hence, we are concerned with objective, rather than subjective, markers of successful aging (cf. P. B. Baltes & M. M. Baltes, this volume). Also, references will be made to the corresponding performances of young adults in the task situations of interest. Obviously, the objectives of the present chapter may be achieved in several different ways, depending largely on one's theoretical orientation. In agreement with many other current researchers (e.g., Bransford, McCarrell, Franks, & Nitsch, 1977; Craik, 1985; Jenkins, 1979; Nilsson, 1984), we conceive of remembering as an activity that reflects an interaction between externally provided information in the form of general or more specific retrieval cues and previously acquired knowledge, skills, and so forth. This orientation rejects the view of memory as a "thing" or a receptacle that can be stimulated, detected, or manipulated as such. As suggested by Craik (1985), "the memory trace is perhaps not a specific structure located at some point (or even diffusely) within the central nervous system, but is rather an altered potential of the system to carry out certain mental activities provided that the context, task, goals, mental set etc. present at the time of initial learning are reinstated, either driven by external information or reconstructed internally by the rememberer" (p. 200).

Within this general framework, Jenkins (1979) argued that a full

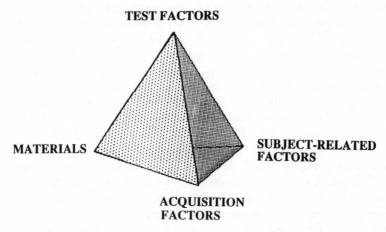

TEST FACTORS

MATERIALS

SUBJECT-RELATED FACTORS

ACQUISITION FACTORS

Figure 5.1. A conceptual framework for the evaluation of memory performance. Each vertex represents a set of variables of a given type. Each edge represents a two-way interaction important to remembering. Each plane represents a three-way interaction, and the whole pyramid represents the four-way interaction among all the variables involved (adapted from Jenkins, 1979).

understanding of memory performance requires consideration of four major sources of variation: acquisition variables (e.g., attention, strategies, level of encoding, elaboration), test variables (e.g., quality and quantity of retrieval information, specificity of transfer), materials (e.g., modality, organizational structure, conceptual difficulty, richness of features), and subject-related variables (e.g., preexperimental knowledge, skills, motivation, interests). A modified version of Jenkins's (1979) tetrahedral model for memory experiments is presented in Figure 5.1.

As is apparent from Figure 5.1, one central assumption in Jenkins's model is that the sources of variation interact vigorously with each other; the implication being that memory is essentially a context-dependent phenomenon. Provided that this relativistic conception of remembering is accurate, it follows that all four sources of variation (and the interactions among them) have to be taken into account when evaluating a particular subject's level of memory performance. Analogously, an attempt to penetrate the issue of memory optimization in aging has to consider the entire Theorist's Tetrahedron in order to be as complete as possible. In this chapter, we thus discuss both external and subject-related factors pertaining to the issue of memory optimization in aging. Although our main concern is with research on healthy older adults, we also discuss the conditions under which successful memory performance may be achieved in a case of pathological aging, namely, Alzheimer's disease. Note that the terms *old* and *older* refer to individuals who are at least 60 years of age. Older subjects typically range between 60 and 80 years of age, whereas young subjects usually are in their late teens and twenties. Also, it is commonplace to match the age-groups tested on various background variables, such as educational level, socioeconomic status, health, and verbal ability.

Memory optimization in normal aging

External factors

Adult age differences favoring young adults are routinely observed in standard episodic memory tasks, which require conscious retrieval of information encountered in the laboratory (see Kausler, 1982; Poon, 1985; Salthouse, 1982, 1985, for reviews). However, the magnitude of this age-related deficit in episodic remembering varies greatly as a function of multiple external (e.g., type of test, pacing, richness of materials, instructions) and subject-related (e.g., motivation, interests, verbal ability, task-relevant expertise) factors. With respect to external factors, an empirical rule possible to derive from the literature is that tasks that involve little contextual support (e.g., free recall of unrelated verbal materials) reveal pronounced age differences in favor of young adults, whereas tasks in which the experimenter, the task, or the materials guide the learner show reduced or even eliminated age differences in memory performance (Bäckman, 1985a, 1989b; Craik, 1983; Craik & Rabinowitz, 1984). Hence, it appears that there is an age difference in the need of contextual support for optimization of episodic memory performance: The old need more than the young (cf. Winocur, 1982). The younger adults' lesser need of support in this context may be attributed to their superior ability in self-initiated recoding operations (Bäckman, 1986; Craik, 1983, 1985). Following Jenkins's (1979) framework for remembering, the category of external factors may be decomposed into acquisition factors, test factors, and materials. Illustrative examples from these three subcategories pertaining to the issue of optimal memory performance in old age are presented in the following subsections.

Acquisition factors. The most common method used to explore the role of acquisition factors for the level of memory performance of older adults is to contrast performance under two conditions: (1) where no specific instructions are provided as to how to encode the to-be-remembered (TBR) information and (2) where pretask encoding suggestions are supplied. A typical result from experiments in which this general procedure has been adopted is that marked age differences in favor of young adults are obtained in the standard instruction condition, whereas the age-related effects are attenuated in the condition involving explicit guidelines for the use of acquisition strategies. Such data have been obtained when organizational instructions (e.g., Hultsch, 1969, 1971), imagery instructions (e.g., Canestrari, 1968; Treat, Poon, & Fozard, 1978), or instructions to use verbal mediators (e.g., Hulicka & Grossman, 1967; Hulicka, Sterns, & Grossman, 1967) have been supplied by the experimenter prior to presentation of the TBR items in free recall and paired-associate learning tasks.

Other acquisition variables relevant in this context are those of rate of presentation and number of study trials. Manipulating presentation rate, several investigators (e.g., Adamowicz, 1976; Arenberg, 1965, 1967; Kinsbourne & Berryhill, 1972; Monge & Hultsch, 1971) have found that older adults benefit selectively with respect to recall of different types of verbal materials when task pacing decreases. Note, however, that others have found that altering presentation rate affects young and older age-groups in a similar manner (e.g., Craik & Rabinowitz, 1985; A. D. Smith, 1976), whereas still others have reported a differential benefit for young adults under less paced task conditions (e.g., Belmont, Freeseman, & Mitchell, 1988; Charness, 1981c). Conceivably, the crucial issue is which cognitive operations can be executed at a given presentation rate. Varying the number of study trials, Crew (1977) found a marked and selective recall improvement by older adults as a function of increasing exposure to the verbal TBR items. R. L. Cohen, Sandler, and Schroeder (1987) extended the finding that older adults are sensitive to this acquisition variable by showing that it applies to both word recall and recall of subject-performed action events.

Further, in two studies (Bäckman & Karlsson, 1987; Kausler & Hakami, 1983a) it was found that older adults increased their level of recall compared with control conditions, when problem-solving activity was required during encoding, whereas young adults were unaffected by this manipulation. Mitchell, Hunt, and Schmitt (1986) showed that generation of TBR items within a sentence context as opposed to simply reading the items (Slamecka & Graf, 1978) resulted in a substantially higher cued recall performance by both young and older age-groups. Conceivably, the added activity during acquisition in the form of problem solving acts as a cognitive support system (cf. Bransford, 1979).

It thus appears that there is an age-related difference in the need of encoding support to perform optimally in these experimental situations; whereas older adults generally exhibit high levels of memory performance (sometimes equivalent to that of their younger counterparts) following supportive encoding conditions, young adults appear to be less sensitive to these types of manipulations. This state of affairs has been interpreted as a demonstration of a production deficiency in older adults; that is, the encoding operations that are beneficial to memory performance are available but not always spontaneously accessible among the aged (e.g., Kausler, 1970; Reese, 1976; A. D. Smith, 1980).

It may be the case, though, that these empirical generalizations are not applicable across the entire adult life span. In a recent study, Bäckman and Karlsson (1986) showed that although a group of 73-year-olds improved their recall performance markedly when receiving organizational instructions compared with standard instructions, a group of 82-year-olds failed to show such an improvement. This pattern of results suggests that there may be qualitative differences between different cohorts of healthy older adults in the ability to utilize support.

Test factors. Although memory performance may be assessed explicitly as well as implicitly (that is, with or without conscious recollection) and although accuracy as well as speed of response may constitute the dependent measure, the literature on episodic memory and aging indicates that two types of contrasts between memory tests have dominated this field of research: free recall versus recognition and free recall versus cued recall.

In a classical study, Schonfield and Robertson (1966) found that although memory performance as assessed by free recall deteriorated across the adult life span, there were no age-related differences when copy cues were supplied as retrieval support in a recognition test. The finding that age differences are eliminated or attenuated when memory is assessed by means of recognition testing has been replicated in a number of subsequent studies (e.g., Erber, 1974; Howell, 1972; Kausler & Hakami, 1983b). In a similar vein, the provision of category cues (e.g., superordinate semantic categories) at the time of testing has been found to attenuate or eliminate age-related differences observed in free recall of organizable verbal materials (e.g., Bäckman & Karlsson, 1986; Hultsch, 1975; Laurence, 1967). In a recent study, Craik and McDowd (1987) compared cued recall and recognition in young and older adults. These investigators found no age-related differences in recognition, whereas the young outperformed the old in cued recall. This result was interpreted as supportive of the notion that cued recall requires more processing resources than does recognition and that such resources are depleted in late adulthood.

The observed effects of retrieval manipulations on the level of memory performance of older adults resemble those of the encoding manipulations described earlier: Older adults' memory performance in these task situations appears to be optimized when retrieval conditions are most supportive, whereas the amount and quality of retrieval information seems to be less important in early adulthood.

Acquisition × test interactions. Compatibility between the conditions prevailing during acquisition and test is regarded as a prerequisite for good memory performance in many prominent conceptions of remembering, such as the encoding-specificity principle (e.g., Tulving, 1983; Tulving & Thomson, 1973) and the transfer-appropriate processing notion (e.g., Adams et al., 1988; Morris, Bransford, & Franks, 1977). In brief, the contention is that the retrievability of a particular item is largely a function of the degree to which the cue information matches the underlying mental representation of the TBR event.

A number of studies have explored the viability of this general principle with regard to memory performance in old age. The results obtained from these studies are quite straightforward: Older adults exhibit excellent performance (and age-related differences are absent) when conditions are similar (and supportive) at encoding and retrieval. Such results have been obtained when category cues (Ceci & Tabor, 1981; A. D. Smith, 1977) or strong semantic associates (Shaps & Nilsson, 1980) are presented along with the TBR items at both stages of remembering. Similarly, several investigations within the levels-of-processing framework employing recognition tests preceded by various forms of orienting tasks have reported remarkably high levels of performance among older adults and no age-related performance differences (Erber, Herman, & Botwinick, 1980; Mason, 1979; White, described in Craik, 1977). Employing a self-generation task in which subjects are provided with their own descriptors of the TBR items as retrieval cues, Bäckman, Mäntylä, and Erngrund (1984) and Bäckman and Mäntylä (1988) reported high levels of recall in young and older adults, although the young performed somewhat better than the old. Note that all studies cited involving dual contextual support (and compatibility between encoding and retrieval conditions) also report a superiority in memory performance of younger adults in a variety of control tasks in which conditions are less supportive.

Contextual reinstatement is not the only way in which cue–trace compatibility may be achieved. An alternative approach is to provide retrieval cues that are less affected by fluctuations in the physical and cognitive environments (Mäntylä, 1986; Mäntylä & Nilsson, 1988). The main characteristic of this cue-distinctiveness approach is that cue–trace compatibility is accomplished by focusing the encoding activity on properties of the TBR information that are distinctive in the sense that their meaning is essentially the same even if the context is changed. Mäntylä and Bäckman (1989) had young and older subjects generate either general or distinctive descriptors of TBR words. Results indicated that distinctiveness of encoding was positively related to recall performance and that older adults improved memory performance disproportionately when distinctive cues were provided at retrieval.

Materials. Research indicates that the nature of the TBR materials is a very important determinant of memory performance in old age. Specifically, it appears that stimulus dimensions like modality, contextual richness, and organizability largely determine older adults' level of memory performance and the absence or presence of an age-related performance deficit.

In three studies from our own laboratory (Bäckman, 1985b; Bäckman & Nilsson, 1984, 1985), we demonstrated that the superiority of young adults routinely observed in traditional verbal free-recall tasks was eliminated when the assignment consisted of remembering series of subject-performed tasks or SPTs (R. L. Cohen, 1981). In this type of experiment, subjects are asked to perform various real-life action events (e.g., bounce the ball, break the match) for purposes of later recall. The high levels of performance shown by older adults in remembering SPTs is attributed to the facts that encoding of SPTs (1) is multimodal, in the sense that several sensory systems are involved; and (2) may be based on a variety of features (e.g., verbal, color, shape, texture, sound, motor). These properties distinguish SPTs from standard verbal memory tasks, in which the encoding is typically unimodal and only verbal features are nominally present. Bäckman (1985b) found that the active motor manipulation seems to be of special importance for older adults' success in this memory task (see also G. Cohen & Faulkner, in press; West, 1986). Although the initial results of adult age equivalence for SPTs were recently replicated (Dick, Kean, & Sands, 1989), it should be noted that other recent investigations (R. L. Cohen et al., 1987; Guttentag & Hunt, 1988; Lichty, Kausler, & Martinez, 1986) have found age-related differences favoring the young in SPT recall. Differences among studies with respect to presentation rate, list length, and item organizability may be responsible for the mixed results.

Regarding the modality variable, Arenberg (1968) and Bäckman (1986) obtained attenuated age differences in memory for bimodally (visually and auditorily) presented items and pronounced age differences for unimodally (visually or auditorily) presented items. Commenting on the relationship between such findings and the results from the SPT studies, Bäckman (1986) concluded that age differences in free recall appear to be marked when the presentation is unimodal, reduced when the presentation is bimodal, and greatly reduced (or eliminated) when the presentation is multimodal. Phrased somewhat differently, in these experimental situations there seems to be a straightforward relationship between memory optimization in old age and the number of modalities activated during encoding.

Two studies on recall of television programs (Cavanaugh, 1983, 1984) lend further support to the notion that the nature of the TBR materials is a critical factor for the level of memory performance in old age. In these studies, Cavanaugh found high levels of propositional recall in older adults and that performance differences between high-verbal young and older adults were small or nonexistent. Interestingly, the encoding of a television program would seem to resemble that of SPTs in the sense that a variety of features (e.g., color, shape, movement) are available in addition to verbal features. Moreover, the plot of the program provides an organizational structure for the encoding of the event. These types of contextual support may constitute critical prerequisites for older adults' high level of television recall.

Research on spatial memory and a number of studies on text recall in adulthood illustrate the importance of inherent organizational structure in the materials for the goodness of memory in old age. Waddell and Rogoff (1981) found that levels of spatial recall doubled in older adults when the materials (objects) were presented in a contextually organized panorama compared with a noncontextually organized stimulus array, whereas middle-aged women performed equally well under both these conditions. Analogously, age-related differences were present in the latter case but not in the former. The lack of adult age-related differences in recall of contextually well organized objects has been replicated in subsequent, follow-up studies (Waddell, 1983; Waddell & Rogoff, 1987). Sharps and Gollin (1987) reported that young adults outperformed older adults in memory of object locations when objects were displayed on a map, whereas no age-related differences were found when objects were displayed in a real-life environment (a real room). The authors attributed this interaction to the higher degree of inherent visual distinctiveness in the room context. Sharps and Gollin (1988) extended this pattern of results to free recall of objects located in space. They found pronounced age-related differences in object memory when contextual cues were lacking (objects presented in a list format or objects presented in a visually bland context). However, this age-related deficit disappeared when visually distinctive cues were added to the spatial context (a colored map, a three-dimensional unpainted model, a three-dimensional painted model, or a large room). Obviously, the results of these two studies suggest that young and older adults are differentially affected by the visual distinctiveness of the context in which spatial and object learning occur and that both nonverbal and verbal memory of older adults may be optimized when encoding conditions are most supportive.

In a similar vein, the results from numerous studies on prose comprehension and text recall in adulthood indicate that age differences in the recall of propositions and in the organization of the text are attenuated or eliminated when the TBR text is well organized; they are exacerbated when the text is less well organized (e.g., Byrd, 1981; S. W. Smith, Rebok, W. R. Smith, Hall, & Alwin, 1983). Thus, it appears that age-related differences in text recall are most likely to occur when subjects have to rely on self-imposed organization of the materials (see Hultsch & Dixon, 1984, for a review).

In sum, then, the nature of the materials (e.g., richness of features, modality, organizational structure) appears to be a very important factor determining the level of memory performance of older adults (and whether age-related performance deficits are observed) across a variety of task situations. In addition, young adults seem to be less sensitive to this factor to perform maximally; in fact, this is the very same pattern of results described previously for acquisition and test factors.

Subject-related factors

A vast number of subject-related factors have to be considered when discussing goodness of remembering in old age, including verbal skills (e.g., Hultsch & Dixon, 1984), task-relevant prior knowledge (e.g., Barrett & Wright, 1981), schooling (Gribbon, Schaie, & Parham, 1980), level of daily activity (e.g., Craik, Byrd, & Swanson, 1987), personality characteristics (e.g., Arbuckle, Gold, & Andres, 1986), and specific memory-related skills (e.g., Yesavage, Lapp, & Skeikh, 1989). With respect to the activity variable, though, it should be noted that the empirical evidence is somewhat mixed. Although Craik et al. (1987) reported a positive relationship between level of daily activity and memory performance of older adults, others (e.g., J. T. Hartley, 1986; Salthouse, Kausler, & Saults, 1988) have failed to find such a relationship. In this section, we focus on two broad categories of subject-related factors, both of which have received considerable attention among investigators: (1) preexperimental knowledge and skills and (2) specific memory-related skills. In addition, we discuss an example of how a subject-related variable (i.e., verbal intelligence) may interact with acquisition and test variables in determining the level of memory performance in old age.

Preexperimental knowledge and skills. Much of the research on the influence of abilities, skills, and knowledge on memory performance in late adulthood has employed texts rather than words or digits as the information to be remembered. An important question that has guided this research is whether adult age–related differences in, for example, the free recall of prose would be attenuated or eliminated given the presence of general (e.g., high verbal ability) or more specific (e.g., task-relevant prior knowledge) expertise among old learners. Note that in the studies addressing this issue, expertise has been conceived of within a normal range of functioning and usually as a variable with which to compare and differentiate within and across age-groups. For example, old and young adult groups may be divided to high- and low-skill subgroups and compared on the free recall of texts. Two categories of skills have received special attention from investigators: (1) the availability of pertinent prior knowledge or schemata and (2) language experience and verbal ability. Relevant research pertaining to these types of skills will be described next.

Preexperimental knowledge. There is ample empirical evidence to suggest that the availability of task-relevant prior knowledge may boost the level of recall in older adults, and sometimes even result in age-related differences favoring older adults. The most common way of manipulating this variable in memory and aging research is to select TBR materials for which the age-groups (e.g., young vs. old) differ in terms of preexperimental knowledge. This may be accomplished by varying the datedness of the TBR information (e.g., dated vs. contemporary), the assumption being that because age and cohort groups have experienced relatively unique cultural and historical events, they may differ with respect to prior knowledge or schemata for some historically relevant topics. Following this principle, Hultsch and Dixon (1983) found that older subjects recalled more propositions from a cohort-relevant text (in this case a biographical sketch of Mary Pickford) than from a biographical sketch of an entertainment figure taken from a more recent cohort (e.g., Steve Martin), whereas the opposite pattern of performance was observed for young adults. The cross-over interaction between age and story also indicated that the old outperformed the young for dated texts, although the young outperformed the old for more contemporary texts; that is, the level of prior knowledge was strongly related to optimization of performance in this situation.

It may be noted that this general pattern of results has been obtained with other types of verbal materials, such as single words (Barrett & Wright, 1981; Erber, Galt, & Botwinick, 1985; Worden & Sherman-Brown, 1983) and names (Bäckman, Herlitz, & Karlsson, 1987; Hanley-

Dunn & McIntosh, 1984). The same effect has also been demonstrated in the context of face recognition memory (Bäckman, 1989a, in press). In addition, the data pattern applies to old–old as well as young–old adults (Bäckman et al., 1987; Bäckman, in press) and to situations in which the speed of retrieval rather than the number of items retrieved constitutes the dependent measure (Poon & Fozard, 1978). The importance of pre-experimental knowledge for the level of memory performance in old age thus appears to be well established.

Verbal skills. With respect to verbal skills as related to text recall in adulthood, the predominant (usually single) indicator has been voca-bulary score. Results from a number of studies suggest that high-verbal older adults may perform at the same level as young adults on various text memory measures, whereas typical age differences favoring the young are observed when the older group is composed of low-verbal subjects (e.g., Harker, J. T. Hartley, & Walsh, 1982; Meyer & Rice, 1981, 1983; Taub, 1979). Although the level of verbal ability may be an important determi-nant for older adults' level of performance in many text recall studies, a number of provisos and qualifications should be pointed out. For exam-ple, the verbal ability variable may interact with task variables, such as level of information (main ideas, details). This is illustrated in a study by Dixon, Hultsch, Simon, and von Eye (1984), who found no age differences in main idea recall and age differences in favor of younger adults in recall of details for high-verbal subjects. For low-verbal subjects, on the other hand, the young outperformed the old across all levels of information (see Spilich, 1983, for similar results). In addition, some authors (e.g., J. T. Hartley, 1986) have found that verbal ability, as indexed by a vocabulary measure alone, is only a weak predictor of text recall and that age-related deficits in overall text recall performance may appear also for high-verbal subjects.

Verbal skill × acquisition × test interactions. On the basis of the tetrahedral model proposed by Jenkins (1979) one should expect that what optimizes memory performance in old age is a joint product of subject-related variables and environmental variables. For example, depending on the level of a particular skill (e.g., verbal), the need of environmental support in order to optimize memory performance may vary. Examples illustrating the complex relationships among internal and external factors pertaining to memory performance in elderly adults are unfortunately sparse in the literature. However, a recent study by Craik et al. (1987) is illustrative. These authors used older adults at various levels of verbal skill and a control group of younger adults as subjects, and varied systematically the environmental support supplied at acquisition (no cues, cues) and test (no cues, cues) in a series of episodic memory tasks. The pattern of results from this study suggests that low-verbal older adults need support at both stages of remembering in order to perform optimally in these situations, whereas high-verbal older adults need support at either acquisition or test to achieve the highest level of performance. The young adults in this study were relatively insensitive to environmental support and performed at about the same level in all task conditions. Viewed from a different perspective, performance differences between the young and the high-verbal older subjects were present only when no cues were provided at encoding and retrieval, whereas the low-verbal older subjects kept up with the other groups only when support was provided at both learning and test. The important implication of this study is that neither environmental variables nor subject-related variables alone can predict the level of memory performance in old age; knowledge about both sets of variables is imperative.

The types of subject-related variables discussed in this section are general memory-related skills and abilities that older individuals possess before entering the laboratory. Next, we describe research on specific memory-related skills in the context of memory training in adulthood.

Specific memory-related skills. Several different approaches have been adopted in the area of memory training and aging. The most straightforward approach calls for simply giving subjects extensive practice on the memory tasks of interest. This variant has, in part, been guided by the hypothesis that the performance decrement of older adults on memory-related tasks is due to diminished intellectual stimulation in the older individual's environment (Labouvie-Vief, 1976, 1977; Labouvie-Vief & Gonda, 1976). Simple practice on memory tasks has been examined by several investigators (e.g., Erber, 1976; Hultsch, 1974; Monge, 1969; Taub, 1973; Taub & Long, 1972) and the results are quite clear-cut: Although considerable increases in memory performance by elderly adults as a function of practice are invariably found, most studies have found either a greater practice effect for the young or equal improvement for old and young subjects. Obviously, such a pattern of results is at variance with a strict environmental deprivation hypothesis to account for age-related memory deficits.

Other approaches may be labeled unifactorial in the sense that they involve training of specific single control processes known to be beneficial to memory performance, such as organization (e.g., Sanders, Murphy, Schmitt, & Walsh, 1980; Schmitt, Murphy, & Sanders, 1981) and visual imagery (e.g., McCarty, 1980; Treat, Poon, & Fozard, 1981; Yesavage,

1983). Again, the results indicate marked improvements of memory performance among older adults following training. However, when age comparisons are available, there are no indications that older adults benefit more than young adults from these forms of intervention. In addition, it appears that there is an age-related difference in the duration of training effects, such that the young are more likely to maintain the beneficial strategies across time (Hellebusch, 1976; Treat et al., 1981).

Employing the method of loci, which may be regarded as a combination of organizational and visual imagery strategies, Robertson-Tchabo, Hausman, and Arenberg (1976) demonstrated that older adults can utilize this method to improve memory, but that optimal performance is achieved only through explicitly cuing them in its continued usage. In another study using the same method, Rose and Yesavage (1983) found better recall after training in young, middle-aged, and old adults but a decrease in the effectiveness of the mnemonic as the age of the subjects increased.

From the perspective that the memory deficits accompanying the adult aging process have several origins, including basic encoding and retrieval operations (e.g., Kausler, 1982; A. D. Smith, 1980), attentional functions (e.g., Bäckman & Nilsson, 1985; Kinsbourne, 1980), and anxiety-related functions (e.g., Bäckman & Molander, 1986; M. F. Elias & P. K. Elias, 1977), it is possible to argue that efforts to alleviate the deficits should be multifactorial as well in order to optimize the effects of training (Bäckman, 1989b). Research efforts aimed at evaluating the benefits of composite programs on memory performance in old age have involved combinations of training in semantic associations and interactive imagery (Yesavage, Rose, and Bower, 1983); categorization, association, and imagery (Zarit, Cole, & Guider, 1981); attention and relaxation (Yesavage & Rose, 1983); imagery and relaxation (Yesavage, 1984); relaxation, attention, and categorization (Lundqvist, Thors, Bäckman, Karlsson, & Nilsson, 1988; Stigsdotter & Bäckman, 1989a, 1989b); and working memory, knowledge acquisition, and the method of loci (Kliegl & Baltes, 1987; Kliegl, Smith, & Baltes, 1986). The overall impression from these studies is that multifactorial training is an extremely effective way of enhancing memory performance in old age, producing effects that may last up to 6 months after completion of training (Lundqvist et al., 1988; Stigsdotter & Bäckman, 1989a, 1989b). However, a word of caution is warranted: Combined approaches using packages of strategies make it difficult, if not impossible, to distinguish the effects of training on the various psychological functions involved (Yesavage et al., 1989). One way to escape this dilemma would be to use large designs including all combinations of the components in the program, whereby additive (and multiplicative) effects could be determined (Bäckman, 1989b).

As is apparent from the research cited, the buildup or strengthening of various memory skills (and related psychological functions) in the laboratory may increase older adults' memory performance up to a level far above their baseline performance. Although the results from memory-training research with older adults thus provide strong evidence of plasticity of memory functioning in old age, we do not yet know whether the observed performance increments are due to activation of skills available (but not spontaneously accessible) in the repertoire of older adults or are a result of the acquisition of new skills (Bäckman & Dixon, 1986, 1989; Dixon & Bäckman, 1986, in press). This important issue was addressed in a recent paper by Baltes, Kliegl, and Dittmann-Kohli (1988), who found support for the position that training gains in old age largely reflect the activation of latent cognitive skills rather than the acquisition of new skills as far as performance in fluid intelligence tasks is concerned. Whether that outcome generalizes to the area of memory training remains an issue for future investigation.

A characteristic feature of the results from memory-training research in adulthood and old age is that although older adults typically exhibit large performance gains as a function of training, the gains are equally large, or even larger, for their younger counterparts. The latter outcome should, in fact, be expected from a research perspective labeled testing-the-limits, used for examining different aspects of plasticity and its boundary conditions (Baltes, 1987; Baltes, Dittmann-Kohli, & Dixon, 1984). Within this perspective, three aspects of plasticity are distinguished: (1) baseline performance, which denotes an individual's initial performance level on a given task, that is, without intervention or other forms of cognitive or contextual support; (2) baseline reserve capacity, which indicates the upper level of an individual's performance potential at a given point in time, that is when all available resources are taxed in order to optimize the level of performance (note that an individual's baseline reserve capacity in a given task may be revealed not only through self-initiated efforts but also when performance conditions are supportive); and (3) developmental reserve capacity, which denotes an increase in an individual's baseline reserve capacity as a result of intervention or developmental progression. A key assumption within this perspective is that developmental differences (e.g., between young and older adults) should be magnified near maximum levels of performance (e.g., Baltes, 1987). In agreement with that postulate, the results from a series of extensive memory-training studies (Kliegl & Baltes, 1987; Kliegl et al., 1986) suggest that although substantial developmental reserve capacity is evident in early as well as later adulthood, there is more room for improvement from intervention in young adults than in older adults, especially when subjects are tested under difficult conditions (see also Poon, Walsh-Sweeney, & Fozard, 1980; Roberts, 1983; Rose & Yesavage, 1983).

Age-related differences in utilization of contextual and cognitive support for remembering

A data pattern showing that the young benefit more than the old from training would seem to run counter to the bulk of single-assessment experimental studies, in which young and older adults have been compared in memory tasks involving varying amounts of contextual or cognitive support; in those types of studies, for a wide variety of memory tasks and materials, older adults have been shown to improve more than young adults when conditions are most supportive (see Bäckman, 1985a, 1989b, for reviews). However, similar to other empirical regularities in the memory literature (R. L. Cohen, 1985), there are exceptions to this pattern of results. For example, research on levels of processing in relation to age (e.g., Eysenck, 1974; Simon, 1979) and on the effects of preexperimental knowledge on adult memory (e.g., Bäckman et al., 1987) indicate that as the encoding task is changed to direct subjects' attention to more relevant aspects of the TBR materials or when the task becomes more meaningful, young adults will make earlier use of the increased compatibility with their knowledge structures and so improve their memory performance earlier than older adults. Commenting on this apparent ambiguity in the literature, Craik et al. (1987) suggested that the difference in improvement in memory peformance between young and older adults as a result of an increase in the meaningfulness of the materials or of other types of environmental support will depend on multiple interactions among tasks, materials, and subjects. That is, although the young may be quicker than the old in utilizing some forms of orienting tasks or guided instructions to improve memory, once conditions are such that the young are already achieving a good encoding for the material in question, further environmental support is likely to be of greater benefit for the old.

Hence, the relationship between the adult age of the rememberer and the extent to which memory performance increases as a function of various forms of support (ranging from pretask encoding suggestions to extensive training) is anything but straightforward. Figure 5.2 displays four prototypical cases depicting different relationships between age and the magnitude of memory improvement in a facilitative condition denoted B compared with a baseline condition denoted A. There is an increase in the amount of contextual support provided in Condition B across panels, such that Panel 1 represents studies in which little support is provided, Panel 2 represents studies in which somewhat more support is provided, and so

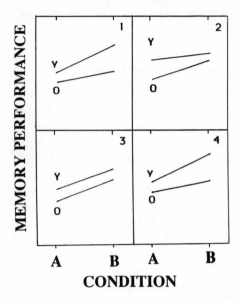

Figure 5.2. Four prototypical cases depicting the relationship between the age of the remember (young vs. old) and the performance gain in different facilitative conditions (B) compared with baseline (A).

forth. It is important to keep in mind that the four graphs displayed in Figure 5.2 should be viewed as schematic illustrations of performance patterns for various combinations of age-group and task rather than as representations of empirical invariances. Thus, it is recognized that, for example, age-related differences in baseline performance may be large, moderate, small, or absent depending on multiple external and subject-related factors. The functions in Figure 5.2 are shown simply to illustrate patterns in the data to be discussed.

Panel 1 in this figure summarizes those cases in which young adults benefit disproportionately from semantic orienting tasks (e.g., Craik, 1977; Eysenck, 1974; Simon, 1979), preexperimental knowledge (e.g., Bäckman et al., 1987), or increased item meaningfulness (Heron & Craik, 1964; Salthouse, 1982). One way of interpreting this data pattern is that young adults have quicker access to the cognitive resources that enable utilization of these forms of support for remembering (Salthouse, 1980, 1982, 1985), or, in other words, they are faster in making use of their baseline reserve capacity (Baltes, 1987; Kliegl & Baltes, 1987). In Panel 2, on the other hand, the interaction pattern is such that the old exhibit a pronounced improvement in memory performance from baseline in the supportive condition, whereas the young perform at about the same level in both conditions. This case is exemplified by all those studies described initially in this chapter, which demonstrate large age differences in standard instruction free-recall or paired-associate learning tasks and reduced or eliminated age differences in tasks where pretask encoding suggestions, explicit guidelines for the use of strategies, or additional retrieval cues are provided, as well as in tasks for which the TBR material is rich in terms of features and has an inherent organizational structure (Bäckman, 1989b). The interpretation of this pattern of outcome is that older adults possess sufficient reserve capacity to enable improved memory performance when the act of remembering is guided by various forms of environmental support (Craik, 1983). Young adults, on the other hand, may already have achieved an optimal encoding of the TBR information in the standard condition, and hence additional support tends to be redundant. In other words, the young adults, given their current level of skill, may have reached their "functional ceiling" in the particular Task A without the provision of encoding and/or retrieval support.

Panel 3 represents those studies in which there is an equivalent gain in the supportive condition for young and older adults. Many of the memory-training studies reviewed earlier represent cases in point. In training studies employing relatively short intervention programs (see Poon et al., 1980; Roberts, 1983; Yesavage, 1985, for reviews), the typical result is a similar increase in memory performance after training for young and older adults. On the basis of such a pattern of results it is tempting to conclude that there are no adult age–related differences in developmental reserve capacity as far as memory functioning is concerned. As indicated in Panel 4, however, this inference may be premature. Similar to Panel 1, the interaction pattern displayed in this panel indicates a larger gain in the supportive condition for young than for older adults. The pattern of outcome seen in Panel 4 has been reported in some memory-training studies (see, e.g., Kliegl & Baltes, 1987; Kliegl et al., 1986; Poon et al., 1980; Rose & Yesavage, 1983). The common denominator of these studies appears to be that the intervention programs are fairly extensive and/or that memory performance is assessed under relatively difficult task conditions (e.g., in terms of pacing). Note that although the same interaction pattern is seen in Panels 1 and 4, the supportive conditions prevailing in the studies represented in these two panels are quite different; in fact, they represent two extreme points on a continuum of contextual support. Whereas relatively little support is supplied in the single-assessment studies portrayed in Panel 1, a substantial amount of support in the form of extensive training is provided in the studies represented in Panel 4.

The general conclusion to be drawn from basic and applied research on memory in adulthood and old age is that sizable plasticity of memory functioning is evident in both young and older adults but that there are age-related differences with respect to the utilization of baseline reserve capacity (see Figure 5.2, Panels 1 and 2) as well as in developmental reserve capacity (see Figure 5.2, Panel 4).

The problem of unequal baselines

Although this analysis may accurately reflect some empirical regularities in the literature on memory and aging, a word of caution is warranted. As indicated in Figure 5.2, age-related differences favoring the young in the standard (baseline) condition are legion. Interpretation of interactions (or the lack of interactions) is risky when groups differ in baseline performance; we do not always know whether there is equivalence of measurement across the entire range of the dependent variable of interest, or the exact form of the process–variable function (e.g., organization versus number of propositions correctly recalled) in each age-group (Loftus, 1978; Salthouse, 1985). Several solutions to this problem have been suggested. First, transformations (e.g., arcsin) may be imposed to maximize the difference in a variable at the extremely low and high ends of the data set to minimize restriction of range near the floor and ceiling of measurement. As noted by Salthouse (1985), however, this and related procedures are justifiable only if the exact form of the process-variable relationship is known for the groups examined; otherwise, an inappropriate transformation is likely to be imposed, and meaningless data will be obtained.

Second, subjects may be preselected and matched on the basis of some characteristic (e.g., memory skill), or criterion tasks known to be relatively insensitive to the aging process may be employed. Although this strategy may have its advantages, it certainly puts restrictions on the number of memory tasks that can be used and may also limit the generalizability of results to those older adults who possess superior memory skills.

Third, some investigators have chosen to match the groups on baseline performance by, for example, presenting the older adults with shorter memory lists, decreasing the retention interval, or decreasing the task pacing for the old (cf. Diesfeldt, 1984). A particularly interesting variant is to adjust the task conditions separately for each individual subject in each age-group (e.g., Salthouse, Rogan, & Prill, 1984; Somberg & Salthouse, 1982), resulting in a more precise equating of performance in the baseline condition. However, the matching approach also has its disadvantages. We cannot be sure that the task stays the same and that the same cognitive processes are tapped when the encoding and/or retrieval conditions are altered. In other words, the process under scrutiny may be affected by manipulating the task conditions.

Finally, Baltes, Reese, and Nesselroade (1977) proposed a method, labeled control by systematic variation, to overcome the problems of unequal baselines. Here, the relevant independent variable (e.g., rate of presentation) is administered at several levels (e.g., rapid, medium, slow) to the samples of each age-group, and the focus is on the relationships between the criterion measure (e.g., number of words recalled) and the independent variable within the age-groups, rather than on the nominal performance levels.

Reviewing these different approaches, Salthouse (1985) concluded that the strategy devised by Baltes et al. (1977) is preferable to the others, because (1) the entire independent-dependent variable function can be examined to determine whether the manipulated variable had similar effects in the age-groups under study; and (2) provided that the functions are similar, comparisons may be made at selected levels of the independent variable across the age-groups, thereby equating for level of performance on a rational basis. However, one practical problem with this approach is that it requires rather extensive data collection to achieve its benefits. In fact, several simultaneous experiments have to be conducted, because the independent variable has to be crossed with each of the relevant levels of the dependent variable.

The research reviewed on the role of subject-related variables for memory performance in old age indicates that preexperimental skills and abilities as well as specific memory skills engineered in the laboratory constitute important sources for memory optimization in aging. As discussed, though, there appear to be age-related differences with respect to the pattern of plasticity of memory functioning: Some performance conditions are more beneficial to the old than to the young, although most forms of contextual and cognitive support bring about memory enhancement across the entire adult life span. However, as will be discussed in the next section, there are reasons to believe that the empirical results that speak to memory optimization in normal aging are not easily generalized to individuals suffering from dementia diseases, such as Alzheimer's disease.

Memory optimization in Alzheimer's disease

There are a number of different dementia diseases that may affect the aged individual. The most common of these are Alzheimer's disease (AD), multi-infarct dementia, and a mixed form of AD and multi-infarct dementia. A severe episodic memory dysfunction constitutes one of the earliest and most prominent signs of AD (R. G. Morris & Kopelman, 1986). In this section, we discuss empirical research relevant to the issue of memory optimization in AD, a disease believed to account for about 50% of all dementia cases (Tomlinson, 1980). To optimize the possibility of comparing memory functioning in AD with that in normal aging, we discuss potential plasticity of memory performance in AD as related to the same types of subject-related and external factors as those considered in the case of normal aging. In addition, memory optimization in AD is discussed in relation to performance increments following intervention and as related to performance increments in particular tasks compared with control tasks. Further, comparisons will be made with the corresponding performances of healthy older adults when such data are available.

Subject-related factors

Although the empirical evidence is sparse, it seems reasonable to assume that a vast number of subject-related variables may influence memory performance in AD patients (e.g., education, prior knowledge, verbal skills). However, it is likely that the subject-related factor that influences memory performance in AD the most is the disease itself and its level of severity. With few exceptions, the more severe the dementing illness is, according to various global-screening instruments (e.g., Mini–Mental State Examination; M. F. Folstein, S. E. Folstein, & McHugh, 1975), the poorer the memory performance (see Poon, 1986, for a review). Accordingly, in research on memory functioning in AD it is of utmost importance to state the requirement for diagnosis as well as to provide information concerning the severity of dementia (R. G. Morris & Kopelman, 1986). Authors of studies reviewed in this chapter have employed strict diagnostic criteria for including patients, unless otherwise stated. Moreover, the AD patients studied are in most cases classified as mildly or moderately demented. Similar to the case of normal aging, two sets of subject-related variables are considered in relation to memory optimization in AD: (1) preexperimental knowledge and skills and (2) specific memory-related skills.

Preexperimental knowledge and skills. Very few studies have explicitly studied the effects of preserved prior knowledge on memory in AD patients. However, in a case study, Martin (1987) showed that an AD patient who had superior premorbid drawing skills was able to draw descriptive pieces of art quite proficiently, although unable to draw simple spatial configurations. Such results are in line with clinical observations suggesting that remote memory is relatively well preserved in AD patients. However, studies have shown a consistent deficit in the recall (Wilson, Kaszniak, & Fox, 1981) and recognition (Sagar, N. J. Cohen, Corkin, & Growdon, 1985) of major public events and of famous individuals from the remote and recent past in AD patients, although mildly demented individuals have been found to possess more semantic knowledge from the 1940s than from today (Beatty, Salmon, Butters, Heindel, & Granholm, 1988).

In a recent face recognition experiment (Bäckman & Herlitz, in press), we sought to examine whether AD patients are able to utilize semantic knowledge to improve episodic remembering. Results replicated those of Beatty et al. (1988), indicating that AD patients, similar to their healthy aged counterparts, possess greater knowledge (both objectively and subjectively) of people famous during the 1940s than of people famous today. However, despite this advantage of dated over contemporary information in semantic memory, AD patients performed at the same level for dated and contemporary public figures in an episodic face recognition test.

Memory training. There have been few attempts to systematically explore whether AD patients are sensitive to memory training. Some studies (e.g., Beck et al., 1985) have reported a lack of effect of concentration, attention, and memory training on AD patients' memory performance. However, others (Hill, Evankovich, Sheikh, & Yesavage, 1987; S. H. Zarit, J. M. Zarit, & Reever, 1982) have demonstrated that it is possible to increase the level of memory performance in patients with mild primary degenerative dementia by means of visual imagery mnemonics. It should be noted, though, that research by Yesavage and colleagues (Yesavage, 1982; Yesavage, Westphal, & Rush, 1981) suggests that improvement can be accomplished by training only in very mild cases of dementia and has minimal practical impact (see also S. H. Zarit et al., 1982).

External factors

Materials. In contrast to their healthy aged counterparts, AD patients typically show no effects of type of material on memory performance. These patients perform equally well with verbal and facial information (Wilson, Kaszniak, Bacon, Fox, & Kelly, 1982) and with rare and common words (Wilson, Bacon, Kramer, Fox, & Kaszniak, 1983). Similarly, patients diagnosed as having primary degenerative dementia perform equally well on organized and nonorganized word lists (Weingartner et al., 1982) and show no picture-superiority effect (Rissenberg & Glanzer,

1986). Moreover, Butters et al. (1983) varied the amount of contextual support received during encoding of pictorial and spatial information, but this manipulation did not enhance memory performance in AD patients.

By contrast, Nebes, Martin, and Horn (1984) demonstrated that AD patients can use their knowledge of regularities of the English language to enhance episodic recall of words or letters, thereby showing the same qualitative pattern of data as normal older adults although performing at a lower level. This finding suggests that some aspects of the organizational structure of language are preserved in AD. Also, Rissenberg and Glanzer (1987) demonstrated an effect of concrete versus abstract words in a free-recall task among AD patients. However, the authors interpreted this result as due to the patients' verbal difficulty in generating abstract words rather than as a "true" effect of item concreteness.

Acquisition factors. As mentioned, the most common way to explore the effects of acquisition factors on memory is to study the way in which subjects spontaneously process a given type of information compared with the way it is processed when experimenter-provided instructions are supplied. Weingartner et al. (1982) found that a group of progressive idiopathic dementia patients were unable to spontaneously discover the semantic organization of a word list and utilize this information to improve recall. In a similar vein, Diesfeldt (1984) explicitly pointed out the semantic categories in a word list to a group of moderately demented patients, without thereby improving their level of recall compared with a standard condition. Corkin (1982) investigated the effects of level of processing (Craik & Lockhart, 1972) in mildly, moderately, and severely demented AD patients. The expected advantage for semantically encoded verbal information occurred for a group of normal older adults, whereas the AD groups performed at the same low level in all conditions. This result was replicated and extended to facial information for mildly demented AD patients (Wilson et al., 1982). Similarly, patients with AD are able to make relatively less use of verbal imagery in recognition compared with normal older adults (Kaszniak, Wilson, & Fox, 1981). Also, the "generation effect" (i.e., a superiority in recall of items that are generated by the subject compared with items provided by the experimenter during study) has not been obtained in AD, although this effect is as strong among normal older adults as among young adults (Mitchell et al., 1986).

A possible exception to this lack of sensitivity to manipulations at acquisition in AD may be the variable of presentation rate. A prolonged presentation has been found to increase AD patients' memory performance (Corkin et al., 1984). Research on the effects of number of study trials has yielded conflicting results. Moffat (in press) demonstrated a beneficial effect of increased number of study trials in AD using the spaced-retrieval technique, whereas Strauss, Weingartner, and Thompson (1985) did not find such an effect. Thus, a slow presentation rate may boost memory performance in AD, whereas it is too early to draw any conclusions concerning beneficial effects of increased number of study trials.

Taken together, research on acquisition factors suggests that progressive idiopathic demented patients and AD patients are unable to spontaneously detect and utilize semantic categories to improve memory and they are unable to benefit from explicit instructions at encoding. This pattern of outcome suggests a qualitative difference between patients and normal older adults in the ability to utilize environmental support at encoding to improve memory performance. Note, however, that AD patients' ability to improve memory by means of increased exposure to the TBR items (Corkin et al., 1984; Moffat, in press) may be an exception to this pattern.

Test factors. It is well known that the retrieval processes of AD patients function less well than those of age-matched controls. Performance on both verbal (Miller, 1975, 1978; Wilson et al., 1982) and facial (Wilson et al., 1982) recognition memory tasks is impaired in AD and tends to decrease as the number of distractors increases (Miller, 1978). Signal detection analysis indicates that this deficit is due to a problem in the memory discrimination between target and distractor stimuli rather than to response bias (Wilson et al., 1982). In a similar vein, studies on cued recall have demonstrated that the provision of category cues at test does not improve the level of recall of AD patients compared with free-recall testing (Davis & Mumford, 1984; Diesfeldt, 1984). However, there are test situations in which AD patients exhibit good memory performance and a qualitatively similar pattern of data to age-matched controls, although the evidence is somewhat inconclusive. In these test situations subjects are provided with partial information at retrieval (e.g., the first letters of a study word). Some investigators (Miller, 1975; R. G. Morris, Wheatley, & Britton, 1983) have found that AD patients improve markedly when provided with partial cues compared with free recall, performing at the same level as normal older adults in the partial-cuing condition. Others (Davis & Mumford, 1984) have reported that although AD patients perform better when receiving partial cues than on free recall, they do not reach the level of performance of healthy older adults. Still others (Salmon, Shimamura, Butters, Squire, & Smith, 1988; Shimamura, Salmon, Squire, & Butters, 1987) have demonstrated a pronounced deficit among AD patients in this task situation, although patients suffering from Huntington's disease and Korsakoff's disease exhibited intact abilities. Obviously, further experimentation is needed in order to trace the sources of the discrepant findings from research on the effects of partial cues on memory performance in AD.

Acquisition × test interactions. There are also experiments showing that AD patients are able to improve their level of performance in standard episodic memory tasks. This improvement is typically observable in tasks that provide favorable conditions during both encoding and retrieval. Diesfeldt (1984) demonstrated that the level of recall in a group of progressive idiopathic dementia patients increased when explanations of the category structure during encoding were combined with category cuing at retrieval. Explanation of the category structure given at the time of presentation or cuing with category names at retrieval did not alone enhance recall. Buschke (1984), using the selective reminding procedure (Buschke, 1973), showed that when mildly demented AD patients process the materials effectively during learning by means of tactile exploration of the TBR objects, they are also able to benefit from cues at retrieval.

As noted, Corkin (1982) failed to find beneficial effects of deep semantic orienting tasks compared with shallow orienting tasks in AD patients. A reason for this result might be that no support was given at the time of retrieval. Martin, Brouwers, Cox, and Fedio (1985) instructed mildly demented AD patients and normal older adults to provide a rhyme to the TBR object (shallow encoding), tell where the TBR object could be found (deep encoding), and pantomime a movement or a series of movements associated with its use (deep encoding). AD patients showed superior recall when selectively cued in the two semantic encoding conditions as compared with the shallow encoding condition. Although consistently recalling fewer words than the controls under all conditions, the AD patients produced a qualitatively similar pattern of recall as that exhibited by normal older subjects. The conclusion to be drawn from these studies is that substantial environmental support at both encoding and retrieval is imperative in order to achieve good memory performance in AD.

Materials × test interactions. Finally, it has been shown that mildly, moderately, and severely demented AD patients perform better on cued recall of SPTs than on cued recall of verbally presented sentences (Karlsson et al., 1989). Thus, AD patients appear to be able to utilize a multimodal and contextually rich encoding environment when receiving category cues at retrieval. Herlitz (1989) further investigated cue utilization in AD. Subjects were here presented with organizable words and objects under five different encoding conditions: nouns; objects; objects with a semantic orienting question; objects with self-generated motoric acts; and SPTs.

Results showed that normal older adults were able to utilize cues in all conditions. Mildly and moderately demented patients utilized cues in all conditions, except in the verbal condition, whereas severely demented patients were able to utilize cues only in the motoric condition. Thus, it seems that the ability to utilize category cues through a motoric encoding is preserved later in the disease than the ability to utilize cues through a semantic encoding. Note that neither a multimodal and rich input nor category cues at test were sufficient to enhance the level of recall in AD – both forms of contextual support were necessary. The result that a multimodal input does not boost free recall of AD patients was also reported by Dick et al. (1989). These data should be seen in contrast to the results from the groups of normal older adults in the Karlsson et al. (1989), Dick et al. (1989), and Herlitz (1989) studies, which showed an improvement of recall following either supportive encoding conditions or supportive retrieval conditions.

Concluding remarks

Reviewing the literature on memory processes in AD, it is apparent that the results differ from those on normal older adults. First, several memory processes that are extensively illuminated in normal older adults have not yet been examined in AD patients. Second, in those cases where data are available on AD patients, replications are sparse. With these provisos in mind, there is empirical evidence to suggest that there are differences between AD patients and normal older adults with regard to what factors promote good memory performance. Whereas normal older adults can utilize several different forms of contextual and cognitive support at encoding and retrieval, AD patients routinely fail to do so. Conceivably, the severe deficits in language functions, spatial abilities, and abstract thinking associated with AD put restrictions on these patients' cognitive reserve capacity. However, there are exceptions to this grim picture: When support is provided at both stages of remembering, AD patients do exhibit reliable increments in memory performance. In addition, there are some indications that AD patients can improve memory performance after being trained in using visual imagery mnemonics, when task pacing decreases, and when the organizational task structure increases.

The issue of ecological relevance

During recent years, several theorists (e.g., Baddeley, 1988; Kausler, 1983; Neisser, 1982) have argued that many of the most commonly used paradigms in memory research (e.g., recall or recognition of unrelated words or digits) are not very representative of the encoding and retrieval requirements of the natural environment. Consequently, pleas have been made both to study remembering in real-life settings and to employ more ecologically relevant tasks and materials. This position has been adopted by many investigators of cognitive aging, a key argument being that because standard psychometric tests and digit or word memory tasks are overrepresented in the laboratory, the typical finding of an age-related performance decline may not be a valid indicator of the overall cognitive readiness, adaptiveness, or everyday performance of older adults (e.g., Baltes & Willis, 1979; Berg & Sternberg, 1985; Labouvie-Vief, 1982, 1985). The extensive research on text recall in adulthood during recent years is an example of this awareness, in part motivated by the expectation that age-related performance differences would be small or absent in more ecologically relevant tasks.

Analyzing the studies reviewed in this chapter, it would seem that some have employed quite artificial types of materials (e.g., word lists, paired associates), whereas others have employed materials more representative of what adults may encounter in everyday life (e.g., action events, texts, television programs). Although the critique of standard laboratory memory tasks may be justified in many respects and the use of tasks that more closely approximate real-world remembering is welcomed, it appears that knowledge about whether the task or materials are ecologically relevant or not is of little help for predicting the level of performance among older adults and the presence or absence of age-related performance differences. For one thing, many efforts to develop measures of "practical cognition" or "practical problem solving" have not resulted in the expected elimination of age differences or even the attenuation of age differences (Denney, 1989; A. A. Hartley, 1989; Salthouse, 1982). In addition, the pattern of performance from traditional episodic memory tasks and ecologically more relevant tasks can be described in quite similar terms: When appropriate cognitive operations are supported or induced by the task or the materials at acquisition and/or test, age-related differences are reduced or eliminated. In contrast, in cases where appropriate operations are less driven by the environment and the individual must necessarily initiate and organize such operations, age-related differences favoring the young are present (Bäckman, 1985a, 1989b; Craik, 1983).

Utilization of compensatory task conditions versus self-initiated compensation

The bulk of demonstrations of good memory performance in old age described in this chapter may be viewed as cases of *utilization of compensa-*

tory task conditions (Bäckman, 1986, 1989b; Bäckman & Dixon, 1986, 1989; Rohwer, 1976). That is, the older individual utilizes contextual or cognitive support in various task situations in order to optimize memory performance. Although the area of aging and episodic remembering presents a large number of situations in which older adults evidence utilization of compensatory task conditions, this domain of inquiry reveals very few direct empirical demonstrations of *self-initiated compensatory efforts* undertaken by older adults. One possible reason for this bias may be that standard episodic memory tasks do not consequently entail (or invoke) the execution of self-initiated compensatory behaviors, because these types of tasks typically involve only a learning and a test phase. This somewhat restricted task situation may limit the repertoire of compensatory skills that may be available or required for successful performance.

However, in many other areas of research in which the concept of compensation has been extensively used (e.g., sensory handicaps, brain injury), the focus has been on self-initiated compensation rather than on utilization of compensatory task conditions (Bäckman, 1989b; Bäckman & Dixon, 1989). In those fields of research, compensation is usually inferred when a loss in one ability or component thereof is balanced by a concomitant growth in another (Salthouse, 1987). In fact, evidence for this form of compensation in older adults has been obtained in other domains of cognitive aging research, such as skilled performance in chess (Charness, 1981a, 1981b) and typing (Salthouse, 1984). In these studies, older adults' compensatory behavior is accomplished through a greater use of different forms of task-specific conceptually driven processes.

As noted, the evidence for self-initiated compensation is somewhat scanty in the area of memory and aging. However, some research on the use of memory aids in everyday life and a recent study on prospective memory serve as illustrative examples. Cavanaugh, Grady, and Perlmutter (1983) reported a greater use of internal (e.g., organization, rehearsal) as well as external (e.g., lists, calendars) memory aids in older compared with younger adults, whereas Dixon and Hultsch (1983) and Dixon and Bäckman (in press) found this to be true only for external aids. This pattern of results may reflect an attempt by older adults to compensate for objective or perceived memory difficulties. Sinnott (1986) found that younger and older adults remembered contextually meaningful information that was needed for future action (i.e., prospective TBR items) equally well (see also Poon & Schaffer, 1982). On the other hand, the young outperformed the old for less meaningful and incidental information. According to Sinnott (1986) the high performance of older adults for prospective memory items may reflect an adaptive compensatory mechanism; that is, as basic memory capacities decline, the older individual may invest more time and effort in remembering information that has obvious social links (e.g., visits, telephone calls). Thereby, the individual's commitment as a social being may be maintained, but possibly at the expense of further decline in some basic cognitive capacities (cf. Baltes, Dittmann-Kohli, & Dixon, 1984).

Summary

The present analysis of memory optimization in aging is guided by the belief that four major sources of variation must be considered to achieve the best understanding of the issue of interest: acquisition factors, test factors, materials, and subject-related factors (Jenkins, 1979). A summary of representative empirical studies illustrating successful memory performance among older adults in relation to these four factors is presented in Table 5.1.

Concerning acquisition factors, test factors, and materials, the empirical generalization is that memory performance of older adults is optimized across a wide variety of situations of remembering when their memory operations are supported by different forms of contextual or cognitive support at encoding and retrieval. Analogously, adult age–related differences in memory are reduced or eliminated when the environment guides the old learner in initiating appropriate operations of remembering compared with when no such guidance is provided. An implication of this pattern of outcome is that young adults are in lesser need of environmental support in order to remember successfully in the bulk of experimental situations requiring conscious recollection of previously acquired information.

However, there are two qualifications attendant on these generalizations. First, there are, indeed, differences between groups of older adults in terms of the need of environmental support to achieve good memory performance and the ability to utilize support to improve memory. These differences may be described in a quite simple way: When the memory capabilities of the old adult are low due to, for example, a low level of education and verbal skill (e.g., Craik et al., 1987; Dixon et al., 1984), very old age (e.g., Bäckman & Karlsson, 1986; Nilsson et al., 1987), or, in the extreme case, dementia (e.g., R. G. Morris & Kopelman, 1986; Poon, 1986), there is an increase in the amount and quality of environmental support needed to maximize memory performance; in addition, some forms of guidance that can be utilized by, for example, high-verbal young–old adults may be of little use when memory functions are severely compromised. Hence, it may be concluded that there are significant differences in cognitive reserve capacity among older adults at different

Table 5.1. *Factors that promote successful memory performance in normal aging and Alzheimer's disease*

Type of factor	Source	
	Normal aging	Alzheimer's disease
External		
Acquisition		
Organizational instructions	Hultsch, 1969, 1971	(−) Diesfeldt, 1984
Imagery instructions	Canestrari, 1968; Treat, Poon, & Fozard, 1981	
Verbal mediators	Hulicka & Grossman, 1967; Hulicka, Sterns, & Grossman, 1967	
Increased study time	Arenberg, 1965; Kinsbourne & Berryhill, 1972	(+) Corkin et al., 1984
Increased number of study trials	Crew, 1977; R. L. Cohen, Sandler, & Schroeder, 1987	(+) Moffat, 1989; (−) Strauss, Weingartner, & Thompson, 1985
Self-generation activity	Mitchell, Hunt, & Schmitt 1986	
Problem-solving activity	Kausler & Hakami, 1983a; Bäckman & Karlsson, 1987	(−) Mitchell, Hunt, & Schmitt, 1986
Test		
Copy cues	Schonfield & Robertson, 1966; Craik & McDowd, 1987	(−) Miller, 1975, 1978; (−) Wilson, Kaszniak, Bacon, Fox, & Kelly, 1982
Category cues	Laurence, 1967; Hultsch, 1975	(−) Davis & Mumford, 1984; (−) Diesfeldt, 1984
Partial cues	R. G. Morris, Wheatley, & Britton, 1983; Davis & Mumford, 1984	(+) Miller, 1975; (+) R. G. Morris, Wheatley, & Britton, 1983; (−) Shimamura, Salmon, Squire, & Butters, 1987; (−) Salmon, Shimamura, Butters, & S. Smith, 1988

Table 5.1. *(cont.)*

	Source	
Type of factor	Normal aging	Alzheimer's disease
Acquisition × Test		
Semantic cues at learning and test	A. D. Smith, 1977; Ceci & Tabor, 1981	(+) Diesfeldt, 1984
Orienting tasks and retrieval support	Mason, 1979; Erber, Herman, & Botwinick, 1980	(+) Buschke, 1984; (+) Martin, Brouwers, Cox, & Fedio, 1985
Self-generated retrieval cues	Bäckman, Mäntylä, & Erngrund, 1984; Bäckman & Mäntylä, 1988	
Distinctive retrieval cues	Mäntylä & Bäckman, 1989	
Materials		
Word familiarity	Wilson, Bacon, Kramer, Fox, & Kaszniak, 1983	(−) Wilson et al., 1983
Inherent verbal organization	Byrd, 1981; S. W. Smith, Rebok, W. R. Smith, Hall, & Alwin, 1983	(−) Weingartner et al., 1982; (+) Nebes, Martin, & Horn, 1984
Inherent spatial organization	Waddell & Rogoff, 1981, 1987	
Richness of features	Cavanaugh, 1983, 1984; Rissenberg & Glanzer, 1986	(−) Butters et al., 1983; (−) Rissenberg & Glanzer, 1986
Multimodality	Bäckman & Nilsson, 1984, 1985; Dick, Kean, & Sands, 1989	(−) Karlsson et al., 1989; (−) Dick et al., 1989; (−) Herlitz, 1989
Visual distinctiveness	Sharps & Gollin, 1987, 1988	
Materials × Test		
Multimodality and category cues	Karlsson et al., 1989; Herlitz, 1989	(+) Karlsson et al., 1989; (+) Herlitz, 1989
Internal		
Preexperimental Knowledge		
Task-specific knowledge	Barrett & Wright, 1981; Hultsch & Dixon, 1983	(−) Bäckman & Herlitz, in press
Verbal ability	Meyer & Rice, 1981; Dixon, Hultsch, Simon, & von Eye, 1984	

Memory-Related Skills

Organization
Sanders, Murphy, Schmitt, & Walsh, 1980; Schmitt, Murphy, & Sanders, 1981

Imagery
Treat, Poon, & Fozard, 1981; Yesavage, 1983
(+) S. H. Zarit, J. M. Zarit, & Reever, 1982; (+) Hill, Evankovich, Sheikh, & Yesavage, 1987

Method of loci
Robertson-Tchabo, Hausman, & Arenberg, 1976; Rose & Yesavage, 1983

Semantic associations + interactive imagery
Yesavage, Rose, & Bower, 1983

Categorization + association + imagery
S. H. Zarit, Cole, & Guider, 1981

Attention + concentration + organization
(−) Beck et al., 1985

Attention + relaxation
Yesavage & Rose, 1983

Imagery + relaxation
Yesavage, 1984

Categorization + attention + relaxation
Lundqvist, Thors, Bäckman, Karlsson, & Nilsson, 1988; Stigsdotter & Bäckman, 1989a, 1989b

Working memory + general knowledge + the method of loci
Kliegl, J. Smith, & Baltes, 1986; Kliegl & Baltes, 1987

Note: For normal older adults all factors listed promote successful memory performance. For AD patients positive outcomes are denoted by a (+), negative outcomes are denoted by a (−), and those factors for which no data are available are left unmarked.

levels of verbal skill, between young–old and old–old adults, and between healthy older adults and patients suffering from dementia diseases. Second, there are cases in which young adults benefit more than the old when the encoding process is guided by orienting tasks, instructions, and so forth (see Craik, 1977; Salthouse, 1982, for reviews). This outcome may reflect the fact that the young are faster than the old in making use of their cognitive reserve capacity (Craik et al., 1987; Kliegl & Baltes, 1987).

A number of subject-related variables ranging from personality traits to task-specific memory skills have been found to be related to goodness of remembering in old age. Of particular interest in this chapter were preexperimental knowledge and abilities and experimentally induced (or activated) memory skills. As to the former category, a high level of verbal skill as well as pertinent prior knowledge related to the content of the TBR information has been found to be of great importance for older adults' success in recalling and recognizing information. Interestingly, the ability to utilize premorbid skills to improve memory appears to be intact in very old age (Bäckman et al., 1987). This result runs counter to the pattern of data described earlier concerning the ability to utilize environmental support in different groups of older adults. This discrepancy may be resolved by recognizing that older adults with low memory capabilities are especially penalized in memory tasks requiring deliberate cognitive operations, as opposed to tasks tapping more automatic or automatized operations (Hasher & Zacks, 1979). A major difference between utilization of, for example, organizational or imagery instructions, on the one hand, and preexperimental knowledge, on the other, is that of demands of deliberate processing: In order to utilize the provision of experimenter-provided instructions, the subject has to deliberately impose strategies on the TBR information. In contrast, when presented with information for which adequate preexperimental knowledge exists, the activation of the subject's knowledge base is likely to be more automatic (van Dijk & Kintsch, 1983).

Research employing unifactorial as well as composite memory-training programs has overall demonstrated large performance gains in older adults following intervention. However, when age comparisons are available, it is clear that the old do not benefit more than the young from training; performance gains tend to be proportional or greater for young than for older adults (e.g., Kliegl & Baltes, 1987; Roberts, 1983; Yesavage et al., 1989). Comparing this pattern of results with that of single-assessment experimental studies on memory and aging, we arrived at the conclusion that the relationship between the age of the learner and the extent to which performance increases as a function of support (ranging from pretask encoding suggestions to extensive training) is rather complex. The young may be quicker in utilizing some forms of support and in achieving an optimal encoding of the TBR information. Because the elderly do not seem to achieve optimal encoding as quickly, they are likely to show positive effects from support longer than the young. That is, baseline reserve capacity is substantial in both age-groups, but there are age-related differences in the way it is utilized. The parallel gains from training in young and older adults observed in some studies would seem to indicate age equivalence with respect to developmental reserve capacity. However, after extensive training and when memory performance is assessed under difficult conditions, the young typically exhibit larger performance gains from training than the old, suggesting a greater developmental reserve capacity in early than in late adulthood (see e.g., Baltes, 1987). In this context, it is important to keep in mind those methodological problems associated with the evaluation of performance gains when age-groups differ in baseline performance, as well as those associated with the procedures aimed at overcoming the problems of unequal baselines.

Finally, we discussed two general issues related to cognitive aging: the representativeness of research paradigms used and the relation between utilization of compensatory task conditions and self-initiated compensatory behaviors. With respect to the former issue, we argue that knowledge concerning whether the memory task is ecologically relevant or not is of little help in predicting the level of memory performance of older adults (and the presence or absence of age-related performance differences). Further, our analysis of the literature indicated that although self-initiated compensatory behaviors may be seen in many groups of individuals affected by various kinds of cognitive deficits, such behaviors are rare in the literature on memory and aging. In contrast, this literature is heavily populated with demonstrations of older adults' utilization of compensatory task conditions. Possibly, this state of affairs reflects the fact that standard episodic memory tasks, due to the somewhat restricted task situations, do not easily invoke the utilization of self-initiated compensatory skills.

NOTE

Preparation of this chapter was supported by grants from the Bank of Sweden Tercentenary Foundation (No. 85/69) and the Commission for Social Research, Swedish Ministry of Health and Social Affairs (No. F85/2023 and No. G 88/20), awarded to the first author and by a predoctoral fellowship from the University of Umeå to the third author.

We are grateful to Alan D. Baddeley, Fergus I. M. Craik, David F. Hultsch, Donald H. Kausler, and three anonymous reviewers for providing constructive comments on an earlier version.

REFERENCES

Adamowicz, J. L. (1976). Visual short term memory and aging. *Journal of Gerontology, 31,* 39–46.

Adams, L. T., Kasserman, J. E., Yearwood, A. A., Perfetto, G. A., Bransford, J. D., & Franks, J. J. (1988). Memory access: The effects of fact-oriented versus problem-oriented acquisition. *Memory & Cognition, 16,* 167–175.

Arbuckle, T. Y., Gold, D., & Andres, D. (1986). Cognitive functioning of older people in relation to social and personality variables. *Psychology and Aging, 1,* 55–62.

Arenberg, D. (1965). Anticipation interval and age differences in verbal learning. *Journal of Abnormal Psychology, 70,* 419–425.

Arenberg, D. (1967). Age differences in retroaction. *Journal of Gerontology, 22,* 88–91.

Arenberg, D. (1968). Input modality in short-term retention of old and young adults. *Journal of Gerontology, 23,* 462–465.

Bäckman, L. (1985a). Compensation and recoding: A framework for aging and memory research. *Scandinavian Journal of Psychology, 26,* 193–207.

Bäckman, L. (1985b). Further evidence for the lack of adult age differences on free recall of subject-performed task: The importance of motor action. *Human Learning, 4,* 79–87.

Bäckman, L. (1986). Adult age differences in cross-modal recoding and mental tempo, and older adults' utilization of compensatory task conditions. *Experimental Aging Research, 12,* 135–140.

Bäckman, L. (1989a). Effects of pre-experimental knowledge on recognition memory in adulthood. In A. F. Bennett & K. M. McConkey (Eds.), *Cognition in individual and social contexts* (pp. 267–281). Amsterdam: Elsevier.

Bäckman, L. (1989b). Varieties of memory compensation by older adults in episodic remembering. In L. W. Poon, D. C. Rubin, & B. A. Wilson (Eds.), *Everyday cognition in adulthood and late life* (pp. 509–544). New York: Cambridge University Press.

Bäckman, L. (in press). Recognition memory across the adult life span: The role of prior knowledge. *Memory & Cognition.*

Bäckman, L., & Dixon, R. A. (1986, September). Compensation and adaptive cognitive functioning in adulthood. In M. M. Baltes & D. L. Featherman (Chairs), *Optimal living for aging.* Symposium conducted at the Second European Conference on Developmental Psychology, Rome, Italy.

Bäckman, L., & Dixon, R. A. (1989). *Compensation.* Manuscript submitted for publication.

Bäckman, L., & Herlitz, A. (in press). The relationship between prior knowledge and face recognition memory in normal aging and Alzheimer's disease. *Journal of Gerontology: Psychological Sciences.*

Bäckman, L., Herlitz, A., & Karlsson, T. (1987). Pre-experimental knowledge facilitates episodic recall in young, young–old, and old–old adults. *Experimental Aging Research, 13,* 89–91.

Bäckman, L., & Karlsson, T. (1986). Episodic remembering in young adults, 73-year-olds, and 82-year-olds. *Scandinavian Journal of Psychology, 27,* 320–325.

Bäckman, L., & Karlsson, T. (1987). Effects of word fragment completion on free recall: A selective improvement of older adults. *Comprehensive Gerontology, 1,* 4–7.

Bäckman, L., & Mäntylä, T. (1988). Effectiveness of self-generated cues in younger and older adults: The role of retention interval. *Internal Journal of Aging and Human Development, 26,* 241–248.

Bäckman, L., & Mäntylä, T., & Erngrund, K. (1984). Optimal recall in early and late adulthood. *Scandinavian Journal of Psychology, 25,* 306–314.

Bäckman, L., & Molander, B. (1986). Effects of adult age and level of skill on the ability to cope with high-stress conditions in a precision sport. *Psychology and Aging, 1,* 334–336.

Bäckman, L., & Nilsson, L.-G. (1984). Aging effects in free recall: An exception to the rule. *Human Learning, 3,* 53–69.

Bäckman, L., & Nilsson, L.-G. (1985). Prerequisites for lack of age differences in memory performance. *Experimental Aging Research, 11,* 67–73.

Baddeley, A. D. (1988). But what the hell is it for? In M. M. Gruneberg, P. E. Morris, & R. N. Sykes (Eds.), *Practical aspects of memory: Current research and issues* (Vol. 1, pp. 3–18). Chichester: Wiley.

Baltes, P. B. (1987). Theoretical propositions of life-span developmental psychology: On the dynamics between growth and decline. *Developmental Psychology, 23,* 611–623.

Baltes, P. B., Dittmann-Kohli, F., & Dixon, R. A. (1984). New perspectives on the development of intelligence in adulthood: Toward a dual-process conception and a model of selective optimization with compensation. In P. B. Baltes & O. G. Brim, Jr. (Eds.), *Life-span development and behavior* (Vol. 6, pp. 33–76). New York: Academic Press.

Baltes, P. B., Kliegl, R., & Dittmann-Kohli, F. (1988). On the locus of training gains in research on the plasticity of fluid intelligence in old age. *Journal of Educational Psychology, 80,* 392–400.

Baltes, P. B., Reese, H. W., & Nesselroade, J. R. (1977). *Life-span developmental psychology: Introduction to research methods.* Belmont, CA: Wadsworth.

Baltes, P. B., & Willis, S. L. (1979). The critical importance of appropriate methodology in the study of aging: The sample case of psychometric intelligence. In F. Hoffmeister & C. Muller (Eds.), *Brain function in old age* (pp. 164–187). Heidelberg: Springer-Verlag.

Barrett, T. R., & Wright, M. (1981). Age-related facilitation in recall following semantic processing. *Journal of Gerontology, 36,* 194–199.

Beatty, W. W., Salmon, D. P., Butters, N., Heindel, W. C., & Granholm, E. L. (1988). Retrograde amnesia in patients with Alzheimer's disease or Huntington's disease. *Neurobiology of Aging, 9,* 181–186.

Beck, C. K., Heacock, P., Thatcher, R., Mercer, S. O., Sparkman, C., & Roberts, M. A. (1985, July). *Cognitive skills remediation with Alzheimer's patients.* Paper presented at the 13th International Congress of Gerontology, New York, NY.

Belmont, J. M., Freeseman, L. J., & Mitchell, D. W. (1988). Memory as problem solving: The cases of young and elderly adults. In M. M. Gruneberg, P. E.

Morris, & R. N. Sykes (Eds.), *Practical aspects of memory: Current research and issues* (Vol. 2, pp. 84–89). Chichester: Wiley.

Berg, C. A., & Sternberg, R. J. (1985). A triarchic theory of intellectual development during adulthood. *Developmental Review, 5,* 334–370.

Bransford, J. D. (1979). *Human cognition: Learning, understanding, and remembering.* Belmont, CA: Wadsworth.

Bransford, J. D., McCarrell, N. S., Franks, J. J., & Nitsch, K. E. (1977). Towards unexplaining memory. In R. Shaw & J. D. Bransford (Eds.), *Perceiving, acting, and knowing* (pp. 431–466). Hillsdale, NJ: Lawrence Erlbaum.

Buschke, H. (1973). Selective reminding for analysis of memory and learning. *Journal of Verbal Learning and Verbal Behavior, 12,* 543–550.

Buschke, H. (1984). Cued recall in amnesia. *Journal of Clinical Neuropsychology, 6,* 433–440.

Butters, N., Albert, M. S., Sax, D. S., Militios, P., Nagode, J., & Sterste, A. (1983). The effect of verbal mediators on the picture memory of brain-damaged patients. *Neuropsychologia, 21,* 307–323.

Byrd, M. (1981). *Age differences in memory for prose passages.* Unpublished doctoral dissertation, University of Toronto, Toronto.

Canestrari, R. E. (1968). Age changes in acquisition. In G. Talland (Ed.), *Human aging and behavior* (pp. 169–187). New York: Academic Press.

Cavanaugh, J. C. (1983). Comprehension and retention of television programs by 20- and 60-year-olds. *Journal of Gerontology, 38,* 190–196.

Cavanaugh, J. C. (1984). Effects of presentation format on adults' retention of television programs. *Experimental Aging Research, 10,* 51–53.

Cavanaugh, J. C., Grady, J. G., & Perlmutter, M. (1983). Forgetting and use of memory aids in 20-and 70-year-olds' everyday life. *International Journal of Aging and Human Development, 17,* 113–122.

Ceci, S. J., & Tabor, L. (1981). Flexibility and memory: Are the elderly really less flexible? *Experimental Aging Research, 7,* 147–158.

Charness, N. (1981a). Aging and skilled problem solving. *Journal of Experimental Psychology: General, 110,* 21–38.

Charness, N. (1981b). Search in chess: Age and skill differences. *Journal of Experimental Psychology: Human Perception and Performance, 7,* 467–476.

Charness, N. (1981c). Visual short-term memory and aging in chess players. *Journal of Gerontology, 36,* 615–619.

Cohen, G., & Faulkner, D. (1989). The effects of aging on perceived and generated memories. In L. W. Poon, D. C. Rubin, & B. A. Wilson (Eds.), *Everyday cognition in adulthood and late life* (pp. 222–243). New York: Cambridge University Press.

Cohen, R. L. (1981). On the generality of some memory laws. *Scandinavian Journal of Psychology, 22,* 267–282.

Cohen, R. L. (1985). On the generality of the laws of memory. In L.-G. Nilsson & T. Archer (Eds.), *Perspectives on learning and memory* (pp. 247–277). Hillsdale, NJ: Lawrence Erlbaum.

Cohen, R. L., Sandler, S. P., & Schroeder, K. (1987). Aging and memory for words and action events: Effects of item repetition and list length. *Psychology and Aging, 2,* 280–285.

Corkin, S. (1982). Some relationships between global amnesias and the memory impairments in Alzheimer's disease. In S. Corkin, K. L. Davies, J. H.

Growdon, E. Usdin, & R. J. Wurtman (Eds.), *Alzheimer's disease: A report of progress* (*Aging*, Vol. 19, pp. 149–164). New York: Raven Press.

Corkin, S., Growdon, J. H., Nissen, M. J., Huff, F. J., Freed, D. M., & Sagar, H. J. (1984). Recent advances in the neuropsychological study of Alzheimer's disease. In R. J. Wurtman, S. Corkin, & J. H. Growdon (Eds.), *Alzheimer's disease: Advances in basic research and therapies. Proceedings of the third meeting of the International Study Group: On the treatment of memory disorders associated with aging* (pp. 75–93). Cambridge, MA: Center for Brain Sciences and Metabolism Trust.

Craik, F. I. M. (1977). Age differences in human memory. In J. E. Birren & K. W. Schaie (Eds.), *Handbook of the psychology of aging* (pp. 384–420). New York: Van Nostrand Reinhold.

Craik, F. I. M. (1983). On the transfer of information from temporary to permanent memory. *Philosophical Transactions of the Royal Society of London, 302*, 341–359.

Craik, F. I. M. (1985). Paradigms in human memory research. In L.-G. Nilsson & T. Archer (Eds.), *Perspectives on learning and memory* (pp. 247–277). Hillsdale, NJ: Lawrence Erlbaum.

Craik, F. I. M., Byrd, M., & Swanson, J. M. (1987). Patterns of memory loss in three elderly samples. *Psychology and Aging, 2*, 79–86.

Craik, F. I. M., & Lockhart, R. S. (1972). Levels of processing: A framework of memory research. *Journal of Verbal Learning and Verbal Behavior, 11*, 671–684.

Craik, F. I. M., & McDowd, J. M. (1987). Age differences in recall and recognition. *Jounnal of Experimental Psychology: Learning, Memory, and Cognition, 13*, 474–479.

Craik, F. I. M. & Rabinowitz, J. C. (1984). Age differences in the acquisition and use of verbal information. In H. Bouma & D. G. Bouwhuis (Eds.), *Attention and performance* (Vol. 10, pp. 471–500). London: Lawrence Erlbaum.

Craik, F. I. M., & Rabinowitz, J. C. (1985). The effects of presentation rate and encoding task on age-related memory deficits. *Journal of Gerontology, 40*, 309–315.

Crew, F. F. (1977). *Age differences in retention after varying study and test trials.* Unpublished master's thesis, Georgia Institute of Technology, Atlanta, GA.

Davis, P. E., & Mumford, S. J. (1984). Cued recall and the nature of the memory disorder in dementia. *British Journal of Psychiatry, 144*, 383–386.

Denney, N. W. (1989). Everyday problem solving: Methodological issues, research findings, and a model. In L. W. Poon, D. C. Rubin, & B. A. Wilson (Eds.), *Everyday cognition in adulthood and late life* (pp. 330–351). New York: Cambridge University Press.

Dick, M. B., Kean, M.-L., & Sands, D. (1989). Memory for action events in Alzheimer-type dementia: Further evidence for an encoding failure. *Brain and Cognition, 9*, 71–87.

Diesfeldt, H. F. A. (1984). The importance of encoding instructions and retrieval cues in the assessment of memory in senile dementia. *Archives of Gerontology and Geriatrics, 3*, 51–57.

Dixon, R. A., & Bäckman, L. (1986, August). The functional role of compensation in life-span cognitive development. In S. G. Paris & R. A. Dixon (Chairs), *Contextualism and life-span cognitive development.* Symposium conducted at the American Psychological Association. Washington, DC.

Dixon, R. A., & Bäckman, L. (in press). Reading and memory for prose in adulthood. In S. R. Yussen & M. C. Smith (Eds.), *Reading across the life span*. New York: Springer.

Dixon, R. A., & Hultsch, D. F. (1983). Structure and development of meta-memory in adulthood. *Journal of Gerontology, 38*, 682–688.

Dixon, R. A., Hultsch, D. F., Simon, E. W., & von Eye, A. (1984). Verbal ability and text structure effects on adult age differences in text recall. *Journal of Verbal Learning and Verbal Behavior, 23*, 569–578.

Elias, M. F., & Elias, P. K. (1977). Motivation and activity. In J. E. Birren & K. W. Schaie (Eds.), *Handbook of the psychology of aging* (pp. 357–383). New York: Van Nostrand Reinhold.

Erber, J. T. (1974). Age differences in recognition memory. *Journal of Gerontology, 29*, 177–181.

Erber, J. T. (1976). Age differences in learning and memory on a digit-symbol substitution task. *Experimental Aging Research, 2*, 45–53.

Erber, J. T., Galt, D., & Botwinick, J. (1985). Age differences in the effects of contextual framework and word-familiarity on episodic memory. *Experimental Aging Research, 11*, 101–103.

Erber, J. T., Herman, T. G., & Botwinick, J. (1980). Age differences in memory as a function of depth of processing. *Experimental Aging Research, 6*, 341–348.

Eysenck, M. W. (1974). Age differences in incidental learning. *Developmental Psychology, 10*, 936–941.

Folstein, M. F., Folstein, S. E., & McHugh, P. R. (1975). "Mini–Mental State": A practical method for grading the cognitive state of patients for the clinician. *Journal of Psychiatric Reserarch, 12*, 189–198.

Gribbon, K., Schaie, K. W., & Parham, I. A. (1980). Complexity of life style and maintenance of intellectual abilities. *Journal of Social Issues, 36*, 47–61.

Guttentag, R. E., & Hunt, R. R. (1988). Adult age differences in memory for imagined and performed actions. *Journal of Gerontology: Psychological Sciences, 43*, 107–108.

Hanley-Dunn, P., & McIntosh, J. L. (1984). Meaningfulness and recall of names by young and old adults. *Journal of Gerontology, 39*, 583–585.

Harker, J. O., Hartley, J. T., & Walsh, D. A. (1982). Understanding discourse – a life span approach. In B. A. Huston (Ed.), *Advances in reading/language research* (Vol. 1, pp. 155–202). Greenwich, CT: JAI Press.

Hartley, A. A. (1989). The cognitive ecology of problem solving. In L. W. Poon, D. C. Rubin, & B. A. Wilson (Eds.), *Everyday cognition in adulthood and late life* (pp. 300–329). New York: Cambridge University Press.

Hartley, J. T. (1986). Reader and text variables as determinants of discourse memory in adulthood. *Psychology and Aging, 1*, 150–158.

Hasher, L., & Zacks, R. T. (1979). Automatic and effortful processes in memory. *Journal of Experimental Psychology: General, 108*, 356–388.

Hellebusch, S. J. (1976). *On improving learning and memory in the aged: The effects of mnemonics on strategy, transfer, and generalization*. Unpublished doctoral dissertation, University of Notre Dame, Notre Dame, IN.

Herlitz, A. (1989). Cue utilization in Alzheimer's disease. In A. F. Bennett & K. M. McConkey (Eds), *Cognition in individual and social contexts* (pp. 569–576). Amsterdam: Elsevier.

Heron, A., & Craik, F.I.M. (1964). Age differences in cumulative learning of meaningful and meaningless material. *Scandinavian Journal of Psychology, 5,* 209–217.

Hill, R. D., Evankovich, K. D., Sheikh, J. I., & Yesavage, J. A. (1987). Imagery mnemonic training in a patient with primary degenerative dementia. *Psychology and Aging, 2,* 204–205.

Howell, S. C. (1972). Familiarity and complexity in perceptual recognition. *Journal of Gerontology, 27,* 364–371.

Hulicka, I. M., & Grossman, J. L. (1967). Age group comparisons for the use of mediators in paired-associate learning. *Journal of Gerontology, 22,* 46–51.

Hulicka, I. M., Sterns, H., & Grossman, J. L. (1967). Age group comparisons of paired-associate learning. *Journal of Gerontology, 22,* 274–280.

Hultsch, D. F. (1969). Adult age differences in the organization of free recall. *Developmental Psychology, 1,* 673–678.

Hultsch, D. F. (1971). Adult age differences in free classification and free recall. *Developmental Psychology, 4,* 338–342.

Hultsch, D. F. (1974). Learning to learn in adulthood. *Journal of Gerontology, 29,* 302–308.

Hultsch, D. F. (1975). Adult age differences in retrieval: Trace-dependent and cue-dependent forgetting. *Developmental Psychology, 11,* 197–201.

Hultsch, D. F., & Dixon, R. A. (1983). The role of pre-experimental knowledge in text processing in adulthood. *Experimental Aging Research, 9,* 17–22.

Hultsch, D. F., & Dixon, R. A. (1984). Text processing in adulthood. In P. B. Baltes & O. G. Brim, Jr. (Eds.), *Life span development and behavior* (Vol. 6, pp. 77–108). New York: Academic Press.

Jenkins, J. J. (1979). Four points to remember: A tetrahedral model of memory experiments. In L. S. Cermak & F.I.M. Craik (Eds.), *Levels of processing in human memory* (pp. 429–446). Hillsdale, NJ: Lawrence Erlbaum.

Karlsson, T., Bäckman, L., Herlitz, A., Nilsson, L.-G., Winblad, B., & Österlind, P.-O. (1989). Memory improvement at different stages of Alzheimer's disease. *Neuropsychologia, 27,* 737–742.

Kaszniak, A. W., Wilson, R. S., & Fox, J. H. (1981). Effects of imagery and meaningfulness on free recall and recognition memory in presenile and senile dementia. *International Journal of Neuroscience, 12,* 264.

Kausler, D. H. (1970). Retention-forgetting as a nomological network for developmental research. In L. R. Goulet & P. B. Baltes (Eds.) *Life-span developmental psychology* (pp. 305–353). New York: Academic Press.

Kausler, D. H. (1982). *Experimental psychology and human aging.* New York: Wiley.

Kausler, D. H. (1983). *Episodic memory and human aging.* Paper presented at the 91st Annual Meeting of the American Psychological Association, Anaheim, CA.

Kausler, D. H., & Hakami, M. K. (1983a). Memory for activities: Adult age differences and intentionality. *Developmental Psychology, 19,* 889–894.

Kausler, D. H., & Hakami, M. K. (1983b). Memory for topics of conversation: Adult age differences and intentionality. *Experimental Aging Research, 9,* 153–158.

Kinsbourne, M. (1980). Attentional dysfunctions and the elderly: Theoretical models and research perspectives. In L. W. Poon, J. L. Fozard, L. S. Cermak, D. Arenberg, & L. W. Thompson (Eds.), *New directions in memory and aging* (pp. 113–129). Hillsdale, NJ: Lawrence Erlbaum.

Kinsbourne, M., & Berryhill, J. L. (1972). The nature of the interaction between pacing and the age decrement in learning. *Journal of Gerontology, 27,* 471–477.

Kliegl, R., & Baltes, P. B. (1987). Theory-guided analysis of development and aging mechanisms through testing-the-limits and research on expertise. In C. Schooler & K. W. Schaie (Eds.), *Cognitive functioning and social structure over the life course* (pp. 95–119). New York: Ablex.

Kliegl, R., Smith, J., & Baltes, P. B. (1986). Testing-the-limits, expertise, and memory in adulthood and old age. In F. Klix & H. Hagendorf (Eds.), *Human memory and cognitive capabilities: Mechanics and performances* (pp. 395–407). Amsterdam: North-Holland.

Labouvie-Vief, G. (1976). Towards optimizing cognitive competence in later life. *Educational Gerontology, 1,* 75–92.

Labouvie-Vief, G. (1977). Adult cognitive development: In search of alternative interpretations. *Merrill-Palmer Quarterly, 23,* 227–263.

Labouvie-Vief, G. (1982). Dynamic development and mature autonomy: A theoretical prologue. *Human Development, 25,* 161–191.

Labouvie-Vief, G. (1985). Intelligence and cognition. In J. E. Birren & K. W. Schaie (Eds.), *Handbook of the psychology of aging* (pp. 500–530). New York: Van Nostrand Reinhold.

Labouvie-Vief, G., & Gonda, J. N. (1976). Cognitive strategy training and intellectual performance in the elderly. *Journal of Gerontology, 31,* 327–332.

Laurence, M. W. (1967). Memory loss with age: A test of two strategies for its retardation. *Psychonomic Science, 9,* 209–210.

Lichty, W., Kausler, D. H., & Martinez, D. (1986). Adult age differences in memory for motor versus cognitive activities. *Experimental Aging Research, 12,* 227–230.

Loftus, G. R. (1978). On the interpretation of interactions. *Memory & Cognition, 6,* 312–319.

Lundqvist, A., Thors, A., Bäckman, L., Karlsson, T., & Nilsson, L. -G. (1988). Maintenance of acquired memory skill in older adults. In C. Perris & M. Eisemann (Eds.), *Cognitive psychotherapy: An update* (pp. 95–99). Umeå: DOPUU Press.

Luria, A. R. (1968). *The mind of a mnemonist* (L. Solotaroff, Trans.). New York: Avon Books. (Original work published 1965)

Mäntylä, T. (1986). Optimizing cue effectiveness: Recall of 500 and 600 incidentally learned words. *Journal of Experimental Psychology: Learning, Memory, and Cognition, 12,* 66–71.

Mäntylä, T., & Bäckman, L. (1989). *Cue distinctiveness and age-related retrieval failures.* Manuscript submitted for publication.

Mäntylä, T., & Nilsson, L.-G. (1988). Cue distinctiveness and forgetting: Effectiveness of self-generated retrieval cues in delayed recall. *Journal of Experimental Psychology: Learning, Memory, and Cognition, 14,* 502–509.

Martin, A. (1987). Representation of semantic and spatial knowlege in Alzheimer's patients: Implications for models of preserved learning in amnesia. *Journal of Clinical and Experimental Neuropsychology, 9,* 191–224.

Martin, A., Brouwers, P., Cox, C., & Fedio, P. (1985). On the nature of the verbal memory deficit in Alzheimer's disease. *Brain and Language, 25,* 323–341.

Mason, S. E. (1979). Effects of orienting tasks on the recall and recognition performance of subjects differing in age. *Developmental Psychology, 15,* 467–469.

McCarty, D. L. (1980). Investigation of a visual imagery mnemonic device for acquiring face–name associations. *Journal of Experimental Psychology: Human Learning and Memory, 6,* 145–155.

Meyer, B. J. F., & Rice, G. E. (1981). Information recalled from prose by young, middle, and old adult readers. *Experimental Aging Research, 7*, 253–268.

Meyer, B. J. F., & Rice, G. E. (1983). Learning and memory for text across the adult life span. In J. Fine & R. O. Freedle (Eds.), *Developmental studies in discourse* (pp. 291–306). Norwood, NJ: Ablex.

Miller, E. (1975). Impaired recall and the memory disturbance in presenile dementia. *British Journal of Social and Clinical Psychology, 14*, 73–79.

Miller, E. (1978). Retrieval from long-term memory in presenile dementia: Two tests of an hypothesis. *British Journal of Social and Clinical Psychology, 17*, 143–148.

Mitchell, D. B., Hunt, R., & Schmitt, F. A. (1986). The generation effect and reality monitoring: Evidence from dementia and normal aging. *Journal of Gerontology, 41*, 79–94.

Moffat, N. J. (1989). Home based cognitive rehabilitation with the elderly. In L. W. Poon, D. C. Rubin, & B. A. Wilson (Eds.), *Everyday cognition in adulthood and late life* (pp. 659–680). New York: Cambridge University Press.

Monge, R. H. (1969). Learning in the adult years: Set or rigidity. *Human Development, 12*, 131–140.

Monge, R. H., & Hultsch, D. F. (1971). Paired-associate learning as a function of adult age and the length of the anticipation and inspection intervals. *Journal of Gerontology, 26*, 157–162.

Morris, C. D., Bransford, J. D., & Franks, J. J. (1977). Levels of processing versus transfer appropriate processing. *Journal of Verbal Learning and Verbal Behavior, 16*, 519–533.

Morris, R. G., & Kopelman, M. D. (1986). The memory deficits in Alzheimer-type dementia: A review. *Quarterly Journal of Experimental Psychology, 38A*, 575–602.

Morris, R. G., Wheatley, J., & Britton, P. (1983). Retrieval from long-term memory in senile dementia: Cued recall revisited. *British Journal of Clinical Psychology, 22*, 141–142.

Nebes, R. D., Martin, D. C., & Horn, L. C. (1984). Sparing of semantic memory in Alzheimer's disease. *Journal of Abnormal Psychology, 93*, 321–330.

Neisser, U. (1982). Memory: What are the important questions? In U. Neisser (Ed.), *Memory observed: Remembering in natural contexts* (pp. 3–19). San Francisco: Freeman.

Nilsson, L.-G. (1984). New functionalism in memory research. In K. Lagerspetz & P. Niemi (Eds.), *Psychology in the 1990's* (pp. 185–224). Amsterdam: North-Holland.

Nilsson, L.-G., Bäckman, L., Herlitz, A., Karlsson, T., Österlind, P.-O., & Winblad, B. (1987). Patterns of memory performance in young–old and old–old adults: A selective review. *Comprehensive Gerontology, 1*, 49–53.

Poon, L. W. (1985). Differences in human memory with aging: Nature, causes, and clinical implications. In J. E. Birren & K. W. Schaie (Eds.), *Handbook of the psychology of aging* (pp. 427–462). New York: Van Nostrand Reinhold.

Poon, L. W. (Ed.). (1986). *Handbook for clinical memory assessment of older adults.* Washington, DC: American Psychological Association.

Poon, L. W., & Fozard, J. L. (1978). Speed of retrieval from long-term memory in relation to age, familiarity, and datedness of information. *Journal of Gerontology, 33*, 711–717.

Poon, L. W., & Schaffer, G. (1982). *Prospective memory in young and elderly adults.*

Paper presented at the 90th Annual Meeting of the American Psychological Association, Washington, DC.

Poon, L. W., Walsh-Sweeney, L., & Fozard, J. L. (1980). Memory skill training for the elderly: Salient issues on the use of imagery. In L. W. Poon, J. L. Fozard, L. S. Cermak, D. Arenberg, & L. W. Thompson (Eds.), *New directions in memory and aging* (pp. 461–484). Hillsdale, NJ: Lawrence Erlbaum.

Reese, H. W. (1976). Models of memory development. *Human Development, 19*, 291–303.

Rissenberg, M., & Glanzer, M. (1986). Picture superiority in free recall: The effects of normal aging and primary degenerative dementia. *Journal of Gerontology, 41*, 64–71.

Rissenberg, M., & Glanzer, M. (1987). Free recall and word finding ability in normal aging and senile dementila of the Alzheimer's type: The effect of item concreteness. *Journal of Gerontology, 42*, 318–322.

Roberts, P. (1983). Memory strategy instruction with the elderly: What should memory training be the training of? In M. Pressley & J. E. Levin (Eds.), *Cognitive strategy research: Psychological foundations* (pp. 75–100). New York: Springer.

Robertson-Tchabo, E. A., Hausman, C. P., & Arenberg, D. (1976). A classical mnemonic for older learners: A trip that works! *Educational Gerontology, 1*, 215–226.

Rohwer, W. D., Jr. (1976). An introduction to research on individual and developmental differences in learning. In W. K. Estes (Ed.), *Handbook of learning and cognitive processes* (Vol. 3, pp. 71–101). Hillsdale, NJ: Lawrence Erlbaum.

Rose, T. A., & Yesavage, J. A. (1983). Differential effects of a list-learning mnemonic in three age groups. *Gerontology, 29*, 293–298.

Sagar, H. J., Cohen, N. J., Corkin, S., & Growdon, J. H. (1985). Dissociations among processes in remote memory. *Annals of the New York Academy of Sciences, 444*, 533–535.

Salmon, D. P., Shimamura, A. P., Butters, N., & Smith, S. (1988). Lexical and semantic priming deficits in patients with Alzheimer's disease. *Journal of Clinical and Experimental Neuropsychology, 10*, 477–494.

Salthouse, T. A. (1980). Age and memory: Strategies for localizing the loss. In L. W. Poon, J. L. Fozard, L. S. Cermak, D. Arenberg, & L. W. Thompson (Eds.), *New directions in memory and aging* (pp. 47–65). Hillsdale, NJ: Lawrence Erlbaum.

Salthouse, T. A. (1982). *Adult cognition: An experimental psychology of human aging*. New York: Springer.

Salthouse, T. A. (1984). Effects of age and skill in typing. *Journal of Experimental Psychology: General, 113*, 345–371.

Salthouse, T. A. (1985). *A theory of cognitive aging*. Amsterdam: Elsevier.

Salthouse, T. A. (1987). Age, experience, and compensation. In C. Schooler & K. W. Schaie (Eds.), *Cognitive functioning and social structure over the life course* (pp. 142–150). New York: Ablex.

Salthouse, T. A., Kausler, D. H., & Saults, J. S. (1988). Investigation of student status, background variables, and feasibility of standard tasks in cognitive aging research. *Psychology and Aging, 3*, 29–37.

Salthouse, T. A., Rogan, J. D., & Prill, K. (1984). Division of attention: Age differences on a visually presented memory task. *Memory & Cognition, 12*, 613–620.

Sanders, R. E., Murphy, M. D., Schmitt, F. A., & Walsh, K. K. (1980). Age differences in free recall rehearsal strategies. *Journal of Gerontology, 35,* 550–558.

Schmitt, F. A., Murphy, M. D., & Sanders, R. E. (1981). Training older adults' free-recall strategies. *Journal of Gerontology, 36,* 329–337.

Schonfield, D., & Robertson, E. A. (1966). Memory storage and aging. *Canadian Journal of Psychology, 20,* 228–236.

Shaps, L., & Nilsson, L.-G. (1980). Encoding and retrieval operations in relation to age. *Developmental Psychology, 16,* 636–643.

Sharps, M. J., & Gollin, E. S. (1987). Memory for object locations in young and elderly adults. *Journal of Gerontology: Psychological Sciences, 42,* 336–341.

Sharps, M. J., & Gollin, E. S. (1988). Aging and free recall of objects located in space. *Journal of Gerontology: Psychological Sciences, 43,* 8–11.

Shimamura, A. P., Salmon, D. P., Squire, L. R., & Butters, N. (1987). Memory dysfunction and word priming in dementia and amnesia. *Behavioral Neuroscience 101,* 347–351.

Simon, E. W. (1979). Depth and elaboration of processing in relation to age. *Journal of Experimental Psychology: Human Learning and Memory, 5,* 115–124.

Sinnott, J. D. (1986). Prospective/intentional and incidental everyday memory: Effects of age and passage of time. *Psychology and Aging, 1,* 110–116.

Slamecka, N. J., & Graf, P. (1978). The generation effect: Delineation of a phenomenon. *Journal of Experimental Psychology: Human Learning and Memory, 5,* 607–617.

Smith, A. D. (1976). Aging and the total presentation time hypothesis. *Developmental Psychology, 12,* 87–88.

Smith, A. D. (1977). Adult age differences in cued recall. *Developmental Psychology, 13,* 326–331.

Smith, A. D. (1980). Age differences in encoding, storage, and retrieval. In L. W. Poon, J. L. Fozard, L. S. Cermak, D. Arenberg, & L. W. Thompson (Eds.), *New directions in memory and aging* (pp. 23–45). Hillsdale, NJ: Lawrence Erlbaum.

Smith, S. W., Rebok, G. W., Smith, W. R., Hall, S. E., & Alwin, M. (1983). Adult age differences in the use of story structure in delayed recall. *Experimental Aging Research, 9,* 191–198.

Somberg, B. L., & Salthouse, T. A. (1982). Divided attention abilities in young and old adults. *Journal of Experimental Psychology: Human Perception and Performance, 8,* 651–663.

Spilich, G. J. (1983). Life-span components of text processing: Structural and procedural differences. *Journal of Verbal Learning and Verbal Behavior, 22,* 231–244.

Stigsdotter, A., & Bäckman, L. (1989a). Comparisons of different forms of memory training in old age. In M. A. Luszcz & T. Nettlebeck (Eds.), *Psychological development: Perspectives across the life-span* (pp. 397–408). Amsterdam: Elsevier.

Stigsdotter, A., & Bäckman, L. (1989b). Multifactorial memory training in old age: How to foster maintenance of improved performance. *Gerontology, 35,* 260–267.

Strauss, M.W., Weingartner, H., & Thompson, K. (1985). Remembering words and how often they occurred in memory-impaired patients. *Memory & Cognition, 13,* 507–510.

Taub, H. A. (1973). Memory span, practice, and aging. *Journal of Gerontology, 28*, 335–338.

Taub, H. A. (1979). Comprehension and memory of prose by young and old adults. *Experimental Aging Research, 5*, 3–13.

Taub, H. A., & Long, M. K. (1972). The effects of practice on short-term memory of young and old subjects. *Journal of Gerontology, 27*, 494–499.

Tomlinson, B. E. (1980). The structural and quantitative aspects of the dementias. In P. J. Roberts (Ed.), *Biochemistry of dementia* (pp. 15–52). Chichester: Wiley.

Treat, N. J., Poon, L. W., & Fozard, J. L. (1978). From clinical and research findings on memory to intervention programs. *Experimental Aging Research, 4*, 235–253.

Treat, N. J., Poon, L. W., & Fozard, J. L. (1981). Age, imagery, and practice in paired-associate learning. *Experimental Aging Research, 7*, 337–342.

Tulving, E. (1983). *Elements of episodic memory.* Oxford: Oxford University Press.

Tulving, E., & Thomson, D. M. (1973). Encoding specificity and retrieval processes in episodic memory. *Psychological Review, 80*, 352–373.

van Dijk, T. A., & Kintsch, W. (1983). *Strategies of discourse comprehension.* New York: Academic Press.

Waddell, K. J. (1983). *Effects of contextual organization and intentionality in adults' spatial memory performance.* Unpublished doctoral dissertation, University of Utah, Salt Lake City.

Waddell, K. J., & Rogoff, B. (1981). Effect of contextual organization on spatial memory of middle-aged and older women. *Developmental Psychology, 17*, 878–885.

Waddell, K. J., & Rogoff, B. (1987). Contextual organization and intentionality in adults' spatial memory. *Developmental Psychology, 23*, 514–520.

Weingartner, H., Kaye, W., Smallberg, S., Cohen, R., Ebert, M. H., Gillin, J. C., & Gold, P. (1982). Determinants of memory failures in dementia. In S. Corkin, K. L. Davies, J. H. Growdon, E. Usdin, & R. J. Wurtman (Eds.), *Alzheimer's disease: A report of progress (Aging,* Vol. 19, pp. 171–176). New York: Raven Press.

West, R. L. (1986). Everyday memory and aging. *Developmental Neuropsychology, 2*, 323–344.

Wilson, R. S., Bacon, L. D., Kramer, R. L., Fox, J. H., & Kaszniak, A. W. (1983). Word frequency effect and recognition memory in dementia of the Alzheimer type. *Journal of Clinical Neuropsychology, 5*, 97–104.

Wilson, R. S., Kaszniak, A. W., Bacon, L. D., Fox, J. H., & Kelly, M. P. (1982). Facial recognition memory in dementia. *Cortex, 18*, 329–336.

Wilson, R. S., Kaszniak, A. W., & Fox, J. H. (1981). Remote memory in senile dementia. *Cortex, 17*, 41–48.

Winocur, G. (1982). The amnesic syndrome: A deficit in cue utilization. In L. S. Cermak (Ed.), *Human memory and amnesia* (pp. 139–166). Hillsdale, NJ: Lawrence Erlbaum.

Worden, P. E., & Sherman-Brown, S. S. (1983). A word-frequency cohort effect in young versus elderly adults' memory for words. *Developmental Psychology, 19*, 521–530.

Yesavage, J. A. (1982). Degree of dementia and improvement with memory training. *Clinical Gerontologist, 1*, 77–81.

Yesavage, J. A. (1983). Imagery pretraining and memory training in the elderly. *Gerontology, 29*, 271–275.

Yesavage, J. A. (1984). Relaxation and memory training in 39 elderly patients. *American Journal of Psychiatry, 141,* 778–781.

Yesavage, J. A. (1985). Nonpharmacologic treatments for memory losses with normal aging. *American Journal of Psychiatry, 142,* 600–605.

Yesavage, J. A., Lapp, D., & Sheikh, J. I. (1989). Mnemonics as modified for use by the elderly. In L. W. Poon, D. C. Rubin, & B. A. Wilson (Eds.), *Everyday cognition in adulthood and late life* (pp. 598–611). New York: Cambridge University Press.

Yesavage, J. A., & Rose, T. A. (1983). Concentration and mnemonic training in elderly with memory complaints: A study of combined therapy and order effects. *Psychiatry Research, 9,* 157–167.

Yesavage, J. A., Rose, T. A., & Bower, G. (1983). Interactive imagery and affective judgements improve face–name learning in the elderly. *Journal of Gerontology, 29,* 197–203.

Yesavage, J. A., Westphal, J., & Rush, L. (1981). Senile dementia: Combined pharmacologic and psychologic treatment. *Journal of the American Geriatrics Society, 29,* 164–171.

Zarit, S. H., Cole, K. D., & Guider, R. L. (1981). Memory training strategies and subjective complaints of memory in the aged. *Gerontologist, 21,* 158–164.

Zarit, S. H., Zarit, J. M., & Reever, K. E. (1982). Memory training for severe memory loss: Effects on senile dementia patients and their families. *Gerontologist, 4,* 373–377.

6 Peak performance and age: An examination of peak performance in sports

K. ANDERS ERICSSON

Introduction

The growing interest in "testing the limits" and "maximum performance" (Baltes, 1987; Kliegl & Baltes, 1987) comes in part from the realization that traditional research does not seem able to obtain valid measures of performance, especially in old subjects. Recent research has shown that the inferior performance of old subjects can be substantially improved by briefly familiarizing them with the test situation, allowing further practice, and giving short-term instruction in efficient strategies for approaching the task (Baltes & Willis, 1982). Furthermore, potential differences in the motivation to perform in young and old subjects is a difficult issue in research on aging.

One approach to dealing with the influence of practice effects is to provide old and young subjects with considerable practice and to examine age differences in results (Kliegl, Smith, & Baltes, 1986; Salthouse & Somberg, 1982). However, even toward the end of extended practice, the performance of both young and old subjects continues to improve and has not reached a stable limit or peak performance. The approach described in this chapter is to seek out subjects who try to attain their best performance in real life. These subjects have spent orders of magnitude more time and effort on improving their performance than could ever be possible within a laboratory setting. *Peak performance* therefore refers to the best possible performance individuals are able to achieve when they are striving for this performance over an unlimited period of time.

In this chapter, I make the following tentative assumptions about peak performance. First, if individuals engage in some activity voluntarily, they must be highly motivated. Second, because practice and training are integral to preparation for "doing one's best," a high level of practice and experience can be assumed in the individuals under study. Third, when no restrictions are imposed on practice, performance is constrained by unmodifiable genetic and biological factors and approaches these pre-determined limits asymptotically. If these assumptions are true, peak performance would provide a particularly interesting measure of the functionality of the underlying biological factors, which would be a likely locus of the effects of aging.

The purpose of this chapter is to evaluate these assumptions about peak performance and to examine the empirical evidence on the relation between peak performance and age. In the next section, I will specify some criteria for the evidence needed to make inferences about peak performance and age. The remainder of the chapter is devoted to an empirical review of the best possible task domain selected on the basis of these criteria for studying peak performance.

The study of peak performance and age

Under optimal conditions, peak performance would be studied using subjects who have steadily tried to attain peak performance during their entire lives, and the results of these performances would be publicly available. The task and the conditions under which the task was to be performed would remain invariant over time for individual subjects as well as across individuals. Finally, it would be desirable – if the perfor-mance is to be reliably evaluated – to provide an objective index of the quality of performance within and across subjects as well as over historical time. In sum, an optimal task domain for studying peak performance and age should contain records on individuals' frequent performances of the same task during the entire life span.

Consider Lehmann's classic book *Age and Achievement* in terms of these criteria. Lehmann (1953) analyzed the age at which people gave their peak performance in sports and made their outstanding contributions to the arts and sciences. In contrast to standard laboratory tasks in which the time to complete the task and the accuracy of response are used to assess performance, Lehmann evaluated performance in the arts and sciences by the quality and originality of the products, such as paintings, symphonies, books, and scientific articles. On the basis of a high general consensus, these products can be classified as major or minor contribu-tions. By noting the date of completion or publication, it is possible to get a rough estimate of the contributor's age at the time the product was generated. Lehmann's (1953) analyses focused on the age distribution for significant scientific and creative contributions.

One problem with Lehmann's (1953) discovery, which states that the peak frequency of significant contributions occurs between 30 and 40 years of age, is the availability of opportunities to make contributions at other, especially later, ages. To alleviate this concern, individuals must be shown to have made uniformly frequent attempts to make significant contributions for other age intervals.

Unfortunately, in scientific and artistic activity it is difficult to distinguish separate attempts. One interesting possibility is to consider each published musical composition, painting, or scientific document as a separate attempt. However, it is questionable whether all products, even minor contributions, are actually attempts to attain peak achievement. A recognized author or composer may well publish works to satisfy economic needs and social demands. Moreover, if artistic and scientific activity is viewed as an acquired skill, it is more appropriate to consider an individual's career as a single attempt to make a general contribution (Ericsson & Crutcher, 1990). The reason is that expert-level performance in any domain apparently requires a preparatory period of a decade or so for the acquisition of prerequisite skills and knowledge. From this standpoint, the study of peak performance would ideally focus on groups of individuals who began to acquire skill and expertise at different ages, and the age of peak performance would then be analyzed as a function of the time they started their careers. However, data on such late beginners are scarce.

Other task domains may better satisfy the criteria for evidence on peak performance and age. Lehmann (1953) pointed out some intriguing similarities between the age of peak achievement in science and the age of peak performance in sports; and indeed the task qualities lacking in scientific activity are present in many sports events. For example, many sports events consist of trials with a definite beginning and end and, in addition, provide reliable and objective measures of performance. The duration of each trial is short, and active athletes complete the event many times during their lives. A majority of the events require minimal instruction and can be performed by untrained as well as expert subjects. Compared with the arts and sciences, smaller differences in strategies between subjects would be expected because of standardized coaching and the assumed simplicity of mediating cognitive processes in highly trained athletes. Finally, sports performance appears to be limited by a genetically determined upper bound. In a recent chapter of the *Annual Review of Psychology* Browne and Mahoney (1984, p. 609) concluded:

There is good evidence that the limits of this physiological capacity to become more efficient with training is determined by genetics. Muscle fiber type (fast-twitch versus slow-twitch percentage) and the maximal amount of oxygen consumed per minute per body weight (called max VO_2) are prime examples. Both are more than 90% determined by heredity for both males and females (Fox & Mathews, 1981).

Hence, peak performance in sports as a function of age is likely to reflect age-related declines in physiological capacity.

The following review examines peak performance in sports as a function of the age of the athletes. The invariance of the relation between peak performance and age is examined across athletes from different cultures as well as across athletes from different times in the history of sports. The results of cross-sectional studies, in which the performance of athletes of different ages is compared at a particular time, are compared with the results of longitudinal studies, in which the performance of the same athletes is examined at several different times. The prevailing assumptions about peak performance are evaluated in light of the stability of the best performances over historical time.

Age and peak performance in sports

There are two major approaches to the study of peak performance and age. The first, originally taken by Lehmann (1953), is to study the age of subjects winning major international competitions, like the Olympic games, or breaking the world record for an event. The second approach is to analyze the best performance of different groups ranging from 25 to over 70 years of age. The latter approach has been facilitated by the recent trend toward establishing special records and races for older age-groups (i.e., master athletes).

Most of the sports originally studied by Lehmann (1953) were interactive sports, such as tennis and boxing, in which the winner is better than the other participating competitors. The fact that the winner's performance is relative to that of a certain group of competitors makes any comparison across historical time difficult, if not impossible. In contrast, such comparisons can easily be made for events in which performance is measured by the time taken to cover a fixed distance. Some track events, such as pole vaulting, have undergone marked changes in technique and equipment and are therefore not suitable for comparisons across time. This chapter focuses on running and swimming, neither of which has been much affected by changes in equipment and technique.

Another important historical change has been the introduction of female athletes in national and international competition. Although the general arguments about peak performance should be equally valid for both men and women, there are obvious sex differences regarding anatomy and physiology that are likely to lead to differences in specific parameters relating age and performance. To simplify matters, I will restrict this review to the performance of men, for which a larger body of empirical evidence is available.

The age of peak performers

The most direct method of estimating the age at which athletes attain peak performance in sports is to calculate the mean age of winners of a prestigious international competition such as the Olympic games. Schultz and Curnow (1988) determined the ages of the winners for the 19 Olympic games from 1896 through 1980. Schultz and Curnow (1988) found that the mean age of Olympic winners for swimming events was similar across different distances (e.g., 100-m, 400-m, and 1,500-m freestyle) and ranged between 19.94 and 21.42 years. In running events, there was a systematic relation between the distance of the event and the mean age of the winner. Mean ages for winners of short- and middle-distance running events ranged from 22.85 years for 100 m to 24.80 years for 1,500 m, with the ages for 200 m and 800 m being intermediate. For long-distance running events (5,000 m, 10,000 m, and marathon), mean ages were between 27.20 and 27.85 years.

The best evidence that the estimates for Olympic winners' mean ages represent the age of peak performance is that mean ages differ for different events. Whatever factors sustain the pursuit of peak performance in long-distance runners until they reach older ages should also apply to swimmers and short-distance runners if their peak performance can be attained at older ages. Although Schultz and Curnow (1988) did not confirm different mean ages for different events with a formal statistical analysis, the standard deviations they reported (ranging from 2.1 to 4.5) imply that the differences are reliable.

Schultz and Curnow (1988) explored the hypothesis that if the estimates of the age for peak performance reflect an age-determined maximum for performance, then they would remain stable over historical time. This analysis is particularly interesting because performance in the Olympic games has dramatically improved during the 84 years of the Olympic games under study (1896–1980). The smallest improvement was 10.6% for 5,000-m running, and the greatest improvement was 53% for 400-m freestyle swimming. To evaluate stability in the age of peak performance, Schultz and Curnow (1988) calculated the mean age of Olympic winners for the first 10 Olympic games (1896–1936) and the 9 last Olympic games (1948–1980). No formal statistical evaluation was made of the stability hypothesis; however, the mean age of the winning freestyle swimmers tended to be about 1 year younger for all distances at the most recent Olympic games. For two of the three long-distance running events, the mean age of the winners was about 3 years older at the most recent games. The mean ages of short- and middle-distance runners were remarkably consistent for both time periods. This pattern of results is consistent with the hypothesis that deviations from the general age of peak performance in sports are increasing with time: The age of winning swimmers is growing even younger, and the age of winning long-distance runners is growing older.

The Olympics are held every 4 years. This means that athletes have only a single opportunity to compete in the Olympics in a particular 4-year period. The year of the Olympic games may not coincide with the age of athletes' best performance. The Olympic games are a special event with a number of unique pressures and distractions that may limit the generalizability of findings from an analysis of Olympic performances. Furthermore, the winner of a gold medal in the Olympic games is selected among the finalists for a running event on the basis of a single race. It is possible that the older ages of the winners of long-distance races are due to the older runners' greater experience and better strategies for controlling the pace of the critical race. Some of these confounding factors could be avoided in an analysis of the ages of athletes by recording the best performances in a certain event for a particular year, during which the athletes would have many opportunities to give their best performance.

In an analysis specially prepared for this chapter, the 10 best performers in five running events in 1986 were identified for seven countries: Australia ("Australiens," 1987), Canada ("Kanadas," 1987), China ("Chinas," 1987), East Germany ("DDR-Bestenliste," 1987), Romania ("Rumäniens," 1987), the Soviet Union ("UDSSR-Männer," 1987), and the United States ("USA-Männer," 1986). The five running distances were 100 m, 400 m, 1,500 m, 5,000 m, and 10,000 m. Using the published year of birth for each athlete, the age of athletes in 1986 could be estimated by subtracting the birth year from 1986. These ages were analyzed in a two-way ANOVA. No reliable interaction between country and event was found, but large main effects of country ($F[6, 304] = 7.18$, $p < .001$) and of running event ($F[4, 304] = 10.54$, $p < .001$) were observed. A post hoc analysis of the effects of country showed that the mean age of Chinese athletes (22.3) was reliably different from those of athletes from the Soviet Union (25.4), Australia (25.1), Canada (25.0), Romania (24.2), and the United States (25.3). Chinese athletes were comparatively young, most likely because organized training and support for competitive sports have been made available only recently in China. Figure 6.1 shows the mean ages of peak performers for each running distance.

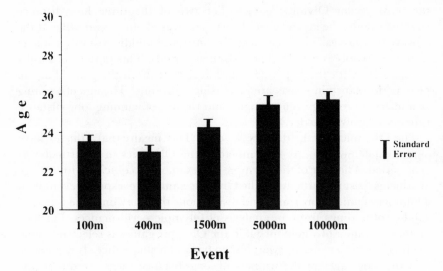

Figure 6.1. Mean age of the 10 best male performers in 1986 from seven countries (Australia, Canada, China, East Germany, Romania, the United States, the USSR) in five running events.

A post hoc analysis showed that the ages for short-distance runners (i.e., 100 m and 400 m) were reliably different from the ages of long-distance runners (i.e., 5,000 m and 10,000 m). These results are consistent with Schultz and Curnow's (1988) findings. The only discrepancy is that the mean ages of long-distance runners were younger than those estimated by Schultz and Curnow (1988), especially for the most recent period of the Olympic games. This discrepancy may be due to the younger ages of competitors with poorer performances, in particular from countries like China and Romania. For the 5,000-m and 10,000-m events, the mean ages of the 10 best athletes from all seven countries were 27.5 and 26.7, respectively, which are reasonably close to Schultz and Curnow's (1988) estimates. The standard deviations associated with these age estimates were less than those obtained by Schultz and Curnow (1988).

In sum, both Schultz and Curnow's (1988) study and the present analysis clearly show that peak performance for different athletic events is attained at systematically different ages. The pattern of age differences for different events was found to be stable both for different countries and across historical time. The results show that peak performance in running and swimming are observed between the ages of about 20 and 30 years.

Peak performance as a function of age: Cross-sectional studies

The effects of age on peak performance have been studied for both swimming (Hartley & Hartley, 1984, 1986; Letzelter, Jungermann, & Freitag, 1986) and running (Joch, 1979; Stones & Kozma, 1981, 1982, 1984). All of these studies include cross-sectional comparisons of the performance of different age-groups of subjects at a particular test occasion. The results for running and swimming are quite similar, and I have selected the study of swimming for two reasons. First, swimmers tend to exhibit peak performance at around 20 years of age, and the youngest age class in master competition is 25–29 years of age in West Germany. In comparison, the youngest age class for master runners starts with athletes who are 40 years old. Second, the studies of swimmers tend to be based on larger samples and sometimes contain information about the average performance of all competitors entering the national masters competition.

The effect of age on peak performance in swimming is quite consistent across studies, and the general results are illustrated by a German study by Letzelter et al. (1986). They identified the best times for participants in the German National Championship for master swimmers, for each age class (5-year intervals starting with 25 years of age and ending with 65 years of age and above) and for each of four events (50-m freestyle, backstroke, breaststroke, and butterfly) for the years from 1971 through 1983. The best times for the events as a function of age are given in Figure 6.2. The results in Figure 6.2 show a very consistent linear decrease with age for all four styles of swimming.

The participants in these championships for master athletes represent a highly select group and can be viewed as peak performers. An analysis of the mean performance of all participants in each age-group provides an informative comparison for the analysis of the best performances in running described in the previous section. This analysis of master swimmers is particularly interesting because the older age-groups have markedly less participants and thus represent a more select group than the younger age-groups.

The average performance of all competitors in each age-group is shown in Figure 6.3. The average performance as a function of age in Figure 6.3 is nonlinear and has a significant quadratic component. Furthermore, Letzelter et al. (1986) reported that the variance of the performance of the oldest subjects is around seven times larger than that of the youngest subjects. This implies considerable heterogeneity in the performance of the oldest subjects.

The degree of overlap in the distribution of performance for different

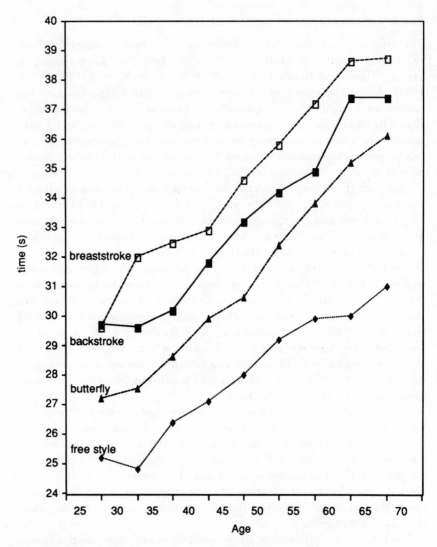

Figure 6.2. Development of professional swimmers' performance: the best times for four swimming events for each age-group (adapted from a figure in Letzelter, Jungermann, & Freitag, 1986, p. 392).

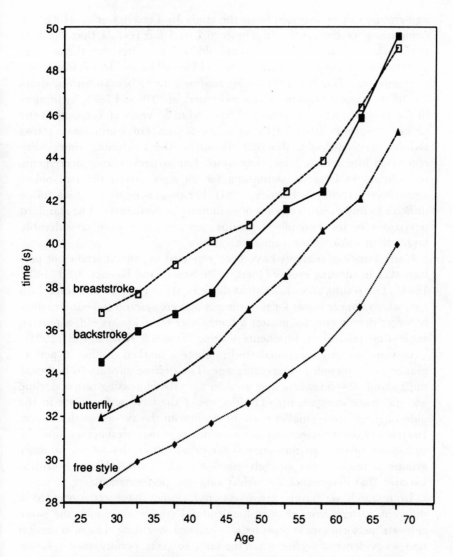

Figure 6.3. Development of professional swimmers' performance: the mean times for four swimming events for each age-group (adapted from a figure in Letzelter, Jungermann, & Freitag, 1986, p. 391).

age-groups can be assessed from the study by Letzelter et al. (1986). A comparison of the results in Figure 6.2 and 6.3 reveals that the best performance of the subjects 65 years old and older matches the average performance of subjects about 40 years old for all four styles of swimming.

Hartley and Hartley (1984, 1986) analyzed the 10 best swimming times for different age-groups of master swimmers in 1976 and 1981. Swimmers in the youngest age-group ranged from 30 to 35 years of age, and in the oldest age-group, from 75 to 79 years of age. For comparison across swimming events with different distances, the swimming times were converted into speeds prior to analysis. Linear performance decrements were found in freestyle swimming for all ages except the two oldest age-groups (Hartley & Hartley, 1984). For these age-groups, it was often difficult to find even 10 reports of swimming performances. The standard deviations of the two oldest groups' performances were considerably larger than those of the young age-groups.

Corresponding analyses have been reported in several studies of performance in running events (Joch, 1979; Stones and Kozma, 1981, 1982, 1984). The results show consistent decrements in peak performance with age, which appear linear for the younger age-groups and show increasingly larger decrements for master athletes over 60–65 years old, a pattern suggesting quadratic components of aging (Stones & Kozma, 1981, 1984).

In sum, the cross-sectional studies show a marked decline in performance as a function of increasing age. The decline appears to be linear until about 60–65 years of age; at older ages the increasing rate of decline has quadratic components. The decline of the best performance in the oldest age-groups is smaller than the decline for the average performance. In spite of extreme selectivity in the members of the oldest age-groups, the variability of their performance is far greater than that of the younger groups, a finding that strongly suggests lack of control over a critical variable that determines the oldest subjects' performances.

In research on aging, cross-sectional studies have often yielded a different pattern from that of longitudinal studies, in which the same subjects' performance is repeatedly measured over time. The next section reviews evidence of decline when the same subjects' performance in sports is monitored over extended time periods.

Peak performance as a function of age: Longitudinal studies

The longitudinal analyses reported in this section are not from well-controlled longitudinal studies of a representative sample of subjects.

Rather, these analyses capitalize on the fact that repeated cross-sectional studies of competitive events often include performances by the same individuals at different time periods – that is, ages. One can argue that individuals who annually participate in championships and sports events represent a healthy group of subjects not affected by serious disease, physical injuries, or other problems that impede physical performance without reflecting the effects of pure aging. The cross-sectional studies previously discussed include such longitudinal studies of individuals with repeated participation.

Letzelter et al. (1986) identified swimmers who had participated in several of the 13 German National Championships for master athletes. A sufficient number of swimmers were found for three age-groups (swimmers were 30–34, 35–39, and 40–44 years of age in 1971). At least 10 swimmers in each of the three age-groups participated in the four events for different swimming styles. As would be expected from Letzelter et al.'s (1986) cross-sectional analysis, reliable differences in performance were found among the three age-groups. However, an analysis of performance across the 13-year period failed to show any reliable decrements in performance with increasing age. Letzelter et al. (1986) argued that the decrements in the cross-sectional analysis reflected not so much biological aging as a decrease in the frequency and intensity of training. The longitudinal analysis indicated that when training is maintained, the decline in performance with increasing age is no longer statistically reliable in their study.

In a similar longitudinal analysis, Hartley and Hartley (1984) found that swimmers participating in both 1976 and 1981 performed worse in 1981, although considerable decrements in performance were apparent only for the age-group of 70 years and older.

If swimmers are able to maintain their performance with increasing age, marked improvements in the average performance of older age-groups should occur over time. Clear evidence for such improvements has been reported by Hartley and Hartley (1984). For performance on track events, Stones and Kozma (1982) found that cross-sectional studies indicated twice as steep a decline with age as did longitudinal studies.

In sum, the longitudinal studies of old athletes and master athletes point to the critical role of practice and maintained training. These athletes appear able to easily maintain or even improve their performance by maintaining or increasing the amount of training and practice. One could argue that world-class athletes are at a stable, optimal level of practice and that increased practice cannot compensate for performance decrements due to aging.

Peak performance of world-class athletes

In this section, empirical evidence for maximal performance by world-class athletes is reviewed. Longitudinal curves showing the best performance per year for three world-class athletes are presented, and the historical development of world-record performance is briefly discussed.

It is relatively rare for a world-class athlete to remain an active competitor in an event for 20 years and longer. Figures 6.4 through 6.7 display the best performance per year as a function of age for three famous athletes (zur Megede, 1968). In Figure 6.4 and 6.5, the running times of the Finnish middle- and long-distance runner Paavo Nurmi are shown for 5,000 m and 10,000 m, respectively. Nurmi gave his best performance for 5,000 m at 27 years of age, as shown in Figure 6.4. An analysis of Nurmi's all-time five best running times for 5,000 m shows that his average age was 27.4 years, with a standard error of .75. He gave his best performance for 10,000 m at 27 years of age, as shown in Figure 6.5, and the average age for his all-time five best performances in this event was 27.2 ± 1.11 years.

Because of the limited availability of longitudinal data, I have relaxed my restriction of considering only running and swimming events and have included two athletes competing in other sports. The longitudinal performance of the German hammer thrower Karl Hein is shown in Figure 6.6. Hein's peak performance occurred at age 30, and the mean ages of his all-time 5 and 10 best performances were $29.8 \pm .2$ and $30.2 \pm .35$ years, respectively. The age-related peak of his performance is clearly evident, as is his remarkable ability to maintain into his fifties a level of performance good enough for participation in national championships.

Finally, the longitudinal performance of the Finnish javelin thrower Matti Järvinen is shown in Figure 6.7. Järvinen's performance as a function of age shows a clear, smooth peak. His all-time best performance was attained at age 27. During his early career, Järvinen broke the world record 10 times, and an alternative estimate of his age of peak performance can be determined by averaging the ages at which he accomplished this feat. That estimate, $23.1 \pm .66$, is clearly inconsistent with the peak age derived from his best life-time performance, shown in Figure 6.7.

It is difficult to make any claims about generalizability on the basis of these three individuals. All three individuals, however, maintain a very high level of performance. Because we lack information about likely changes in training intensity and equipment for javelin and hammer throwing, one should be cautious in viewing changes in performance as a direct reflection of age. Nonetheless, the curves of these three famous athletes clearly indicate a performance peak between 25 and about 30 years of age. This finding is in accordance with the analyses of the mean

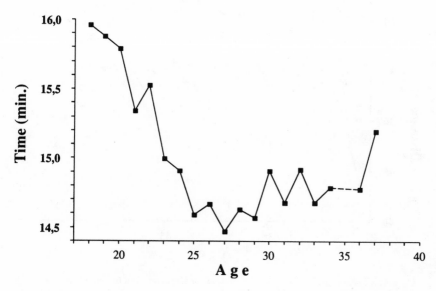

Figure 6.4. The best 5,000-m race time each year for Paavo Nurmi as a function of age.

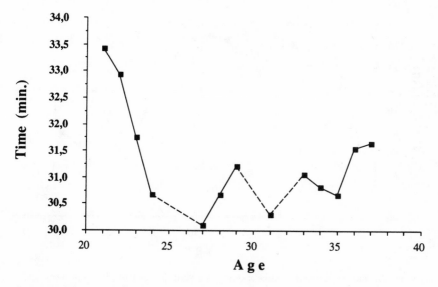

Figure 6.5. The best 10,000-m race time each year for Paavo Nurmi as a function of age.

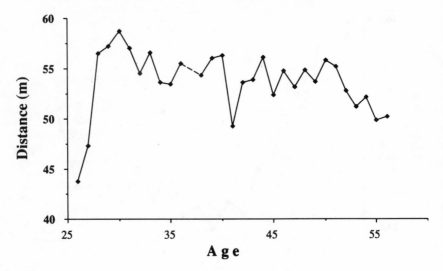

Figure 6.6. The longest hammer throw each year for Karl Hein as a function of age.

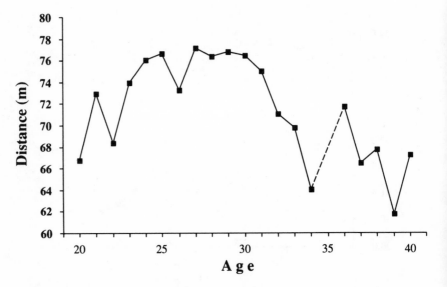

Figure 6.7. The longest javelin throw each year for Matti Järvinen as a function of age.

Table 6.1. *Mean age of individuals exhibiting their best world-record-breaking performance and Pearson and Spearman correlations relating the age of the performer and the date (year) of the performance for five running events*

Event	Number of observations	Mean age	Standard deviation	Standard error of mean	Pearson correlation	Spearman correlation with correction for ties
100 m	45	22.58	2.57	0.38	−0.07	−0.17
400 m	16	23.60	2.94	0.74	0.15	−0.04
1,500 m	35	24.49	2.43	0.41	0.04	0.05
5,000 m	21	26.48	2.38	0.52	−0.05	0.06
10,000 m	17	28.12	4.12	1.00	0.01	−0.11

Note: The data on ages for world-record-breaking performance used in this analysis were compiled by zur Megede (1987).

ages of Olympic winners and elite athletes in the cross-sectional studies discussed earlier. The case analyses also reveal some biases in estimates of age of peak performance based on the age of winners of the Olympic games and the age of individuals breaking the world record in an event. The ideal data would include the age at which the best performance was attained during the athlete's entire career.

An examination of ages of individuals breaking the world record comes close to an analysis of such ideal data, if only the best world record for each athlete is considered. The corresponding mean ages for five running events are shown in Table 6.1. The mean ages in Table 6.1 increase with the distance of the race, as was found in the analyses discussed earlier. Given that the recorded performances span almost a century of active competition in sports, this data set is well suited to an evaluation of stability of age in lifetime best performances over historical time.

In Table 6.1, the Pearson and Spearman correlations between age of performer and the date (year) of the performance are given. There is no indication of a systematic trend in the age of peak performance for any of the five running events. The stability of this measure of peak performance across historical time suggests that it is superior to the measures discussed earlier. However, the standard deviations in Table 6.1 do not appear to be systematically smaller than those for the other two measures. Hence, the age interval when peak performance in running can be attained, appears to be fairly wide, regardless of the measure used to access it. Although individual athletes exhibit an age-related performance peak, there is no evidence that the maximum human performance in any event has been attained.

Remarks on age and peak performance in sports

Contrary to the widely held view that sports performance is rigidly limited by invariant physiological factors, world records and best annual performances on specific events have been steadily improving over time. In their analysis of the Olympic-gold winners, Schultz and Curnow (1988) found that improvements in performance on specific events have ranged between 10% and 50% during the last century of Olympic competition. The increase in amount of preparation and training and improvements in training methods are probably the major factors responsible for improvements in most events. In fact, the greatest improvement has occurred in 400-m freestyle swimming, on which improvements in equipment have had the least influence. From time to time, perceived ultimate limits for human performance have been proposed, for example, the 4-min mile and 9.9 s for the 100-m dash. However, these predicted limits have been surpassed, and exceeding the 4-min mile limit is now the rule rather than the exception for winners in elite competition. These steady improvements in performance do not, of course, rule out the idea of an upper bound on human performance, but they do raise some doubts about the hypothesis that the ultimate physiological limit on performance is inevitably attained through extended practice.

This remarkable improvement in athletic performance over historical time provides an interesting frame of reference for judging the decrements associated with aging. In cross-sectional studies discussed earlier, striking decrements were observed for master athletes as a function of their age in comparison with the performance of younger athletes active today. But what would be the result of comparing the best performance of contemporary master athletes with that of athletes competing in the first Olympic games? This comparison would be unfair, of course, because the Olympic athletes would have had only a single opportunity to attain their best performance. Therefore, I have also included the unofficial world records from 1896. In Table 6.2, the best performances of master athletes in age-groups 50–54, 55–59, 60–64, and 65–69 were taken from Stones and Kozma (1981) and compared with the performances of winners of the Olympic games and the unofficial world records for 1896.

The number of performances matching or surpassing those of the Olympic-gold winners in 1896 is five, three, two, and one for the four age-groups of master athletes. The master athletes never attained a performance better than the world records of 1896. This comparison of

Table 6.2. *Peak performance by Olympic athletes in 1896 and by master athletes in 1979*

Event (measurement units)	Best time in Olympic games of 1896[a]	Unofficial world record in 1896[b]	Age category (years) for master athletes in 1979[c]			
			50–54	55–59	60–64	65–69
100 m (s)	12.0	10.8	11.4	11.6	12.0	13.2
200 m (s)	22.2	21.8	23.6	23.6	24.9	27.9
400 m (s)	54.2	48.2	52.9	54.6	59.1	65.1
800 m (min/s)	2:11.0	1:53.4	2:01.1	2:11.4	2:19.9	2:27.2
1,500 m (min/s)	4:33.2	4:10.4	4:14	4:20.4	4:53.2	4:59.2
Marathon (hr/min/s)	2:58.50	—	2:25:17	2:26:35	2:47:46	2:53:03

[a] Data from "Olympic games," 1985.
[b] Data from zur Megede, 1987.
[c] Data from Stones and Kozma, 1981.

absolute performance across time indicates that contemporary training methods can go a long way toward compensating for age-related declines in performance.

Summary of peak performance and age

The upper limits on performance in sports decline with age, and people tend to exhibit the peak performances of their careers between 20 and 30 years of age. Performance at any age is critically dependent on the amount of practice and training. The large increases in numbers of world records for most events as a function of the time appear to be determined largely by increases in the amount of practice as well as by better methods of practice. The emergence of master athletes who regularly practice at older ages has clearly demonstrated that peak performance at older ages was vastly underestimated and that decrements in performance with increasing age can be dramatically reduced with continued practice.

The crucial role of training and practice in determining limits and age-related decline in performance brings into question the notion set forth at the beginning of this chapter, namely, that through training, athletes approach an asymptote of performance determined by genetic and biological factors. In the next section, I review studies in which the physiological systems and components of subjects exhibiting peak performance were measured and related to their performance. Through direct measurement of mediating physiological mechanisms at different performance levels and after varying amounts of sustained training, it is possible to evaluate the extent to which the function of these mechanisms is influenced and changed by training. The role of training in moderating age-related decline in the function of these mechanisms can be explored with a similar methodology.

Physiological components of peak performance in sports

The most successful efforts to identify physiological correlates of performance have been made with long-distance running. This sport is attractive to study because it involves maintaining a comparatively simple motor activity for extended periods of time. It is also relatively easy to set up a laboratory situation for steady-state running on a treadmill. The details of runners' movement patterns do not seem to be important, because differences in running style among elite and subelite long-distance runners are apparently unimportant in determining performance (Cavanagh, Pollock, & Landa, 1977).

During steady-state running or cycling on an exercise bicycle, the body converts energy into work through the metabolism of oxygen. In the laboratory, it is possible to measure both the maximal ability to take up oxygen (aerobic power) and the efficiency with which oxygen is converted into work at submaximal levels of running. The aerobic power of runners is highly predictive of their long-distance running performance. Correlations between running times and maximal oxygen uptake (aerobic power) range between −.82 and −.91 for several studies for well-trained and experienced runners (Conley & Krahenbuhl, 1980). When the analysis is restricted to highly trained, experienced runners with high aerobic powers, no reliable relation between running performance and aerobic power is found. However, even within such a select group of long-distance runners, individual differences in running economy or efficiency are highly predictive of running performance (Conley & Krahenbuhl, 1980).

Aerobic power is a measure of the overall ability of the body to metabolize oxygen and produce muscular energy. Through examination of the physiological components mediating the circulation of oxygen and its metabolism in the muscles, it might be possible to identify those components that account for the superior aerobic power of elite long-distance runners. Most of the studies have used a cross-sectional approach and have compared the physiological characteristics of elite athletes with those of normal subjects. One of the first findings was that athletes have hearts that are larger than normal (see Morganroth & Maron, 1977). A larger heart provides the capacity to circulate more oxygen-rich blood, which is critical to high aerobic power. The oxygen-rich blood eventually needs to reach the muscles, and studies have shown that subjects' aerobic power is closely related to the number of capillaries supplying each muscle fiber with blood (Saltin, Henriksson, Nygaard, Andersen, & Jansson, 1977). Muscles are composed of muscle fibers with different characteristics. Some muscle fibers, such as slow-twitch muscle fibers, are particularly suited to the sustained activity involved in long-distance running. A high proportion of slow-twitch muscle fibers is highly predictive of good long-distance running performance (see Bouchard, 1986, for a review). The superior aerobic power of athletes can, at least in part, be accounted for by their larger hearts and the larger number of capillaries for each muscle fiber. In a similar manner, it is possible to account for the greater running efficiency of long-distance runners by their higher percentage of slow-twitch muscle fiber.

The nature of these physiological differences suggests that they reflect stable, individual, genetic differences and that elite runners lie at the extreme end of normal variation. Some earlier studies tend to confirm this view by showing extremely high (over 90%) genetic determination (i.e., heritability) for these differences (see Fox & Mathews, 1981, for a review).

It is also clear that short-term training and practice cannot account for the anatomical characteristics of the heart and the composition of the muscle fibers observed in elite long-distance runners. However, as shown in the next section, the training necessary to become an elite long-distance runner is intensive and needs to be maintained for about 10 years. In light of new research findings, the next section considers whether such extreme amounts of training could lead to the necessary anatomical changes.

Training and peak performance in long-distance running

The necessity of intensive and extended training for attaining exceptional levels of performance in sports is generally recognized. Long-distance runners participate in active competition for about 10 years before attaining their peak performance (Wallingford, 1975). Highly trained and experienced long-distance runners were found to have trained for 10 years on the average (Conley & Krahenbuhl, 1980). Elite long-distance athletes usually run twice a day and cover distances from 110 to 240 km every week of the year (Hagan, Smith, & Gettman, 1981; Wallingford, 1975).

The study of the role of training in long-distance running is particularly tractable. Long-distance runners often keep records of both their running times during practice and the distances covered. These practice records can easily be quantified and through regression analysis related to running times on actual races.

Hagan et al. (1981) found that the regularity and amount of practice during 9 weeks prior to a marathon race were strongly related to running times. The length of training runs and the total distance covered per week accounted for nearly half of the variance in actual running times on the marathon (Hagan et al., 1981). In a combined sample of elite long-distance and good middle-distance runners, Fink, Costill, and Pollock (1977) found that the runners' best times for a 6-mile race were highly predictable ($r = -.61$) from the percentage of slow-twitch muscle fibers. However, when the elite long-distance runners were analyzed separately, no relation was found. Furthermore, the daily training for elite long-distance runners ranged from 17.7 km to 32.2 km, whereas the good middle-distance runners trained less than 17.7 km per day. Hence, the amount of daily training could, in the same way, predict running performance and the percentage of slow-twitch muscle fibers.

The strong relations between current and past practice and many physiological tests, such as aerobic power, and between practice and characteristics of the body, such as amount of body fat and percentage of slow-twitch muscle fibers, make any formal analysis of causes virtually impossible on the basis of cross-sectional data. Nevertheless, it is possible to refute the claims presented earlier that physiological characteristics are completely determined by genetics and that these characteristics do not change in response to training. Then, an attempt can be made to attribute the critical physiological differences to effects of extensive practice.

A reexamination of the unmodifiability of physiological differences

Recent research has demonstrated that the human physiological system is far more adaptable than was once believed possible. Changes in the number of capillaries supplying blood to muscle fibers are found to take place as a result of practice (Salmons & Henriksson, 1981). The most extensive research has been conducted on the amount of transformation possible in the characteristics of muscle fibers, and this research is the topic of this section.

Because muscle composition in long-distance runners is distinctly different from that of other types of runners, a better understanding of the factors determining that composition may even explain the older ages for peak performance in long-distance running events. According to Salmons and Henriksson's (1981) recent review, the first clear demonstration that the characteristics of muscle fibers could be completely transformed in response to continuous use was made through electrical stimulation of muscles in animal research. Within the first week of stimulation, increases in capillary density occurred, and within a couple of months fast-twitch muscle fibers were completely transformed into slow-twitch muscle fibers. About 6 weeks after stimulation was stopped, the muscles reverted to the original fast-twitch muscle fibers. A subsequent review by Howald (1982) showed that these results can be generalized to human skeletal muscles. The evidence presented included case studies of top athletes who were forced to stop or reduce training because of injuries. Drastic decrements in the percentage of slow-twitch fibers occurred within 6 months to 1 year. Howald also showed that training studies and studies using electrical stimulation produced a very consistent pattern of results. The transformation from fast-twitch to slow-twitch muscle fibers appeared to be gradual and involved a number of intermediate muscle types. Although studies of limited training rarely demonstrate a complete conversion of fast-twitch to slow-twitch fibers, clear changes to intermediate muscle types are regularly seen.

The only piece of evidence contradicting Howald's (1982) account is the nearly perfect heritability of the percentage of muscle types (Browne & Mahoney, 1984), mentioned previously. To reconcile this evidence with his account of environmental factors influencing the composition of muscles, Howald (1982) reviewed developmental data on the percentage of slow-twitch fibers in children of different ages and found that the activity patterns of different age-groups could account for these differences. Howald (1982) argued that high similarities in muscle composition in monozygotic twins are due not only to genetic factors determining muscle composition directly but also to genetic factors such as leg length and anatomical differences that provide the muscle with a similar pattern of habitual activity. Conversely, more recent genetic studies have been unable to replicate the early high heritability estimates and have indicated a much lower degree of genetic determination (Bouchard, 1986). The role of genetic factors in determining sports performance appears to be considerably less significant than originally believed.

In summarizing the results of a large symposium on genetic factors in sports performance, Bouchard and Malina (1986, p. 184) stated: "It has been established that maximal aerobic power and capacity, anaerobic alactic capacity, and skeletal muscle histochemical and biochemical characteristics are characterized by only a moderate heritability component." Because Howald's (1982) account appears to remain valid, even these estimates are probably high as they include the indirect influence of genetically determined physical attributes such as height.

Examination of the effects of extensive training

If extensive training does affect any of the critical physiological characteristics, those that are affected must closely correspond to specific functions central to the training activities. Hence, characteristics acquired or improved through training may be adaptations to the demands of training. As noted earlier, aerobic power is closely related to long-distance running performance, except in elite long-distance runners, for whom a ceiling effect may be present. Elite long-distance runners differ from other elite runners in their running efficiency at rates lower than maximum. At rates similar to their regular running speeds during races, elite long-distance athletes are able to run more efficiently; that is, they can maintain speed with a minimal consumption of oxygen (Conley & Krahenbuhl, 1980).

One of the most striking examples of adaptation with training is the anatomical differences in the hearts of different types of athletes. Morgan-roth and Maron (1977) reviewed research showing that the mass of the heart was larger in both endurance athletes, such as runners and swimmers, and athletes focusing on strength, such as wrestlers and shot-putters. The increase, however, was due to different factors in the two types of athletes. In athletes focusing on strength, the thickness of the left ventricular wall was increased, but it was normal in endurance athletes. Rapid transport of oxygen-rich blood to the muscles is facilitated by the thicker and stronger wall. This capability is critical for athletes relying on a sudden exhibition of force and strength but is not relevant for the steady state of the endurance athlete. On the other hand, endurance athletes benefit from a larger volume of circulated oxygen-rich blood, and their hearts showed an increased left ventricular diastolic volume, which is normal for wrestlers. This demonstrated match between circulatory demands and anatomical characteristics of the athletes' hearts does not completely rule out self-selection of athletes for specific sports. It is notable, however, that the cardiac characteristics of elite athletes appear to be outside the normal range for untrained athletes. Furthermore, except for the critical characteristics, the athletes' hearts were found to be within the normal range.

In a particularly interesting study, Tesch and Karlsson (1985) examined the size and frequency of fast- and slow-twitch fibers in the muscles of different types of elite athletes as well as of students serving as control subjects. For all subjects, samples of muscle tissue were taken from the deltoid muscle in the back and the vastus muscle in one leg. Tesch and Karlsson (1985) found, as would be expected, that middle- and long-distance runners had a significantly higher percentage of slow-twitch fibers in the leg muscle than did the control subjects, but the runners' back muscles were no different from those of the control subjects. For elite kayakers, the pattern was reversed. There was no difference in the proportions of fibers in kayakers' leg muscles compared with those of the control subjects. From these and other findings, Tesch and Karlsson (1985) argued that differences in the muscles of elite athletes occur only for muscles specifically trained for a sport (legs in running and back muscles in kayaking), with no differences for untrained muscles. The elite athletes studied by Tesch and Karlsson had had a minimum of 4 years of systematic training. This means that the inability of about half of the earlier studies to find changes in the proportion of slow-twitch fibers as a result of short-term training (10–20 weeks) is consistent with the claim that such changes result from years of training and practice.

Whether the physiological attributes of elite endurance runners are acquired through training or are genetically endowed can best be explored in longitudinal studies. Elovainio and Sundberg (1983) tested 10 endurance runners and 18 control subjects at age 14. Five years later, 6 of the 10 runners were still active and had attained elite status as runners. They were retested along with 7 of the control subjects who were matched to the runners in height, weight, and percentage of body fat. At age 14, the endurance runners and control subjects were no different, except that the runners had a somewhat lower maximum heart rate and resting pulse. At age 19, however, the runners had a significantly higher maximal oxygen uptake and larger relative heart volume than did the control subjects. The resting pulse remained lower for the runners, although both groups had a much lower resting pulse at retest than they had 5 years previously. At age 19, the difference in maximal pulse rate was no longer reliable. With respect to the two variables of real interest, maximal oxygen uptake and relative heart volume, there was no difference between the control subjects at two test occasions or between the control subjects and the runners at age 14. However, the elite runners showed a marked improvement from their original level during the 5 years of intense training. This finding strongly suggests that the enhanced level of maximal oxygen intake in elite runners is due to prolonged endurance training.

Effects of aging

The cross-sectional analysis of peak performance and age showed that increasing age was associated with lower performance. However, longitudinal studies revealed that the decline in the performance of master athletes was dramatically reduced. This section examines the extent to which training can reduce the performance decrements observed with age. First, I consider a study that examined the physiological functions of master athletes. Second, I briefly review studies of older subjects who were provided with training.

Hagberg et al. (1985) made detailed physiological assessments of eight master long-distance runners whose ages averaged 56 years. When Hagberg et al. (1985) recruited young runners with comparable performance relative to their age-group, they found that the younger runners not only had faster race times but were also running considerably more during training. To control for amount of training, they recruited a group of young runners in their midtwenties who were matched to the master athletes on the basis of their 10-km race times, training mileage, and running pace during training. Hagberg et al. (1985) also tested a group of healthy, age-matched subjects with no active participation in sports.

The aerobic power of the master athletes was found to be almost twice as high as that of the age-matched controls, but it was also reliably lower than that of the competitive young runners (19%) and the young runners matched for amount of training (9%). A detailed analysis of a number of physiological indicators suggested that the master athletes' lower aerobic power could be attributed primarily to their lower maximum pulse rate, which was 13% lower than that of both of the two groups of young runners. Interestingly enough, the maximum pulse rate of the master athletes was, if anything, lower than that of the age-matched controls with no active participation in sports. Hagberg et al. (1985) reviewed several other studies and found that the maximal heart rate invariably decreased with increasing age. This interesting study demonstrated clearly that aerobic power can be almost twice as high in older individuals actively participating in sports as in old control subjects and implies that many, but not all, physiological functions can be maintained through training.

In a more recent review, Hagberg (1987) discussed the decline of aerobic power with increasing age. In a number of studies, the decline was shown to be 10% per decade after the age of 25 for subjects who did not actively participate in physical exercise and training programs. As late as 1977, it was proposed that the decline in aerobic power was inevitable and unaffected by continued training (Hagberg, 1987). Recent studies have shown, however, that continued exercise has been an important factor in minimizing decline. According to Hagberg (1987), some of the best evidence was provided by Pollock and his colleagues, who reexamined a number of runners after 10 years. Runners who decreased their training during the 10-year interval showed a 13% decline in aerobic power. However, those runners who maintained their training showed a decline in aerobic power of only 2%. Several studies have found that aerobic power decreased only by about 5% in subjects who engaged in high levels of physical activity.

Older adults without a previous history of physical exercise can greatly improve their aerobic power by exercising regularly. Hagberg (1987) cited one study that found average gains of 30% in aerobic power in 61- to 67-year-old adults after they had participated in a year-long exercise program. These old subjects attained improvements in aerobic power with very low training intensities that would not be effective in improving aerobic power in younger subjects. Hence, the low aerobic power of the old subjects before training was not due to aging per se but was an adaptation to an inactive life-style. Whether adults over the age of 70 can improve their aerobic power as a result of training is currently unclear (Hagberg, 1987).

Remarks on peak performance and aging

This section focuses on decrements in peak performance with increasing age. The research reviewed in the previous section showed that with continued training intensity, performance can be maintained with minor decrements up to 60–70 years of age. The analysis of the physiological components of master athletes suggested that maintained training can preserve the functionality of many critical components that normally decline in old age. However, when training is reduced or stopped, marked decrements in performance are observed. It is well known that at any age thé beneficial effects of short-term physical exercise programs are rapidly lost within about 2 months without continued training (Fox & Mathews, 1981). Even for competitive young runners, a 2-week interval without training markedly reduced their performance and aerobic power, and a subsequent 2-week interval of training was insufficient for regaining original performance (Fox & Mathews, 1981). As noted earlier, a large proportion of slow-twitch muscle fibers in elite runners reverts to fast-twitch muscle fibers when training is stopped because of injury. There is evidence that the enlarged hearts of elite athletes do not fully return to normal after the end of active competition (Morganroth & Maron, 1977). It is likely, however, that the former elite athletes may remain more physically active than control subjects. In sum, the capacity of the critical physiological functions appears to be determined by an adaptation to the most recent frequency and intensity of training.

Nevertheless, the available data indicate that the extreme effects of training may be limited to a restricted age range. Elite athletes tend to undergo intensive training between 10 and 30 years of age, and thus the period of intensive training often overlaps with athletes' normal physical development. It may be, then, that the capacity for extreme adaptation as a result of training is dependent upon age. Because master athletes seem to have been active as athletes when they were younger, it is possible that their high performance is related to their ability to maintain a high performance acquired in their youth and not to a capability for attaining such performance for the first time at older ages. As age increases, it is likely that the intensity and amount of training would have to be reduced, and this reduction, combined with effects of aging, would lead to observed decrements in performance due to declines in the function of physiological components. Hagberg et al. (1985) demonstrated that elite runners in their twenties trained considerably more than elite master runners did. Hence any comparisons of peak performance across age-groups most likely reflect not only "pure" age effects but also age effects restricting the intensity and amount of training, as well as possible interactions. Whether reductions in training and general physical activity are the primary causes of the more pronounced decrements in subjects over the age of 70 remains unclear.

Conclusion

In the introduction to this chapter, a simplistic view of peak performance in sports was presented. According to that view, peak performance is attained relatively easily through training and is a "pure" reflection of fixed limits set by genetically determined biological factors.

The alternative conception of peak performance in sports emphasizes the remarkable adaptability of human behavior and the human body. Long-term intensive training appears to lead to adaptations and changes in many physiological structures previously thought to be fixed and uninfluenced by external factors. The focus on adaptation makes it natural to see an individual's current performance as a reflection of current as well as past training demands on the physiological system. With a decrease in the intensity and extent of training, adaptation to smaller demands occurs.

This theoretical framework for explaining peak performance can effectively incorporate the main findings about peak performance and its relation to age. The considerable improvements in world-record performance and average elite performance for many events over the history of athletic competition can be seen as being due primarily to changes in training conditions. The discrepancies between declines assessed with cross-sectional and longitudinal methods can to a large degree be attributed to differences in the intensity of training. Declines in peak performance with age should be seen as a result of pure aging effects on physiological function, decreases in the intensity and extent of training, and possible interaction effects.

The age at which peak performance in sports is attained in different events requires further discussion. That age tends to occur between 20 and 30 years and differs systematically across events. For the events discussed in this chapter, the youngest ages for peak performance are recorded for swimming (around 20), followed by short-distance running (around 23) and finally long-distance running (around 27). These ages for attaining peak performance are consistent with the findings that many physiological functions, such as maximal heart rate, appear to reach maximal capacity in untrained subjects at around 20 years of age. The critical role of long-term intensive training in attaining physiological adaptation of the cardiovascular system and in converting fast-twitch muscle fibers into slow-twitch fibers is consistent with the older mean ages of long-distance runners. The age of peak performance in a given event can then be seen as the optimization of several age-related constraints. This view of peak performance points to the central role of early preparation and training in reaching one's performance limit.

Our knowledge of detailed training histories for peak performers in sports is quite limited. Some of the best evidence comes from a recent study by Bloom and his collaborators, who interviewed about 40 world-class swimmers and tennis players about their lives (Bloom, 1985). Both types of athletes began to participate in their sport at a remarkably early age: The average age for starting to play tennis was 6.5 years (Monsaas,

1985), and for learning to swim, 4.5 years (Kalinowski, 1985). Around the age of 10, both groups of athletes were spending about 15 hours per week playing tennis (Monsaas, 1985) or practicing swimming (Kalinowski, 1985). By the time they were teenagers, the amount of time they spent on their respective sports had further increased to about 20 hours a week.

About 10 years of dedicated preparation appears necessary to attain a world-class level in tennis and swimming (Ericsson & Crutcher, 1990; Kalinowski, 1985; Monsaas, 1985), a conclusion that is consistent with the estimates reported earlier for long-distance runners. These estimates of amount of training and preparation suggest that contemporary peak performers are quite close to a limit in the amount of training and preparation possible. If such a limit exists and is attained, one might argue that stable peak performance is also attained.

What would a limit set by the availability of training and preparation be like? It is clear that increases in the amount and intensity of practice and training do not always lead to better performance. Too much training can lead to physical exhaustion and dramatically increase risks of injury. Extended intensive training can lead to event-related injuries due to systematic wearing out of critical functions. Intensive running occasionally leads to "runner's knee," "runner's heel bumps," shinsplints, Achilles tendonitis, and bone deformities of the foot such as bunions and hammertoes (Subotnick, 1977). Maintaining motivation and avoiding "burnout" are also critical.

Intensive training over months, years, and decades taxes resources such as time and effort that are also required for other needs, interests, and external demands. Many of these factors that influence the amount and intensity of training are likely to change during adulthood and, especially in very old age, are likely to be quite different from what they were during youth. The large number of other interacting demands in life suggests that an optimum amount of intensity and type of training would be very difficult to attain and even more difficult to maintain for extended periods of time. Hence, it is unlikely that the true limits of performance will ever be completely reached.

In the introduction to this chapter, the study of peak performance was proposed as a means for uncovering subjects' stable performance limits through extended practice and thus eliminating the influence of previous experience. The examination of peak performance in sports in this chapter does not support that view. On the contrary, intensive long-term training has been shown to have dramatic effects on the underlying physiological functions previously assumed to be the fixed factors determining the limit of an individual's performance. It is likely that the real limits for these physiological functions are determined by limits on the type, intensity, and amount of training for extended periods of time. The most intriguing and exciting challenge in the study of peak performance is not to determine the performance limit itself but to discover the processes that regulate and sustain the training of subjects trying to achieve their best performance.

More generally, this framework for conceptualizing peak performance in sports ought to be important for understanding the sources of frequently observed decrements in performance with increasing age. Only a small proportion of the decrements in performance of old subjects can be attributed to inevitable deterioration of the efficiency of the mediating physiological components, as shown by studies of master athletes who maintain the duration and intensity of training. The observed decrements in motor performance in old subjects have been shown in this chapter to be closely linked to reductions in intensity of training for old athletes and to lower levels of physical activity among subjects in general. It would therefore be important to consider the possibility that lowered levels of motor performance in old healthy individuals reflect, to a large degree, reduced physiological capacities that are determined by a physiological adaptation to less-demanding physical activities. If one assigns an important role in determining physiological capacities to adaptive mechanisms, it is no longer useful to simply measure these capacities in old subjects. One would need to provide detailed descriptions of the physical activities in the daily lives of old subjects and to study the full range of factors that influence the levels of these activities in a longitudinal design. Only future research will tell whether the complex interactions inherent in adaptive mechanisms will provide a fruitful framework for describing the many empirical results relating age to performance.

NOTE

The thoughtful comments and suggestions on earlier drafts of this chapter from Janet Grassia, Reinhold Kliegl, Clemens Tesch-Römer, and Laura Thompson are gratefully acknowledged. Peter Usinger's skillful help in locating data on peak performance deserves special mention and recognition.

REFERENCES

Australiens Männer 1986. (1987). *Leichtathletik, 26*(6), 174.
Baltes, P. B. (1987). Theoretical propositions of life-span developmental psychology: On the dynamics between growth and decline. *Developmental Psychology, 23*, 611–626.

Baltes, P. B., & Willis, S. L. (1982). Plasticity and enhancement of intellectual functioning in old age. In F. I. M. Craik & E. E. Trehub (Eds.), *Aging and cognitive processes* (pp. 353–389). New York: Plenum Press.

Bloom, B. S. (Ed.). (1985). *Developing talent in young people*. New York: Ballantine Books.

Bouchard, C. (1986). Genetics of aerobic power and capacity. In R. M. Malina & C. Bouchard (Eds.), *Sport and human genetics* (pp. 59–88). Champaign, IL: Human Kinetics.

Bouchard, C., & Malina, R. M. (1986). Concluding remarks. In R. M. Malina & C. Bouchard (Eds.), *Sport and human genetics* (pp. 183–184). Champaign, IL: Human Kinetics.

Browne, M. A., & Mahoney, M. J. (1984). Sport psychology. *Annual Review of Psychology, 35*, 605–625.

Cavanagh, P. R., Pollock, M. L., & Landa, J. (1977). A biomechanical comparison of elite and good distance runners. *Annals of the New York Academy of Sciences, 301*, 328–345.

Chinas Männer 1986. (1987). *Leichtathletik, 26*(13), 398.

Conley, D. L., & Krahenbuhl, G. S. (1980). Running economy and distance running performance of highly trained athletes. *Medicine and Science in Sports and Exercise, 12*, 357–360.

DDR-Bestenliste 1986: Männer. (1987). *Leichtathletik, 26*(11), 328.

Elovainio, R., & Sundberg, S. (1983). A five-year follow-up study on cardiorespiratory function in adolescent elite endurance runners. *Acta Paediatrica Scandinavia, 72*, 351–356.

Ericsson, K. A., & Crutcher, R. J. (1990). The nature of exceptional performance. In P. B. Baltes, D. L. Featherman, & R. M. Lerner (Eds.), *Life-span development and behavior* (Vol. 10, pp. 187–217). Hillsdale, NJ: Lawrence Erlbaum.

Fink, W. J., Costill, D. L., & Pollock, M. L. (1977). Submaximal and maximal working capacity of elite distance runners. Part II: Muscle fiber composition and enzyme activities. *Annals of the New York Academy of Sciences, 301*, 323–327.

Fox, E. L., & Mathews, D. K. (1981). *The physiological basis of physical education and athletics* (3rd ed.). Philadelphia: Saunders.

Hagan, R. D., Smith, M. G., & Gettman, L. R. (1981). Marathon performance in relation to maximal aerobic power and training indices. *Medicine and Science in Sports and Exercise, 13*, 185–189.

Hagberg, J. M. (1987). Effects of training on the decline of VO_{2max} with aging. *Federation Proceedings, 46*, 1830–1833.

Hagberg, J. M., Allen, W. K., Seals, D. R., Hurley, B. F., Ehsani, A. A., & Holloszy, J. O. (1985). A hemodynamic comparison of young and older endurance athletes during exercise. *Journal of Applied Physiology, 58*, 2041–2046.

Hartley, A. A., & Hartley, J. T. (1984). Performance changes in champion swimmers aged 30 to 84 years. *Experimental Aging Research, 10*, 141–147.

Hartley, A. A., & Hartley, J. T. (1986). Age differences and changes in sprint swimming performances of master athletes. *Experimental Aging Research, 12*, 65–70.

Howald, H. (1982). Training-induced morphological and functional changes in skeletal muscle. *International Journal of Sports Medicine, 3*, 1–12.

Joch, W. (1979). Zu den altersabhängigen motorischen Leistungsminderungen

[On age-related decrements in motor performance]. In N. Mueller, H.-E. Roesch, & B. Wischmann (Eds.), *Alter und Leistung* [Age and performance] (pp. 197–203). Hochheim am Main, West Germany: Schors-Verlag.

Kalinowski, A. G. (1985). The development of Olympic swimmers. In B. S. Bloom (Ed.), *Developing talent in young people* (pp. 139–192). New York: Ballantine Books.

Kanadas Männer 1986. (1987). *Leichtathletik, 26*(22), 684.

Kliegl, R., & Baltes, P. B. (1987). Theory-guided analysis of mechanisms of development and aging through testing-the-limits and research on expertise. In C. Schooler & K. W. Schaie (Eds.), *Cognitive functioning and social structure over the life course* (pp. 95–119). Norwood, NJ: Ablex.

Kliegl, R., Smith, J., & Baltes, P. B. (1986). Testing-the-limits, expertise and memory in old age. In F. Klix & H. Hagendorf (Eds.), *Human memory and cognitive capabilities* (pp. 395–407). Amsterdam: North-Holland.

Lehmann, H. C. (1953). *Age and achievement.* Princeton, NJ: Princeton University Press.

Letzelter, M., Jungermann, C., & Freitag, W. (1986). Schwimmleistungen im Alter [Swimming performance in old age]. *Zeitschrift für Gerontologie, 19,* 389–395.

Monsaas, J. A. (1985). Learning to be world-class tennis player. In B. S. Bloom (Ed.), *Developing talent in young people* (pp. 211–269). New York: Ballantine Books.

Morganroth, J., & Maron, B. J. (1977). The athlete's heart syndrome: A new perspective. *Annals of the New York Academy of Sciences, 301,* 931–941.

Olympic games (1985). *The New Encyclopaedia Britannica* (15th ed., Vol. 8, pp. 926–942).

Rumäniens Männer 1986. (1987). *Leichtathletik, 26*(13), 45.

Salmons, S., & Henriksson, J. (1981). The adaptive response of skeletal muscle to increased use. *Muscle and Nerve, 4,* 94–105.

Salthouse, T. A., & Somberg, B. L. (1982). Skilled performance: Effects of adult age and experience on elementary processes. *Journal of Experimental Psychology: General, 111,* 176–207.

Saltin, B., Henriksson, J., Nygaard, E., Andersen, P., & Jansson, E. (1977). Fiber types and metabolic potentials of skeletal muscles in sedentary man and endurance in runners. *Annals of the New York Academy of Sciences, 301,* 3–29.

Schultz, R., & Curnow, C. (1988). Peak performance and age among superathletes: Track and field, swimming, baseball, tennis, and golf. *Journal of Gerontology: Psychological Sciences, 43,* 113–120.

Stones, M. J., & Kozma, A. (1981). Adult age trends in athletic performances. *Experimental Aging Research, 17,* 269–280.

Stones, M. J., & Kozma, A. (1982). Cross-sectional, longitudinal, and secular age trends in athletic performances. *Experimental Aging Research, 8,* 185–188.

Stones, M. J., & Kozma, A. (1984). Longitudinal trends in track and field performances. *Experimental Aging Research, 10,* 107–110.

Subotnick, S. I. (1977). A biomechanical approach to running injuries. *Annals of the New York Academy of Sciences, 301,* 888–899.

Tesch, P. A., & Karlsson, J. (1985). Muscle fiber types and size in trained and untrained muscles of elite athletes. *Journal of Applied Physiology, 59,* 1716–1720.

UDSSR-Männer 1986. (1987). *Leichtathletik, 26*(13), 395–396.

USA-Männer 1986. (1986). *Leichtathletik, 25*(47), 1515–1516.

Wallingford, R. (1975). Long distance running. In A. W. Tayler & F. Landry (Eds.), *The scientific aspects of sports training* (pp. 118–130). Springfield, IL: Thomas.

zur Megede, E. (1968). *Die Geschichte der olympischen Leichtathletik* [History of track and field in the Olympic games] (Vol. 1). Munich: Verlag Bartels & Wernitz.

zur Megede, E. (1987). *Progression of world best performances and official IAAF world records.* Monaco: International Athletic Foundation.

7   Personal control over development and quality of life perspectives in adulthood

JOCHEN BRANDTSTÄDTER AND
BERNHARD BALTES-GÖTZ

Introduction

Construing cohesion and coherence in human development over the life span is often seen as coterminous with the search for causal order (see Overton & Reese, 1981). The search for continuous causal chains in development, however, tends to obscure the fact that the conditions constituting the developmental ecology for an individual are to a large extent the results of actions. Human development is, by nature, dependent on culture; observed developmental patterns reflect tendencies of development-related control extant in a given cultural and historical situation. Developmental research, thus, has to investigate not only the causal nexus but also the actional nexus between developmental phenomena. We have to extend the scope of our explanatory schemes to account not only for the causal mechanisms but also for the systems of action that generate developmental changes, and we have to recognize that observed regularities of development usually have the status of quasi laws that are conditional on the execution (or nonexecution) of certain actions and interventions (see Brandtstädter, 1981, 1984).

Cultural formation of development involves, and is partly mediated by, processes of self-regulation. The adult person shapes his or her development by opting for certain life designs, striving toward developmental goals, as well as by selecting and constructing developmental niches that fit personal interests and competences (Lerner & Lerner, 1983; Super & Harkness, 1986). Individuals, however, are not the sole producers of their development. Any effort to optimize personal development over the life span is subject to cultural and natural constraints and usually generates unpredicted and unintended side effects. Thus, a person's life course always braids together autonomous and heteronomous influences.

197

The subjective weighting of autonomous and heteronomous influences on personal development varies widely in different individuals. Such development-related beliefs, being dependent on personal experience as well as on the interchange of naive and scientific views about the life course, are themselves subject to age-graded and historical changes. Unfortunately, garnered evidence on this issue is scant and inconsistent (see Krampen, 1987; Lachman, 1986; Rodin, 1987; Shupe, 1985). We can nevertheless assume that control beliefs – and especially beliefs related to the control of personal development – deeply influence the ways in which individuals experience, and try to manage, their development in different phases and areas of life. Self-percepts of control over personal development influence the attribution of responsibility for developmental outcomes and achievements, they motivate efforts to counteract anticipated developmental losses, and thus, they should determine the emotional quality of developmental prospects in adulthood and old age.

There are, thus, reasons to consider development-related control beliefs as key variables for optimal development and successful aging (see also Shupe, 1985; Thomae, 1981). This basic assumption, however, needs to be qualified in certain respects. The quality of one's life perspective not only hinges on subjective potentials to attain personally valued developmental options but also crucially depends on the adjustment of developmental aspirations to personal capabilities and contextual constraints. If personal control is defined in terms of subjective potentials to realize personally important goals, it follows that a sense of power and control can also be maintained by accommodating preferences to feasible options and by disengaging from goals that seem inherently inaccessible (Elster, 1983). The potential psychological benefits of adjusting preferences to situational constraints have already been stressed in the traditional distinction between defensive and offensive conceptions of happiness (Tatarkiewicz, 1984), and the problem of finding an appropriate balance between adaptive and counteradaptive attitudes has been a key issue in philosophical conceptions of wisdom and successful living (Kamlah, 1973; Schopenhauer, 1851).

In 1982 we launched a cross-sequential research project centering on the theme of personal self-regulation of development in adulthood (see also Brandtstädter, 1989; Brandtstädter, Krampen, & Greve, 1987; Brandtstädter, Krampen, & Heil, 1986).[1] In the following, we will present findings from this project that bear on conditions and variations of successful aging. Three particular issues will be highlighted. First, patterns of age-related change in development-related control beliefs (autonomous and heteronomous control) will be discussed, and the relationship of these control beliefs to the individual's emotional appraisal of his or her developmental achievements and prospects will be examined. Second, we will present some findings concerning accommodative readjustments in developmental goals and their relationship to depression. Finally, evidence for an age-related shift in strategies of coping and control will be presented. Before turning to results, we will briefly describe our research approach.

Research approach

Sample

The analyses reported below are based on questionnaire data obtained in the first three waves (1983, 1985, 1987) of a longitudinal cohort sequence on a sample of 1,228 participants (married couples). Participants were recruited from an urban area in southwestern Germany. As regards level of income, education, and occupational status, the sample is fairly representative of the general population, with a majority of subjects belonging to the middle class. For cross-sequential comparisons, subjects were grouped into five cohorts (age ranges and number of subjects within birth cohorts refer to first time of measurement): (1) 30–35 years (254), (2) 36–41 (244), (3) 42–47 years (267), (4) 48–53 years (228), and (5) 54–59 years (235). Respondents were remunerated for participation. Over 70% of the initial sample participated at both longitudinal replications, which span a longitudinal interval of 4 years. No systematic dropout effect was observed on the central variables considered in the present study.

Variables

The questionnaire used in this investigation was designed to assess various facets of the individual's cognitive appraisal of his or her developmental situation, with a special focus on development-related control beliefs.[2]

For different goal dimensions of development, participants rated

- the personal importance of each goal;
- the perceived distance from the goal;
- the extent to which developmental progress on each goal dimension depends on personal effort;
- the extent to which development on each goal dimension is affected by uncontrollable factors;
- the subjective reserve potential for goal achievement;
- the anticipated change toward or away from the goal;
- the extent to which goal attainment is seen as supported by the spouse.

These assessments were made with reference to the following developmental goals: (1) health, physical well-being; (2) emotional stability; (3) wisdom, mature understanding of life; (4) self-esteem; (5) social recognition; (6) occupational efficiency; (7) assertiveness, self-assurance; (8) harmonious partnership; (9) empathy; (10) personal independence; (11) family security; (12) prosperity, comfortable standard of living; (13) intellectual efficiency; (14) self-development; (15) physical fitness; (16) satisfying friendship; and (17) commitment to ideals. This selection of goals partly follows Rokeach's (1973) taxonomy of terminal values.

Further parts of the questionnaire referred to emotional and behavioral aspects of self-regulation. For 16 different domains of behavior, each represented by three behavioral facets, subjects had to rate the actual strength or salience of each behavioral aspect, as well as intended behavioral changes. Participants were also asked to describe their feelings with regard to personal development (1) looking back on the past 3 years of life and (2) looking forward to the coming 3 years of life. For the prospective and retrospective modes, two lists of adjective scales were used.

The various ratings were effected on unipolar and bipolar Likert-type scales. The questionnaire battery further comprised reference measures for the assessment of generalized control beliefs (IPC scales according to Levenson, German version: Krampen, 1981), personality traits (Freiburger Persönlichkeits-Inventar, FPI, short version: Fahrenberg, Hampel, & Selg, 1973), marital adjustment (Dyadic Adjustment Scale, DAS: Spanier, 1976), and general life satisfaction (Löhr & Walter, 1974; Wiendieck, 1970).

On the third occasion of measurement (1987), a newly developed questionnaire focusing on processes of disengagement and preference accommodation was added to the set of variables. A brief description of this instrument will be given in a later section.

Construction of aggregated indices of personal development

From the questionnaire data, several aggregated indicators were derived relating to different aspects of the subject's evaluation of his or her personal development. These indicators, as well as the aggregational procedures, are described in Table 7.1. The aggregational approach has some distinct methodological advantages in the present research context. Aggregated measures are less susceptible to floor and ceiling effects than single scales, and they also seem less susceptible to response biases than usual self-reports. Furthermore, the study of differential longitudinal change presupposes highly reliable measurement procedures. This re-

Table 7.1. *Assessment of development-related cognitions and emotions: Construction of aggregated index variables*

Index variable	Basic scales (sample questions)	Aggregation formula	Internal consistency (α)
Autonomous Control over Development (CDA)	For each goal g ($g = 1, \ldots, 17$): • Personal importance of g ("How important is this goal for you personally?") (pi_g) • Self-percepts of control with respect to g ("To what extent is achieving this goal dependent on your own behavior?") (ac_g)	$\sum\limits_g ac_g pi_g$	.89
Heteronomous Control over Development (CDH)	For each goal g: • Perceived impact of uncontrollable factors on development with respect to g ("To what extent is achieving this goal dependent on conditions over which you have no control?") (hc_g) • Personal importance of g (pi_g)	$\sum\limits_g hc_g pi_g$	.89
Personal Control over Development (PCD)	For each goal g: • Self-percepts of control with respect to g (ac_g) • Perceived impact of uncontrollable factors on development with respect to g (hc_g) • Personal importance of g (pi_g)	$\sum\limits_g (ac_g - hc_g)\, pi_g$ ($= \text{CDA} - \text{CDH}$)	.89
Depressive Outlook on Personal Development (DPR)	Selected adjective scales referring to the emotional evaluation of past (P) and future (F) personal development: • P5 ("depressed") • F5 ("discouraged") • P7 ("resigned") • F8 ("being at a loss") • P10 ("powerless") • F13 ("depressed")	Sum of self-ratings on P5, P7, P10, F5, F8, F13	.80

Table 7.1. (cont.)

Index variable	Basic scales (sample questions)	Aggregation formula	Internal consistency (α)
Subjective Developmental Deficit (SDD)	For each goal g: • Perceived distance from g ("How far are you presently from achieving this goal?") (d_g) • Personal importance of g (pi_g)	$\sum_g d_g pi_g$	.88
Anticipated Developmental Gain (ADG)	For each goal g: • Anticipated change toward or away from g ("Suppose you did not change your way of living: To what extent would you come closer to or depart from this goal over the next 3 years?") (ec_g) • Personal importance of g (pi_g)	$\sum_g ec_g pi_g$	.94
Self-corrective Tendency (SCT)	For each behavioral aspect b ($b = 1, \ldots, 48$): • Intended behavioral change with respect to b ("To what extent do you intend to change your behavior or increase your efforts in this respect?") (ct_b)	$\sum_b ct_b$	.97
Perceived Marital Support (PMS)	For each goal g: • Perceived marital support with respect to g ("To what extent does your partner support or hinder you in achieving this goal?") (sp_g) • Personal importance of g (pi_g)	$\sum_g sp_g pi_g$	.94
Subjective Developmental Reserve (SDR)	For each goal g: • Reserve potential for attainment of g ("If you undertook every effort, to what extent could you achieve this goal?") (dr_g) • Personal importance of g (pi_g)	$\sum_g dr_g pi_g$	.91

quirement is more easily met by aggregated variables, because the aggregation procedure eliminates uncorrelated error at the level of basic variables. Internal consistency coefficients obtained for the main sample are given in Table 7.1. Retest reliabilities, estimated over a short time interval (1–13 days) on an independent sample (83 psychology under-graduates), range between .78 (for Subjective Developmental Deficit, SDD) and .85 (for Self-corrective Tendency, SCT). Longitudinal stabil-ity over the 4-year interval was found to be lowest for Subjective De-velopmental Deficit (.45) and highest for Perceived Marital Support, PMS (.67). In the following, we will first turn to the cross-sequential findings for the three indicators relating to self-percepts of control over development.

Development-related control beliefs: Cross-sequential findings

Let us first take a closer look at the findings for Personal Control over Development (PCD). Figure 7.1 depicts the cross-sectional gradients for the first (1983) and third (1987) occasion of measurement as well as the corresponding 4-year longitudinal changes. The pattern of effects was evaluated by a nonorthogonal (5 × 2 × 3) ANOVA involving the factors of Cohort (C), Gender (G), and Time of Measurement (T). Because neither the effect of G nor any of the interactions involving G attain significance, we can retain the assumption that the developmental pattern for Personal Control over Development does not systematically differ for the male and female groups.

The cross-sectional gradients shown in Figure 7.1 suggest that perceived control over personal development diminishes over the age range studied; the main effect of C is highly significant, $F(4, 566) = 8.49$, $p < .001$. In contrast, the longitudinal gradients exhibit a less-consistent pattern (Fig-ure 7.2). In general, they reveal a fair degree of stability on the level of group means; the main effect of T does not attain significance, and cohort differences in longitudinal change as reflected by the T × C interaction fall short of significance, too.

Remember that Personal Control over Development was constructed as the difference between the indicators of Autonomous Control over De-velopment (CDA) and Heteronomous Control over Development (CDH). These two components are not polar opposites but constitute largely independent aspects of perceived control (the correlation at Time 3 is .16). Accordingly, the possibility has to be considered that Autonomous Con-trol over Development and Heternomous Control over Development

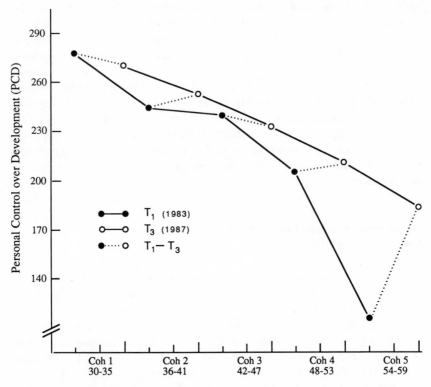

Figure 7.1. Personal Control over Development: Cross-sectional comparisons and 4-year longitudinal changes (occasions 1983 and 1987; age ranges for cohorts refer to first occasion).

when considered separately do not simply exhibit an opposite developmental pattern as would be implied by a unidimensional–bipolar (internal vs. external) conception of control. Figure 7.3 and 7.4 depict cross-sectional differences and 4-year longitudinal changes for these two components. Except for a significant main effect of G on Heteronomous Control ($F[1, 649] = 4.12, p < .05 [f > m]$), no systematic effects related to G were observed.

Longitudinal and cross-sectional findings for Heteronomous Control over Development (Figure 7.3) suggest that in middle and later adulthood, personal development is increasingly seen as influenced by factors outside personal control (main effect for C: $F[4, 649] = 11.41, p < .001$; main effect for T: $F[2, 648] = 4.65, p < .01$). For Cohort 5, the longitudinal findings indicate a turnaround toward lower levels of Heteronomous Control. The apparent decrease of Heteronomous Control in

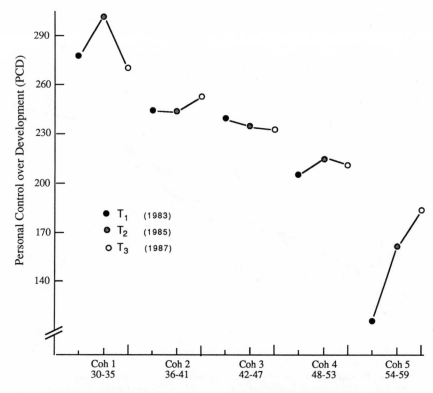

Figure 7.2. Personal Control over Development: Longitudinal gradients for Cohorts 1–5 (occasions 1983, 1985, 1987; age ranges for cohorts refer to first occasion).

later adulthood (which is consistent with the longitudinal increase in Personal Control over Development for the same age range; see Figure 7.2) may be related to the transition to retirement; those who have retired or approach the age of retirement may experience more freedom in planning their lives and personal futures.

The results for Autonomous Control over Development are less clearcut. Whereas cross-sectional differences between age-groups do not reach significance, the 4-year longitudinal gradients for Cohorts 2 to 5 indicate an age-related *increase* in Autonomous Control (main effect for T: $F[2, 668] = 7.53$, $p < .001$).

These findings may be summarized as follows. In middle and later adulthood – at least up to the late fifties – personal development is increasingly seen as affected by heteronomous influences beyond personal control. There is, however, no convincing evidence for a correspond-

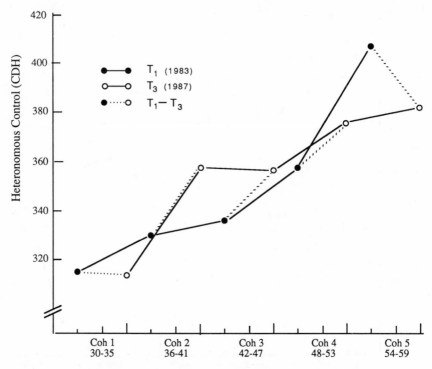

Figure 7.3. Heteronomous Control over Development: Cross-sectional comparisons and 4-year longitudinal changes (occasions 1983 and 1987; age ranges for cohorts refer to first occasion).

ing age-related decrease in autonomous control over personal development, that is, in the perceived dependence of developmental achievements and prospects on personal behavior. On the contrary, longitudinal findings indicate that self-percepts of autonomous control become more pronounced during middle and later adulthood.[3] The finding that longitudinal changes in Autonomous Control and Heteronomous Control have the same directionality may seem counterintuitive at first glance, but it is by no means conceptually incoherent, given the orthogonal feature of these indicators of personal control. As we have argued elsewhere (Brandtstädter, Krampen, & Baltes-Götz, 1989), the impact of external and accidental influences on personal development may be felt more distinctly by the older person, but this experience may also instigate self-regulatory efforts to optimize the course of development in later life. As the results for Personal Control demonstrate, converging changes in autonomous and heteronomous facets of control may cancel each

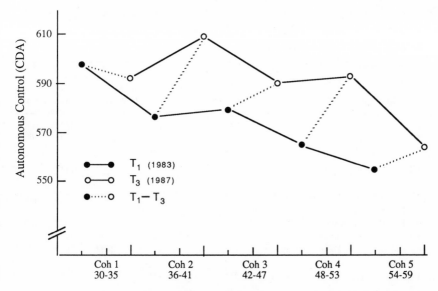

Figure 7.4. Autonomous Control over Development: Cross-sectional comparisons and 4-year longitudinal changes (occasions 1983 and 1987; age ranges for cohorts refer to first occasion).

other out on a global level of assessment, so that a (possibly misleading) picture of stability results.

Control beliefs and subjective quality of personal development

As intimated above, different lines of theoretical argument converge in suggesting that self-percepts of control over development should be closely related to the emotional evaluation of personal developmental prospects. People having a strong sense of autonomous control should be more self-confident and persistent in the face of obstacles, they should be more prone to meet potentially enriching challenges, and at least in the long run, they should be more efficient in achieving their life goals than individuals entertaining doubts about their self-regulatory capacities (Bandura, 1981). Perceived deficits of control over personally significant areas of life, on the other hand, most likely give rise to feelings of futility and alienation. Whether people find their lives meaningful depends on whether they are committed to subjectively meaningful goals, and this commitment, in turn, presupposes self-percepts of control and efficacy (Klinger, 1977). In a similar vein, helplessness theorists consider per-

Table 7.2. *Correlations of Personal Control over Development (PCD), Autonomous Control over Development (CDA), and Heteronomous Control over Development (CDH) with selected reference measures*

Variable	Time 1 (1983)			Time 3 (1987)		
	PCD	CDA	CDH	PCD	CDA	CDH
IPC – Internality	.33**	.28**	−.11**	.28**	.30**	−.04
IPC – Powerful Others	−.31**	−.16**	.23**	−.26**	−.12**	.23**
IPC – Chance Control	−.26**	−.12**	.22**	−.26**	−.08*	.26**
ADG – Anticipated Developmental Gain	.31**	.47**	.11**	.28**	.44**	.11**
SDD – Subjective Developmental Deficit	−.27**	.05	.40**	−.20**	.05	.36**
SCT – Self-corrective Tendency	−.02	.23**	.27**	−.01	.19**	.23**
DPR – Depressive Outlook	−.36**	−.20**	.25**	−.31**	−.17**	.22**
SDR – Subjective Developmental Reserve	.37**	.67**	.24**	.38**	.66**	.22**
PMS – Perceived Marital Support	.28**	.43**	.10**	.26**	.39**	.11**
LS – Life Satisfaction	.28**	.19**	−.15**	.27**	.20**	−.13**
DAS – Dyadic Adjustment	.20**	.10**	−.15**	.14**	.11**	−.06
Age	−.18**	−.06*	.18**	−.14**	−.05	.14**
Sex (*f*)	−.03	−.01	.03	−.01	−.02	−.04
Education	.14**	.05	−.12**	.07	.02	−.07

Note: N (Time 1) ≥ 973; N (Time 3) ≥ 701 (pairwise deletion of missing data).
*p ≤ .05. **p ≤ .01.

ceived loss of control over personally important concerns to be the central etiological factor in the development of depression (e.g., Peterson & Seligman, 1984). Such arguments strongly support the assumption that self-percepts of control over development should generally be associated with a positive and optimistic evaluation of developmental achievements and prospects.

Our results are largely consistent with this basic assumption. Let us begin by looking at the correlational patterns reported in Table 7.2 (because the findings are highly consistent across all three measurement points, we can restrict our discussion to Time 1 and Time 3). Persons scoring high in Personal Control over Development are more satisfied with their lives; they report less marital problems and seem to have a more optimistic (or less depressive) outlook; they also tend to ascribe to themselves lower levels of Subjective Developmental Deficit, as well as greater Subjective Developmental Reserve. As expected, Personal Control over Development is positively related to generalized "internal" control beliefs (IPC-I). The correlational pattern for Autonomous Control over Development is rather similar to that obtained for PCD. In contrast, subjects scoring high in Heteronomous Control experience larger developmental deficits (high Subjective Developmental Deficit) and also report lower levels of life satisfaction and marital adjustment. The correlational patterns exhibit a high degree of stability over the 4-year interval.

As mentioned earlier, participants were asked to describe their feelings with regard to their past and future development. As might already be extrapolated from the findings above, Autonomous Control and Heteronomous Control – although they have little variance overlap – predict diametrically opposed emotional syndromes. Table 7.3 shows multiple correlations of Personal, Autonomous, and Heteronomous Control with self-attributed emotions obtained for the first and third testing occasions. As expected, self-percepts of control are associated with a generally positive and optimistic outlook on personal development. Subjects scoring high in Personal Control or Autonomous Control tend to describe their feelings in terms like *proud, happy, glad,* and *satisfied*; looking toward the future, they feel more *hopeful, calm, confident,* and *venturesome.* Heteronomous Control, in turn, predicts a converse pattern of depression, despondency, and worry. Again, the correlational structures are highly stable or stationary over time.

It is remarkable that similar patterns of covariation emerge when we consider differential longitudinal change over the 4-year interval (Time 3 − Time 1). As Table 7.4 shows, increases in Personal Control or Autonomous Control go with increases in Anticipated Developmental Gain (ADG), Subjective Developmental Reserve, and Perceived Marital Support and are generally accompanied by shifts toward a positive evaluation of past and future personal development. Increases in Heteronomous Control, on the other hand, are symptomatic of a general deterioration of developmental prospects. Though difference scores are generally less reliable than the basic measures, these relationships are conceptually consistent and highly significant. Very similar findings are obtained when base-free, or residualized, change is considered, that is, when we remove from the longitudinal changes the portion that can be linearly predicted from the Time 1 measures. Whereas simple differences, due to regression effects, are generally negatively correlated with initial measurements, residualized change scores are statistically independent of initial status; they thus reflect positional changes within the sample, or "normative" change (as given by Kagan, 1980).

Table 7.3. *Multiple correlations of Personal Control over Development (PCD), Autonomous Control over Development (CDA), and Heteronomous Control over Development (CDH) with ratings of emotional attitude toward past (P) and future (F) personal development*

Predictor variables (self-attributed emotions)	Time 1 (1983)			Time 3 (1987)		
	PCD	CDA	CDH	PCD	CDA	CDH
P – 1 distressed	−.52	−.24	.60	−.63	−.41	.43
P – 2 proud	.40	.58	.12	.36	.44	.02
P – 3 happy	.51	.48	−.23	.45	.39	−.20
P – 4 exhausted	−.62	−.25	.69	−.51	−.28	.46
P – 5 depressed	−.65	.30	.68	−.62	−.30	.60
P – 6 glad	.59	.55	−.27	.57	.50	−.25
P – 7 resigned	−.69	−.43	.61	−.60	−.32	.55
P – 8 indifferent	−.56	−.45	.37	−.21	−.30	.41
P – 9 satisfied	.53	.39	−.38	.50	.45	−.20
P – 10 powerless	−.67	−.34	.70	−.61	−.31	.56
P – 11 angry	−.50	−.21	.57	−.48	−.23	.47
P – 12 grateful	.42	.46	−.10	.43	.50	.06
P – 13 sad	−.61	−.32	.62	−.62	−.36	.49
F – 1 hopeful	.61	.68	−.13	.71	.74	−.15
F – 2 calm	.49	.43	−.26	.55	.52	−.20
F – 3 uneasy	−.54	−.30	.52	−.52	−.30	.44
F – 4 cheerful	.23	.24	−.04	.16	.08	−.15
F – 5 discouraged	−.72	−.43	.66	−.71	−.41	.61
F – 6 worried	−.15	−.06	.13	−.16	−.21	−.04
F – 7 anxious	−.50	−.22	.57	−.63	−.31	.66
F – 8 at a loss	−.54	.33	.48	−.71	−.36	.67
F – 9 fearful	−.54	.23	.62	−.70	−.31	.75
F – 10 confident	.65	.57	−.35	.61	.50	−.34
F – 11 troubled	−.31	−.11	.38	−.57	−.30	.56
F – 12 venturesome	.62	.78	−.06	.71	.83	.00
F – 13 depressed	−.61	−.37	.57	−.69	−.36	.62
R	.45**	.43**	.33**	.40**	.41**	.31**
N	1,057	1,120	1,108	757	813	794

Note: To facilitate interpretation of regression structures, correlations between predictors and multiple regression functions (regression structure coefficients) are given instead of beta weights.

$**p \leq .01$ (listwise deletion of missing data).

Table 7.4. *Multiple correlations of change in Personal Control over Development (PCD), Autonomous Control over Development (CDA), and Heteronomous Control over Development (CDH) with change in selected indicators of successful development*

Predictor variables	Simple differences (Time 3 − Time 1)			Residualized change (Time 3 − Time 1)		
	PCD	CDA	CDH	PCD	CDA	CDH
ADG – Anticipated Developmental Gain	.65	.58	−.07	.64	.63	.14
SDD – Subjective Developmental Deficit	−.40	.10	.77	−.42	.13	.78
SCT – Self-corrective Tendency	−.05	.19	.38	−.13	.18	.46
DPR – Depressive Outlook	−.40	−.10	.46	−.40	−.13	.33
SDR – Subjective Developmental Reserve	.67	.88	.25	.69	.91	.40
PMS – Perceived Marital Support	.59	.59	.06	.55	.59	.22
LS – Life Satisfaction	.37	.17	−.34	.48	.24	−.27
DAS – Dyadic Adjustment	.22	.15	−.10	.23	.17	.00
P – 2 proud	.20	.27	.06	.22	.29	.13
P – 3 happy	.23	.20	−.06	.27	.23	−.02
P – 5 depressed	−.33	−.12	.32	−.31	−.14	.23
P – 9 satisfied	.35	.13	−.38	.33	.19	−.16
P – 11 angry	−.27	−.16	.13	−.22	−.09	.17
P – 12 grateful	.30	.17	−.23	.36	.25	−.04
F – 1 hopeful	.38	.27	−.18	.41	.34	−.02
F – 2 calm	.30	.07	−.34	.38	.24	−.11
F – 5 discouraged	−.40	−.10	.41	−.42	−.17	.31
F – 9 fearful	−.20	.00	.38	−.33	−.08	.36
F – 12 venturesome	.39	.29	−.16	.43	.41	.07
F – 13 depressed	−.29	−.05	.38	−.37	−.12	.30
R	.47**	.58**	.40**	.48**	.62**	.44**
N	408	450	441	408	450	441

Note: Intraindividual changes over a 4-year longitudinal interval (1983–1987). To facilitate interpretation of regression structures, correlations between predictors and multiple regression functions (regression structure coefficients) are given instead of beta weights.
**$p \leq .01$ (listwise deletion of missing data).

Accommodative modes of coping and control

Development-related control activities involve attempts to shape the course of development so that it fits with personal goals and preferences. This mode of control has to be distinguished from the adjustment of goals and preferences to perceived action potentials, developmental resources, and contextual affordances. Whereas the former strategy basically aims at *assimilating* given circumstances to individual life designs, the latter one involves the *accommodation* of one's life design to experienced constraints.[4] This dual-process conception converges to some extent with the distinction between problem-focused and emotion-focused coping (Lazarus & Launier, 1978; Moos & Billings, 1982) or between primary and secondary control (Rothbaum, Weisz, & Snyder, 1982); its theoretical underpinnings are elaborated in greater detail elsewhere (Brandtstädter, 1989; Brandtstädter & Renner, 1990). Where the individual is confronted with aversive changes or losses that are unavoidable or irreversible, disengagement from thwarted developmental options and reorientation toward new and meaningful perspectives are obviously the only means to regain or maintain satisfying developmental prospects (see also Klinger, 1977). Here, the salient process is not the solution but rather the *dissolution* of developmental problems by affective reevaluation, rescaling of aspirations, or search for meaning. This process is often reactive and should not be considered as a deliberately chosen strategy of coping or control (parenthetically, this is one issue on which our position differs from the notion of primary vs. secondary control as introduced by Rothbaum, Weisz, & Snyder, 1982).

It may be instructive to consider briefly a further complex of findings that ties in with these arguments. As mentioned, participants were asked for a variety of developmental goals to rate the subjective importance of and the perceived distance from each goal. Remember that both ratings are involved in the aggregation of Subjective Developmental Deficit (see Table 7.1). Accommodative processes involving disengagement from thwarted goals and rescaling of aspirations should affect the relationship between distance and importance ratings. We found that for nearly all goal dimensions considered, importance ratings covaried negatively with distance ratings (the one noticeable exception was the goal dimension of "health, physical well-being"). For Time 1, intercorrelations ranged between .12 and −.43, with a mean correlation of −.17 over all 17 goal dimensions (with $N = 997$, coefficients beyond −.07 exceed the .01 level of significance). For Time 2 and Time 3, very similar results were obtained. Significant inverse relationships between distance and importance ratings were also observed for longitudinal change scores (Time 3 − Time 1); that is, intraindividual changes toward goals are related to raised importance ratings, but shifts away from goals are accompanied by a devaluation of the respective goals. Presumably, such reevaluations can be considered an accommodative reaction that minimizes experienced developmental deficits and enables the subject to maintain satisfying developmental prospects.

This train of thought led us to assume that the observed regression of importance on distance ratings should be moderated by measures of depression; more specifically, with rising levels of depression (as measured by Depressive Outlook on Personal Development, see Table 7.1), the slope of the regression line should become less negative or even change its sign. This prediction was borne out for 15 out of 17 goal dimensions. Figure 7.5 exemplifies this effect for a selected goal dimension (Goal 16, "satisfying friendship"). The conditional regression functions were obtained by hierarchical regression; the moderating effect of Depressive Outlook on the relationship between rated distance from goal (D) and personal goal importance (I) is documented by the fact that the predicted variance in importance ratings significantly increases when the product variable D × DPR is entered in the multiple regression (for the given example, $F_{change}[1, 1240] = 22.4, p < .01$; Time 1 data). The moderation effects are not very strong but are highly consistent across goal dimensions and times of measurement.

Evidence for an age-related shift in strategies of coping and control

The findings reported in the last section have prompted an extension of the questionnaire battery used in our project. On the third occasion of measurement (1987), we added to the variable set a short questionnaire derived from the theoretical distinction between assimilative and accommodative modes of coping.

Before turning to the cross-sectional results, let us briefly describe the new instrument (for details, see Brandtstädter & Renner, 1990). The questionnaire consists of two independent scales – Flexible Goal Adjustment (FGA) and Tenacious Goal Pursuit (TGP) – each comprising 15 items. FGA assesses the individual's capability or disposition to flexibly revise or disengage from thwarted commitments and aspirations and to build up new and meaningful perspectives for personal development easily (sample items: "In general, I'm not upset very long about an opportunity passed up." "I can adapt quite easily to changes in a situation." "Even if everything goes wrong, I still can find something positive about the situation." "I usually recognize quite easily my own

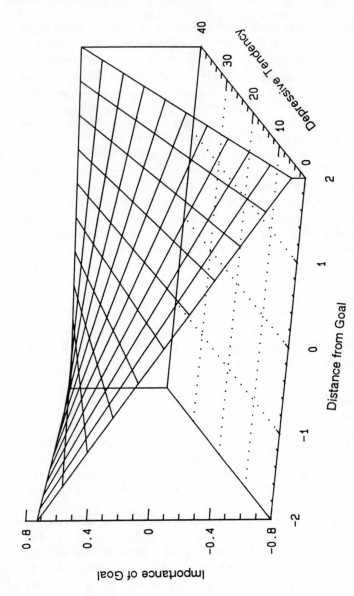

Figure 7.5. Conditional regression of personal goal importance on perceived goal distance at different levels of depression (sample case: Goal 16, "satisfying friendship"). Predictor (distance) and criterion (importance) are scaled in standardized (*z*) units; the moderator variable (depressive tendency) is given in raw units.

limitations."). The TGP scale, on the other hand, taps an offensive style of coping and control that is characterized by a tendency to defend a personal commitment or maintain a chosen course of action even against greatest difficulties (sample items: "The harder a goal is to achieve, the more desirable it often appears to me." "Even if everything seems hopeless, I still look for a way to master the situation."). The psychometric qualities of the scale as well as correlations with selected reference variables were investigated in a pilot study on a sample of 109 men and 97 women (mean age: 34.3 years). Internal consistencies were found to be satisfactory (FGA: $\alpha = .83$; TGP: $\alpha = .80$). FGA and TGP showed little variance overlap ($r = .06$); flexible adjustment of goals and tenacious goal pursuit, thus, do not denote opposite or mutually exclusive dispositions. Consistent with their coping-theoretical interpretation, both scales were found to correlate positively with optimism (as measured by the Life Orientation Test: Scheier & Carver, 1985) and with failure-related action orientation (as measured by the Action Control Scale: see Kuhl, 1985); furthermore, both scales were negatively related to depressive tendencies (Brandtstädter & Renner, 1990).

At present, the question of how the dynamics of coping and control change with the processes of aging is largely unsettled (Lazarus & DeLongis, 1983; McCrae, 1982). However, a fair amount of agreement exists that uncontrollable events and life changes cumulate as we grow older (Baltes, 1973; Brim & Ryff, 1980; Seligman & Elder, 1986), an assumption congruent with our own observation that the perceived impact of heteronomous factors on personal development increases in middle and later adulthood. Thus, it is plausible to expect a gradual shift in emphasis from assimilative or offensive to accommodative strategies of coping and control.

In point of fact, FGA and TGP exhibit clear-cut opposite relationships with age. The correlations found in the pilot study were .34, $p < .01$, for FGA, and $-.18, p < .01$, for TGP (the difference between these dependent correlation coefficients is significant with $p < .001$). The cross-sectional findings for the third wave (1987) replicate this result and lend further empirical support to the assumption of an age-related shift from assimilative to accommodative modes of coping. For TGP, the two-factorial (Cohort × Gender) ANOVA yields highly significant main effects for Cohort, $F(4, 865) = 2.92, p < .05$, and Gender, $F(1, 865) = 14.91, p < .001$. For FGA, too, differences between age-groups are highly significant, $F(4, 862) = 6.09, p < .001$, whereas gender differences fall short of significance. Again the linear regressions of TGP and FGA on age clearly differ in direction (FGA: .14, $p < .01$; TGP: $-.14, p < .01$; the difference is significant with $p < .001$). Figures 7.6 and 7.7 show the pattern of effects.

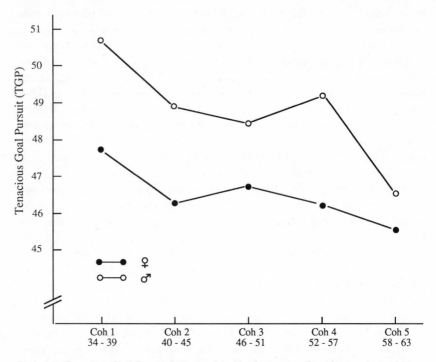

Figure 7.6. Tenacious Goal Pursuit by age and gender (age ranges for cohorts refer to 1987 occasion).

The opposite relationship of FGA and TGP to the age variable is remarkable, given the fact that the scales have little variance in common and show similar relationships to various measures of personality and perceived quality of personal development. The results from this larger study replicate the earlier finding that both scales predict absence of depression (correlation with the Depressive Outlook composite: $-.25$, $p < .01$, for TGP; $-.33$, $p < .01$, for FGA). Furthermore, both scales were found to have significant positive correlations with Personal Control over Development (TGP: .21, $p < .01$; FGA: .21, $p < .01$), Subjective Developmental Reserve (TGP: .21, $p < .01$; FGA: .22, $p < .01$), Anticipated Developmental Gain (TGP: .21, $p < .01$; FGA: .33, $p < .01$), Life Satisfaction (TGP: .29, $p < .01$; FGA: .37, $p < .01$), and FPI/Emotional Stability (TGP: .28, $p < .01$; FGA: .35, $p < .01$). With regard to issues of discriminant validity, it should be noted that the scales are differentially predictive of Perceived Marital Support (TGP: .09, $p < .05$; FGA: .30, $p < .01$), as well as of personality traits such as FPI/Aggression (TGP: .05; FGA: $-.19$, $p < .01$), FPI/Dominance (TGP: $-.05$; FGA: $-.25$, $p <$

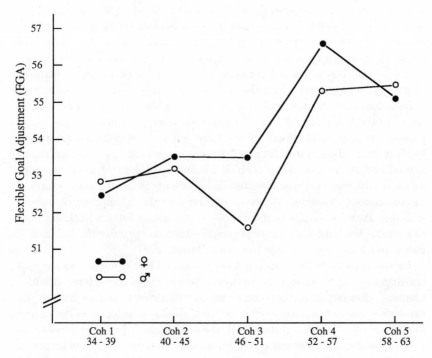

Figure 7.7. Flexible Goal Adjustment by age and gender (age ranges for cohorts refer to 1987 occasion).

.01), and FPI/Calmness (TGP: .21, $p < .01$; FGA: .51, $p < .01$) (differences between correlations are significant with $p < .001$).

Summary and discussion

Development over the life span is shaped by personal actions as well as by uncontrolled influences. Individuals vary in the degree to which they attribute developmental changes to their own actions and efforts or to heteronomous factors beyond personal control. In our research project, these differences were assessed by aggregated indicators of perceived autonomous and heteronomous control over development, which are derived from ratings concerning the influence of controllable and uncontrollable factors on the achievement of personally valued goals of development. Age differences and age-related change in these variables were evaluated in a cross-sequential approach spanning an age range of 30–60 years and a longitudinal interval of 4 years. The findings clearly indicate that the perceived influence of heteronomous factors on personal development increases during middle and later adulthood. This increase may reflect feelings of obsolescence and the growing impact of age-related life transitions and critical events (physical problems, loss of friends and relatives, mandatory retirement, and so on). The increase in Heteronomous Control continues at least up to the late fifties; there are indications of a slight turnaround when the individual approaches retirement.

Believing that the personal biography is to a large extent dependent on uncontrollable factors, however, apparently does not imply for the aging person that personal efforts to optimize one's developmental prospects become futile. In point of fact, there were no indications of a significant age-related decrement in perceived autonomous control over development; on the contrary, the longitudinal gradients indicated some increase in Autonomous Control. We have argued that the felt impact of uncontrollable aversive events that typically cumulate in later adulthood may not inhibit but rather instigate personal efforts to optimize the balance of gains and losses in later life (see also Baltes, 1987).

In the composite of Personal Control over Development, which was constructed as the difference between Autonomous and Heteronomous Control, changes in autonomous and heteronomous control having the same directionality cancel each other out, so that developmental changes are less marked on this global level of assessment. It becomes obvious at this point that the complex developmental changes in self-percepts of control such as those documented in the present study cannot easily be captured by bipolar–unidimensional conceptions of internal versus external control. To date, developmental changes in perceived control have been investigated largely within such a unidimensional framework, and this may be one reason for the amazing inconsistency of findings in this field (see Krampen, 1987; Lachman, 1986; Rodin, 1987).

Some methodological reservations concerning the interpretation of our cross-sequential findings have to be made. As is well known, longitudinal comparisons confound age-related changes with effects related to occasions of measurement, whereas cross-sectional comparisons notoriously confound age with cohort effects. There is no way to simultaneously assess these different but mathematically interdependent sources of developmental variation. We can, however, evaluate how far the obtained data pattern is consistent with a specified a priori structure of effects. Under the assumption that the cross-sequential patterns reflect purely ontogenetic age-graded effects, cross-sectional and longitudinal gradients should satisfy one common function (the converse does not hold, of course). As is clear already from simple inspection, this assumption does not hold for our data. The longitudinal effects often appear more marked than cross-sectional differences, and longitudinal changes over a 2-year interval sometimes exceed 4-year changes. It is noteworthy that Lachman (1986), using a three-item index of personal efficacy, found similarly irregular patterns of cross-sequential effects. Although there are different ways to account for such apparent inconsistencies between cross-sectional and longitudinal gradients, we believe that the observed longitudinal effects not only reflect ontogenetic change but also involve variation related to time of measurement (effects due to history or to testing, as defined by Cook & Campbell, 1979). From a methodological point of view, it should further be noted that our observations come from a sample of married couples. For most of the variables involved in this study, the intradyadic correlation between partners, which reflects effects of homogamy, mutual co-orientation, and so on, is low to moderate (e.g., for the third occasion of measurement, the following intradyadic correlations were observed: for Personal Control over Development: .19, $p < .01$; for Autonomous Control: .29, $p < .01$; for Heteronomous Control: .13, $p < .01$; for TGP: .03; for FGA: .09). A closer scrutiny of these intradyadic effects is beyond the scope of the present chapter; however, we should be aware of possible pitfalls in drawing statistical conclusions from nonindependent observations. When scores for each pair are positively correlated, effects of factors varying within dyads may be underestimated, whereas effects of between-dyad factors may be overestimated (see Kenny, 1988). There are different approaches for checking such biases (e.g., using dyads as units of analysis, randomly omitting one score from each pair of observations). In the present case, such checks clearly show that the main findings and conclusions are not affected by dyadic interdependence.

A further substantive focus of the present investigation was on relationships between development-related control beliefs and aspects of optimal development or successful aging. Broadly considered, the stronger the self-percepts of autonomous control over development and the weaker the influence attributed to heteronomous factors beyond personal control, the more optimistic is the individual's outlook; with decreasing personal control, symptoms of depression and resignation emerge. This pattern of covariation also holds on the level of intraindividual change. The observed relationship of perceived control to aspects of health and well-being is largely consistent with models of learned helplessness (e.g., Peterson & Seligman, 1984) and self-efficacy (e.g., Bandura, 1981), as well as with recent theoretical notions centering on the construct of optimism (e.g., Scheier & Carver, 1985). Thus, it seems promising to extend these notions to the field of personal self-regulation of development.

The reported patterns of concurrent and longitudinal covariation, of course, do not allow for a causal ordering of variables. To examine possible causal priorities, we have applied cross-lagged panel analysis (Kenny, 1979) to the synchronous and lagged (Time 1 – Time 3) correlations between the various indicators of development-related control beliefs and emotional outlook. None of the cross-lagged differentials attained significance. Thus, the assumption of a recursive causal relationship between control beliefs and emotions (see also Peterson & Seligman, 1984) is not supported by our data. This, however, does not invalidate our thesis that the emotional quality of life perspectives crucially depends on one's beliefs about the control one has over life events and personal development. Self-percepts of low control over development, however, should perhaps be considered more appropriately as constitutive, rather than causal, conditions of despondency and depression (see also Brandtstädter, 1987).[5]

We have argued that uncontrollable events that bring about radical changes in the individual's system of developmental options cumulate in later life. Notions of control and helplessness apparently do not help us very much in understanding how individuals emotionally adjust to irreversible changes and losses. The dual-process conception of assimilative and accommodative modes of coping seems more promising in this respect. Whereas assimilative strategies aim at transforming the situation in accordance with personal needs and aspirations, accommodative processes involve adjustment of aspirations to changes in the set of feasible developmental options. Obviously, accommodative modes become relevant to the extent that assimilative, problem-oriented control activities are dysfunctional or futile. Subjects who are highly disposed toward tenacious, assimilative modes of control may even be more vulnerable to depression when faced with events that necessitate acceptance and accommodation (Coyne, Aldwin, & Lazarus, 1981; Janoff-Bulman & Brickman, 1982).

Apparently, a deeper understanding of the processual and developmental dynamics of depression requires the simultaneous consideration of assimilative and accommodative tendencies. In the present study, these different modes of coping and control were assessed on the dispositional level by two independent scales of Tenacious Goal Pursuit and Flexible Goal Adjustment. Both scales predict an optimistic outlook and absence of depressive symptoms. At the same time, they exhibit opposite developmental trends in middle and later adulthood: Tenacious Goal Pursuit decreases with age, and Flexible Goal Adjustment shows a clear increase. So far, this result is based only on cross-sectional comparisons, but it clearly conforms with theoretical expectations. The compensatory shift from assimilative toward more accommodative styles of coping may help to stabilize the subjective balance of developmental gains and losses over the life span; thus, it may account for the fact that age-comparative studies to date have not been able to document a general deterioration of personal satisfaction and well-being in later life (Mayring, 1987). Given these findings, it seems that theoretical postures conceptualizing successful development and aging predominantly in terms of active–offensive modes of control may seriously underrate the functional relevance of accommodative processes for coping with typical problems of aging.

NOTES

1 Entwicklungskontrolle und Entwicklungserleben in Partnerschaften, funded by the German Research Foundation.

2 The listing of variables given here is not exhaustive but includes only a selection of measures pertaining to the specific focus of the present study (see also Table 7.1). For a detailed description of the variable set, see Brandtstädter, Krampen, & Greve, 1987, and Brandtstädter, Krampen, & Heil, 1986.

3 One may ask at this point how far the developmental patterns observed on the global aggregational level can be generalized across the goal domains involved in the aggregation. The global developmental trends observed for Personal, Autonomous, and Heteronomous Control on the aggregational level are in fact differently expressed on the different goal domains. In general, however, domain-specific findings follow the global pattern rather closely. The global structure of cross-sequential effects is most typically expressed on the following goal domains: health, physical well-being; wisdom, mature understanding; assertiveness, self-assurance; intellectual efficiency; self-development; and physical fitness.

4 To prevent misunderstanding, it should be emphasized that the concepts *assimilative* and *accommodative* are used here in a generic sense, without implying the meanings that these terms may have in other (e.g., Piagetian) theoretical contexts.

5 Recently, Seligman and Elder (1986) have argued against the assumption that observed correlations between self-percepts of low efficacy and depression could be due to inherent conceptual links. Their argument, briefly considered, runs as follows: (1) Self-percepts of low control not only predict depression as measured by pertinent inventories but also physical symptoms of depression; (2) there are individuals who are not depressed but who have the insidious attributional style related to self-percepts of low control. Although correct in themselves, these arguments clearly miss the point. As to the first argument, we simply do not see how the observation that a test A predicts both a test B and also external correlates of B could rule out the assumption that the correlation between A and B is tautological or due to conceptual overlapping. The second argument in fact discredits the assumption that depression and low control are conceptually equivalent, but of course it does not invalidate the more sensible assumption that perceptions of low control are a conceptually necessary ingredient of depression.

REFERENCES

Baltes, P. B. (1973). Life-span models of psychological aging: A white elephant? *Gerontologist*, *13*, 475–512.

Baltes, P. B. (1987). Theoretical propositions of life-span developmental psychology: On the dynamics between growth and decline. *Developmental Psychology*, *23*, 611–626.

Bandura, A. (1981). Self-referent thought: A developmental analysis of self-efficacy. In J. H. Flavell & L. Ross (Eds.), *Social cognitive development: Frontiers and possible futures* (pp. 200–239). Cambridge: Cambridge University Press.

Brandtstädter, J. (1981). *Entwicklung in Handlungskontexten: Aussichten für die entwicklungspsychologische Theorienbildung und Anwendung* (Trierer Psychologische Berichte 8, Heft 8). Trier: Universität Trier. (Reprinted in H. Lenk, Ed., 1984, *Handlungstheorien interdisziplinär: Vol. 3, II. Verhaltenswissenschaftliche und psychologische Handlungstheorien*, pp. 848–878. Munich: Fink)

Brandtstädter, J. (1984). Personal and social control over development: Some implications of an action perspective in life-span developmental psychology. In P. B. Baltes & O. G. Brim, Jr. (Eds.), *Life-span development and behavior* (Vol. 6, pp. 1–32). New York: Academic Press.

Brandtstädter, J. (1987). On certainty and universality in human development: Developmental psychology between empiricism and apriorism. In M. Chapman & R. Dixon (Eds.), *Meaning and the growth of understanding: Wittgenstein's significance for developmental psychology* (pp. 69–84). Berlin: Springer.

Brandtstädter, J. (1989). Personal self-regulation of development: Cross-sequential analyses of development-related control beliefs and emotions. *Developmental Psychology*, *25*, 96–108.

Brandtstädter, J., Krampen, G., & Baltes-Götz, B. (1989). Kontrollüberzeugungen im Kontext persönlicher Entwicklung. In G. Krampen (Ed.), *Diagnostik von Attributionen und Kontrollüberzeugungen* (pp. 155–171). Göttingen: Hogrefe.

Brandtstädter, J., Krampen, G., & Greve, W. (1987). Personal control over development: Effects on the perception and emotional evaluation of personal development in adulthood. *International Journal of Behavioral Development*, *10*, 99–120.

Brandtstädter, J., Krampen, G., & Heil, F. E. (1986). Personal control and emotional evaluation of development in partnership relations during adulthood. In M. M. Baltes & P. B. Baltes (Eds.), *The psychology of aging and control* (pp. 265–296). Hillsdale, NJ: Lawrence Erlbaum.

Brandtstädter, J., & Renner, G. (1990). Tenacious goal pursuit and flexible goal adjustment: Explication and age-related analysis of assimilative and accommodative strategies. *Psychology and Aging*, *5*, 58–67.

Brim, O. G., Jr., & Ryff, C. D. (1980). On the properties of life events. In P. B. Baltes & O. G. Brim, Jr. (Eds.), *Life-span development and behavior* (Vol. 3, pp. 368–389). New York: Academic Press.

Cook, T. D., & Campbell, D. T. (1979). Causal inference and the language of experimentation. In T. D. Cook & D. T. Campbell (Eds.), *Quasi-experimentation: Design and analysis issues for field settings* (pp. 1–36). Chicago: Rand McNally.

Coyne, J. L., Aldwin, L., & Lazarus, R. S. (1981). Depression and coping in stressful episodes. *Journal of Abnormal Psychology, 90,* 439–447.

Elster, J. (1983). *Sour grapes: Studies in the subversion of rationality.* Cambridge: Cambridge University Press.

Fahrenberg, J., Hampel, R., & Selg, H. (1973). *Freiburger Persönlichkeits-Inventar (F-P-I)* (2nd ed.). Göttingen: Hogrefe.

Janoff-Bulman, R., & Brickman, P. (1982). Expectations and what people learn from failure. In N. T. Feather (Ed.), *Expectations and actions: Expectancy-value models in psychology* (pp. 207–237). Hillsdale, NJ: Lawrence Erlbaum.

Kagan, J. (1980). Perspectives on continuity. In O. G. Brim, Jr., & J. Kagan (Eds.), *Constancy and change in human development* (pp. 26–74). Cambridge: Harvard University Press.

Kamlah, W. (1973). *Philosophische Anthropologie: Sprachkritische Grundlegung und Ethik.* Mannheim: BI Taschenbücher.

Kenny, D. A. (1979). *Correlation and causality.* New York: Wiley.

Kenny, D. A. (1988). The analysis of data from two-person relationships. In S. W. Duck (Ed.), *Handbook of personal relationships* (pp. 57–77). New York: Wiley.

Klinger, E. (1977). *Meaning and void.* Minneapolis: University of Minnesota Press.

Krampen, G. (1981). *IPC-Fragebogen zu Kontrollüberzeugungen.* Göttingen: Hogrefe.

Krampen, G. (1987). Entwicklung von Kontrollüberzeugungen: Thesen zu Forschungsstand und Perspektiven. *Zeitschrift für Entwicklungspsychologie und Pädagogische Psychologie, 19,* 195–227.

Kuhl, J. (1985). Volitional mediators of cognition-behavior consistency: Self-regulatory processes and action versus state orientation. In J. Kuhl & J. Beckmann (Eds.), *Action control: From cognition to behavior* (pp. 101–128). Berlin: Springer.

Lachman, M. E. (1986). Personal control in later life: Stability, change, and cognitive correlatives. In M. M. Baltes & P. B. Baltes (Eds.), *The psychology of control and aging* (pp. 207–236). Hillsdale, NJ: Lawrence Erlbaum.

Lazarus, R. S., & DeLongis, A. (1983). Psychological stress and coping in aging. *American Psychologist, 38,* 245–254.

Lazarus, R. S., & Launier, R. (1978). Stress-related transactions between person and environment. In L. A. Pervin & M. Lewis (Eds.), *Perspectives in interactional psychology* (pp. 287–327). New York: Plenum Press.

Lerner, J. V., & Lerner, R. M. (1983). Temperament and adaption across life: Theoretical and empirical issues. In P. B. Baltes & O. G. Brim, Jr. (Eds.), *Life-span development and behavior* (Vol. 5, pp. 198–228). New York: Academic Press.

Löhr, G., & Walter, A. (1974). Die LZ-Skala: Zur Erfassung der subjektiven Lebenszufriedenheit im Alter. *Diagnostica, 20,* 83–91.

Mayring, P. (1987). Subjektives Wohlbefinden im Alter: Stand der Forschung und theoretische Weiterentwicklung. *Zeitschrift für Gerontologie, 20,* 367–376.

McCrae, R. R. (1982). Age differences in the use of coping mechanisms. *Journal of Gerontology, 37,* 454–460.

Moos, R. H., & Billings, A. G. (1982). Conceptualizing and measuring coping resources and processes. In L. Goldberger & S. Breznitz (Eds.), *Handbook of stress: Theoretical and clinical aspects* (pp. 212–230). New York: Free Press.

Overton, W. F., & Reese, H. W. (1981). Conceptual prerequisites for an understanding of stability–change and continuity–discontinuity. *International Journal of Behavioral Development, 4,* 99–123.

Peterson, C., & Seligman, M. E. P. (1984). Causal explanations as a risk factor for depression: Theory and evidence. *Psychological Review, 91*, 347–374.

Rodin, J. (1987). Personal control through the life course. In R. P. Abeles (Ed.), *Life-span perspective and social psychology* (pp. 103–119). Hillsdale, NJ: Lawrence Erlbaum.

Rokeach, M. (1973). *The nature of human values*. New York: Free Press.

Rothbaum, F., Weisz, J. R., & Snyder, S. S. (1982). Changing the world and changing the self: A two-process model of perceived control. *Journal of Personality and Social Psychology, 42*, 5–37.

Scheier, M. F., & Carver, L. S. (1985). Optimism, coping, and health: Assessment and implications of generalized outcome expectancies. *Health Psychology, 4*, 219–247.

Schopenhauer, A. (1851). *Parerga und Paralipomena: Kleine philosophische Schriften*. Berlin: A. W. Hayn.

Seligman, M. E. P., & Elder, G. H., Jr. (1986). Learned helplessness and life-span development. In A. B. Sørensen, F. E. Weinert, & L. Sherrod (Eds.), *Human development and the life course: Multidisciplinary perspectives* (pp. 377–428). Hillsdale, NJ: Lawrence Erlbaum.

Shupe, D. R. (1985). Perceived control, helplessness, and choice: Their relationship to health and aging. In J. E. Birren & J. Livingston (Eds.), *Cognition, stress, and aging* (pp. 174–197). Englewood Cliffs, NJ: Prentice-Hall.

Spanier, G. B. (1976). Measuring dyadic adjustment: New scales for assessing the quality of marriage and similar dyads. *Journal of Marriage and the Family, 38*, 15–28.

Super, C. M., & Harkness, S. (1986). The developmental niche. *International Journal of Behavioral Development, 9*, 545–570.

Tatarkiewicz, W. (1984). *Über das Glück*. Stuttgart: Klett.

Thomae, H. (1981). Expected unchangeability of life stress in old age: A contribution to a cognitive theory of aging. *Human Development, 24*, 229–239.

Wiendieck, G. (1970). Entwicklung einer Skala zur Messung der Lebenszufriedenheit im höheren Erwachsenenalter. *Zeitschrift für Gerontologie, 3*, 215–224.

8 Successful mastery of bereavement and widowhood: A life-course perspective

CAMILLE B. WORTMAN AND
ROXANE COHEN SILVER

Introduction

Because increasing age is typically accompanied by the loss of important social relationships, the study of coping with loss is particularly relevant for understanding successful aging. Moreover, loss of a spouse is generally considered to be one of the most serious threats to health, well-being, and productivity during the middle and later years (see Clayton, 1979; Osterweis, Solomon, & Green, 1984; M. Stroebe & W. Stroebe, 1983; W. Stroebe & M. Stroebe, 1987; and Vachon, 1976, for reviews). In the United States alone, approximately 800,000 people are widowed each year (Osterweis et al., 1984). In fact, there are presently more than 10 million widows and 3 million widowers in the United States, and the number of bereaved continues to increase (Ball, 1976–1977). The period of widowhood is often lengthy, particularly for women. Only one quarter of widows remarry within 5 years of the loss of their spouse, and the average woman remains widowed for the rest of her life, typically about 19.5 years (Carter & Glick, 1976).

Successful mastery of this major transition is an important feature of the aging experience. The marital pair may have such closely interwoven lives that the loss of one partner may cut across the very meaning of the other's existence (Raphael, 1983). Widowhood is associated with higher mortality for both sexes, although the excess risk is much greater for men, especially during the first 6 months of bereavement (M. Stroebe & W. Stroebe, 1983; W. Stroebe & M. Stroebe, 1987). Concerning physical health, there is evidence that the bereaved consult physicians more often (Parkes, 1964), consume more alcohol, tobacco, and tranquilizers (Osterweis et al., 1984; Parkes & Brown, 1972), and exhibit higher rates of symptoms and illness than controls (Palmore, Cleveland, Nowlin, Ramm, & Siegler, 1979). Investigators have found that many bereaved show marked emotional distress, particularly depression (Carey, 1977; Glick, Weiss, & Parkes, 1974; Maddison & Viola, 1968; Maddison & Walker, 1967; Parkes, 1964; Parkes & Brown, 1972; Parkes & Weiss, 1983; Vachon, Sheldon et al., 1982). In fact, a recent review has reported that 10% to 20% of the bereaved, or 80,000 to 160,000 each year, are sufficiently symptomatic a year or more after their loss to suggest clinical depression (Osterweis et al., 1984). There is also some evidence to suggest that the bereaved are more likely than matched controls to consult professionals for help with emotional problems (Parkes & Brown, 1972) and are at increased risk for suicide (Bock & Webber, 1972; Carter & Glick, 1976; Gove, 1972; MacMahon & Pugh, 1965).

Despite considerable research activity in the area of bereavement, there are many gaps in current knowledge. In a recent comprehensive review completed by the Institute of Medicine (Osterweis et al., 1984), it was concluded that "inadequacies in the data base, such as the narrow scope of research, lack of good multidisciplinary studies, and some pervasive methodological problems, have hampered the development of definitive conclusions" (p. 9). There is a clear need for more information regarding factors that may place individuals at risk following bereavement – particularly the role of gender, race, socioeconomic status, and age (Osterweis et al., 1984; M. Stroebe & W. Stroebe, 1983; W. Stroebe & M. Stroebe, 1987). At the present time, the literature is limited almost exclusively to studies of white, predominantly middle-class persons (see Osterweis et al., 1984). In addition, little is known about how the elderly cope with bereavement. Many of the most important and influential studies of widowhood have focused exclusively on young widows (see Gallagher, Thompson, & Peterson, 1981/1982). The few studies that have focused on the elderly bereaved have involved small and unrepresentative samples (e.g., Heyman & Gianturco, 1973). Another major unresolved issue concerns how long the effects of conjugal bereavement typically last. There is surprisingly little empirical data on the effects of such a loss beyond 1 or 2 years (see Lehman, Wortman, & Williams, 1987, for a review).

In this chapter, we take a close look at the question of successful mastery of the bereavement experience. We begin by reviewing current theories of grief and loss in order to identify the prevailing view about what constitutes successful mastery of the loss of one's spouse. We then discuss how it is widely believed that following such a loss, individuals will go through a period of intense distress, the absence of which is assumed to be indicative of a problem. In order to adapt successfully, it is maintained that individuals must engage in active attempts to "work through" or process the loss. Following a relatively short period of time, individuals are expected to have moved through the grieving process, to have resolved the loss, and to have returned to their earlier level of functioning.

Drawing from our own research and that of others, we then identify what we believe to be a number of problems with the current views of successful mastery of the bereavement experience. First, the empirical evidence suggests that there is far greater variability in response to the loss of a spouse than the prevailing view would imply, with some people showing relatively little distress following the loss and others experiencing enduring problems. Second, little attention has been devoted to identifying those factors that may account for this variability or to clarifying the theoretical mechanisms through which bereavement might influence health and well-being. Third, we believe current work on bereavement would be enriched by considering the topic of effective mastery of bereavement from a life-course perspective. The tasks to be mastered following the loss of one's spouse, as well as the resources available to cope with these tasks, vary markedly from one point in the life cycle to the next. In addition, the current view of successful bereavement equates mastery with homeostasis, or return to normal functioning. Insufficient attention has been paid to a view of mastery that includes the possibility of growth or positive change. We conclude the chapter with a description of ongoing prospective work that we hope will address the limitations we have raised. Finally, we discuss theoretical and empirical questions that are currently being pursued in our ongoing research.

Theories of grief and loss

Several different theoretical formulations have influenced current conceptions concerning successful mastery of a major loss (see Bowlby, 1980; Osterweis et al., 1984; and Raphael, 1983, for reviews).[1] One of the most influential approaches to loss has been the classic psychoanalytic model of bereavement, which is based on Freud's important paper "Mourning and Melancholia" (1917/1957). Freud maintained that the major task of mourning is the gradual surrender of psychological attachment to the deceased. Freud believed that relinquishment of the love object involves an internal struggle, because the individual experiences intense yearning for the lost loved one, yet is faced with the reality of the loved one's absence. This struggle is inevitably painful and involves turbulent emotions. Initially, the individual may deny that the loss has occurred, become preoccupied with thoughts of the deceased, and lose interest in the outside world. However, as thoughts and memories are reviewed, ties to the deceased person are gradually withdrawn. At the conclusion of the mourning period, the bereaved individual is said to have "worked through" the loss and to have freed himself or herself from an intense attachment to an unavailable person. According to Freud, when the process has been completed, the bereaved person regains sufficient emotional energy to invest in new relationships.

A second influential theoretical orientation to loss is the attachment model of grief originally developed by John Bowlby (1961, 1973, 1980). In this formulation, Bowlby drew heavily from psychodynamic thought, from the developmental literature on young children's reactions to separation, and from work on the mourning behavior of animals. Bowlby maintained that during the course of normal development, individuals form instinctive affectional bonds or attachments, initially between child and parent and later between adults. Bowlby maintained that when such bonds are threatened, powerful attachment behaviors are activated, such as clinging, crying, and angry protest. He argued that bereavement can be conceptualized as an unwilling separation that gives rise to many forms of attachment behavior. Unlike Freud, Bowlby suggested that the function of this behavior is not withdrawal from the lost object but rather reunion. In short, he argued that behaviors arising from separation anxiety, such as pining and restlessness, are critically important features of grief.

Drawing in part from these theoretical notions and in part from available research, Bowlby (1980) maintained that effective mastery of bereavement involves passing through four stages, or phases, of mourning. Initially, individuals are expected to go through a phase of numbness or feeling stunned. This first phase is then followed by a phase of yearning and searching, where the bereaved may show manifestations of a strong urge to find, recover, and reunite with the lost person. During this period, the individual may experience anger at the loss, as well as general restlessness and irritability. Bowlby argued that, over time, those behaviors aimed at reestablishing the attachment bond usually cease, and individuals enter the third phase of the mourning process. According to Bowlby, this phase is characterized by giving up the attempts to recover the deceased. The bereaved person typically experiences depression and feels a disinclination to look to the future. Eventually, individuals enter the final phase, in which they are able to break down their attachment to the lost loved one and start to establish new ties to others. In this phase of reorganization or recovery, there is a gradual return of former interests.

In the bereavement literature, a number of other theorists have also proposed models that, like Bowlby's, involve phases or stages of reaction to loss (see, e.g., Horowitz, 1976, 1985). Perhaps the most well known of such models is the one proposed by Kubler-Ross (1969) in her highly influential book *On Death and Dying*. Although offered to explain dying patients' reactions to their own impending death, Kubler-Ross identified five stages of emotional response to anticipated loss: denial, anger, bargaining, depression, and ultimately acceptance. Over the past two decades, descriptions of stage models of reactions to loss have also appeared in numerous textbooks and articles written by and for physicians, nurses, therapists, social workers, ministers, and patients and their families (see Silver & Wortman, 1980). As a result, these models have become firmly entrenched among health care professionals. There is evidence that professionals sometimes use the stages as a kind of yardstick to assess progress and evaluate how a given individual is doing. Yet, as research has begun to accumulate, it has become clear that although stage models of response to loss are held widely, there is little empirical evidence to support them (see Silver & Wortman, 1980, for a review). In fact, the authoritative Institute of Medicine review of bereavement research cautioned against the use of the phrase *stages of response* when considering the grieving process. It noted that this phrase "might lead people to expect the bereaved to proceed from one clearly identifiable reaction to another in a more orderly fashion than usually occurs. It might also result in ... hasty assessments of where individuals are, or ought to be in the grieving process" (Osterweis et al., 1984, p. 48). This report concluded that although individuals appear not to go through discrete stages in an orderly fashion, grief may best be understood as a series of overlapping clusters of reactions or "phases" over time (see also W. Stroebe & M. Stroebe, 1987).

Prevailing views of the grieving process

The current view of grief recognizes that reliance on the stages concept alone is too simplistic. However, many health care professionals still regard grief as a process that all individuals must go through if they are to successfully master their loss (see, e.g., Donovon & Girton, 1984; Jette, 1983). Individuals are expected to experience intense distress as they come to accept the reality of the loss. By working through their grief, they are expected to resolve the loss and over time, return to their earlier level of functioning. We will now discuss each of these components of the grieving process in more detail.

Distress is inevitable, and failure to experience distress is indicative of pathology

In theories and clinical lore about the grieving process, it is widely believed that when a person suffers an important loss, he or she will react with distress or depression. The models described earlier are based on the assumption that, at some point, individuals will confront the reality of their loss and go through a period of depression. As the Institute of Medicine report expressed it, there is a "near-universal occurrence of intense emotional distress following bereavement, with features similar in nature and intensity to those of clinical depression" (Osterweis et al., 1984, p. 18.) Similarly, Shuchter (1986) has indicated that "virtually everyone whose spouse dies exhibits some signs and symptoms of depression" (p. 170).

The literature is clear in suggesting that depression is a necessary precondition for subsequent mastery of the loss and that those who fail to respond with intense distress are reacting abnormally.[2] In one of the earliest statements on the matter, Deutsch (1937) maintained "first, that the death of a beloved person *must* produce reactive expression of feeling in the normal course of events; second, that omission of such reactive responses is to be considered just as much a variation from the normal as excess in time and intensity" (p. 13). Bowlby (1980) identified "prolonged absence of conscious grieving" (p. 138) as one of two possible types of disordered mourning, along with chronic mourning. Similarly, Marris (1958) argued that "grieving is a process which 'must work itself out' . . . if the process is aborted from too hasty a readjustment . . . the bereaved may never recover" (p. 33). In the Institute of Medicine report, "absent grief" was also classified as one of two types of "pathologic" mourning (Osterweis et al., 1984, p. 65). This report emphasized that it is commonly assumed, particularly by clinicians, "that the absence of grieving phenomena following bereavement represents some form of personality pathology" (p. 18). Although the authors of this report note that there is little empirical evidence in support of this assumption, they nonetheless conclude that "professional help may be warranted for persons who show no evidence of having begun grieving" (p. 65).

An important component of this view is that it assumes that if individuals fail to experience distress shortly after a loss, problems or symptoms of distress will erupt at a later point. As Bowlby (1980) maintained, individuals who have failed to mourn may suddenly, inexplicably become acutely depressed at a later time. Marris (1958) commented that "much later, in response to a less important or trivial loss, the death of a more distant relative, a pet . . . the bereaved person is overwhelmed by intense grief" (p. 27). Rando (1984) has likened grief to a wound, for which, if "not appropriately cleaned and tended to, time will not be helpful. It will only mark the progress of festering infection" (p. 114). According to Rando, "There is no way to go over, around, or under grief . . . we must go through it. Grievers must be helped to understand that grief cannot be delayed indefinitely, for it will erupt in some way, directly or indirectly" (pp. 97–98). It is also widely believed that the failure to grieve will result in subsequent health problems. Bowlby (1980) suggested that those who fail to grieve are apt to be afflicted with a variety of physical ailments. The Institute of Medicine report reviews the work of several investigators who have suggested that those who fail to grieve may unconsciously become depressed and that this depression may be masked by a variety of physical symptoms (see Osterweis et al., 1984).

The belief that distress should occur following loss is so powerful that it often leads to negative attributions toward those who do not show evidence of it. One such attribution is that the person is denying the loss. As one author has maintained: "A person should be depressed because something significant has happened, and not to respond as such is denial. Such obvious denial is rare except in the case of a retarded person or in the very young" (Siller, 1969, p. 292). A second conclusion sometimes drawn is that the person is emotionally too weak to initiate the grieving process. Drawing from clinical experience with patients undergoing psychiatric treatment, Deutsch (1937) maintained that grief-related affect was sometimes omitted among individuals who were not emotionally strong enough to begin grieving. Perhaps the most common attribution made about individuals who fail to grieve is that they were not really attached to the person who died. For example, Raphael (1983) has suggested that among those who do not show signs of grief, the preexisting relationship may have been "purely narcissistic with little recognition of the real person who was lost" (pp. 205–206).

Working through the loss is important

Thus, it is widely assumed that a period of depression will occur once the person confronts the reality of the loss. At this point, it is commonly believed that in order to master the loss successfully, the person must work through what has happened (see Brown & Stoudemire, 1983; Doyle, 1980). It is maintained that individuals need to focus on and process the loss and that attempts to deny its implications, or block feelings or thoughts about it, will ultimately be unproductive. As Bowlby (1980) wrote, "Only if the person can tolerate the pining, the more or less constant searching, the seemingly endless examination of how and why the loss occurred and the anger at anyone who might have been responsible, not sparing even the dead person, can he [or she] gradually come to recognize and accept that the loss is in truth permanent and that his [or her] life must be shaped anew" (p. 93). Similarly, Parkes and Weiss (1983) have argued that for a state of emotional acceptance to be reached, "there must be a repeated confrontation with every element of the loss until the intensity of the distress is diminished" (p. 157). Marris (1958) has maintained that "if the bereaved cannot work through this process of grieving they may suffer lasting emotional damage" (p. 29). Rando (1984) concurred with this assessment, stating that "for the griever who has not attended to his [or her] grief, the pain is as acute and fresh ten years later as it was the day after" (p. 114).

An element of working through a loss that has received considerable attention from clinicians is the importance of breaking down one's attachment to the lost object. This view contends that grief work is completed only when the bereaved individual withdraws energy from the lost person and frees himself or herself from intense attachment to an unavailable individual. According to this perspective, if this process fails to occur, individuals will be unable to invest their energy in living. As Rando (1984) wrote, "The single most crucial task in grief is 'untying the ties that bind' the griever to the deceased individual. This does not mean that the deceased is forgotten or not loved; rather, it means that the emotional energy that the mourner had invested in the deceased is modified to allow the mourner to turn it towards others for emotional satisfaction" (p. 19).

A state of resolution and recovery must be reached following loss

As a result of working through their loss, it is assumed that individuals will ultimately achieve a state of resolution regarding it. One important type of resolution involves accepting the loss intellectually. Parkes and Weiss (1983) argue that people must come up with a rationale for the loss; they must be able to understand what has happened and make sense of it (see also Moos & Schaefer, 1986). This theme has also played an important role in the work of Marris (1958), who has suggested that bereavement is painful, in large part, because it deprives one's life of meaning. Similarly, Craig (1977), in her writings on the loss of a child, has maintained that an essential part of grief work is to resolve the meaninglessness of the crisis (see also Miles & Crandall, 1983).

A second type of resolution involves accepting the loss emotionally. Emotional acceptance is thought to be reached when the person no longer feels the need to avoid reminders of the loss in order to function. The lost person can be recalled, and reminders can be confronted, without intense emotional pain (Parkes & Weiss, 1983). In fact, it has been suggested that once resolution is achieved, memories of the deceased will evoke a sense of well-being (Rubin, 1985). It is generally assumed that much of the grief work in which the bereaved engage, such as reviewing the events of the death or the course of the illness or accident, will aid in resolution.

The final task believed to be involved in the successful mastery of bereavement concerns recovery of functioning. As Rubin (1982) has expressed it, the task is to "reestablish homeostatic functioning in all areas" (p. 277). Almost every stage model of coping with loss postulates a final stage of adaptation, which has been called recovery (Klinger, 1975, 1977), acceptance (Kubler-Ross, 1969), or reorganization (Bowlby, 1980). "Chronic grief" or failure to recover is identified as a major type of "pathological" mourning in virtually every major treatise on the bereavement process (see, e.g., Bowlby, 1980; Osterweis et al., 1984; Parkes & Weiss, 1983). Of course, none of these authors postulate precisely how much time should elapse before recovery from the loss of a spouse. Yet an individual who has recovered would not be expected to experience intense emotional distress or difficulties in role functioning after an extended period of time. Bereaved individuals typically comment that within a year or so after the loss, they are expected to be finished with the mourning process and be "back to normal" (Wortman & Silver, 1987).

Empirical studies on successful mastery of bereavement: A reevaluation of prevailing views

In our judgment, there are a number of problems with the prevailing view regarding what constitutes effective mastery of widowhood. We first review studies indicating that the major assumptions underlying this view are unsubstantiated by empirical evidence. In fact, variability is far more common than might be expected. Second, we maintain that it is impossible to evaluate the extent to which a person has mastered the bereavement experience without focusing on factors that might account for this variability, such as the circumstances surrounding the loss and the nature of the marital relationship. Third, we argue that there is great utility in applying a life-course perspective when considering what successful mastery of the bereavement experience might entail. Finally, we suggest that prevailing conceptions of successful mastery would benefit from a broader definition of mastery that focused not only on recovery, or return to homeostasis, but also considered the role of positive growth or change.

Is distress inevitable following bereavement, and is failure to experience distress indicative of pathology?

Among people who have encountered a major loss, is it true that distress is universally experienced? Will distress or depression "leak out" at a later date among those who fail to exhibit distress in the first several weeks or months following a loss, as clinical lore would suggest? Surprisingly, these assumptions have rarely been subjected to empirical tests. Their investigation requires longitudinal research where individuals are examined in the weeks or months after a major loss and followed for a period of several months or years. Over the past 2 years, we have made an effort to identify a number of methodologically sound data sets that meet the requirements to permit testing these assumptions. To date, we have examined five such data sets (see Wortman & Silver, 1990, for a more detailed discussion). Four of these were originally collected by other researchers and focus on the loss of a spouse (Bornstein, Clayton, Halikas, Maurice, & Robins, 1973; Lund et al., 1986; Vachon, Rogers, et al., 1982; Zisook & Shuchter, 1986). One was collected by the present authors and focuses on the loss of a child to the Sudden Infant Death Syndrome (SIDS). Except where otherwise noted, each of the studies we have examined uses standardized outcome measures and structured interviews of relatively large, unbiased samples.

In each of these studies, respondents were interviewed within the first month following the loss of their spouse or child, and then again at one or more subsequent intervals. The Time 2 assessment occurred anywhere from 13 months to 25 months following the loss. A few studies included multiple assessments over a period of years, so they provide an opportunity to determine whether those who show little depression shortly after the loss manifest depression at any time thereafter.

Specific information about the data sets is provided in Table 8.1. As this table illustrates, each of the investigative teams chose to define distress in a different way. For example, two studies relied on the Zung (1965) depression scale, and another used the psychiatric diagnostic criteria in effect at that time (Feighner et al., 1972). For each study, the investigators determined a cutoff score to classify respondents as high or low in distress, based on deviations from normative samples. (For example, Lund et al. [1986] used a cutoff score of 60 or greater on the Zung scale.) Using cutoffs established by each investigative team, an effort was made to examine the patterns of grieving among respondents in each study. Four basic patterns were identified: high–low ("normal" grief), which involves moving from high distress to low distress over time; low–low (attenuated or "absent" grief), which involves scoring low in distress at both time points; high–high ("chronic" grief), which involves scoring high in distress at both time points; and low–high ("delayed" grief), which involves scoring low in distress initially and high at a later point.

Table 8.1 summarizes the percentages of individuals who fell within each of the patterns of grieving. On the basis of these data, a number of points are apparent. First, it is clear that attenuated, or "absent," grief is very common. The number of individuals who fail to show high distress at either time point ranges from over one quarter of the sample to over

Table 8.1. *Patterns of response to loss*

Study	N	Respondents' mean age	Method of assessing distress	Patterns of grieving (%) (Time 1 = approx. 1 month; Time 2 = 13–25 months)			
				High–Low ("normal")	Low–Low ("absent")	High–High ("chronic")	Low–High ("delayed")
Silver & Wortman, 1990[a]	125	25	SCL-90 depression subscale	41.0	26.2	30.3	2.5
Bornstein, Clayton, Halikas, Maurice, & Robins, 1973[b]	109	61	Feighner et al. (1972) criteria for depression[c]	29.3	56.5	13.0	1.0
Vachon, Rogers, et al., 1982[b]	162	54	GHQ (General Health Questionnaire) (5 and above)	41.4	30.3	26.3	2.0
Lund et al., 1986[b]	117	67.6	Zung depression scale (60 or greater)[d]	9.4	77.8	7.7	5.1
Zisook & Shuchter, 1986[b]	48	50	Zung depression scale (50 or greater)	20.0	65.0	15.0	0.0

[a]Respondents had lost a child to SIDS.
[b]Respondents had lost a spouse.
[c]To be classified as depressed, respondents must admit to low mood and experience at least four of eight additional symptoms, including weight loss, sleep difficulties, fatigue, agitation, loss of interest, difficulty in concentrating, feelings of guilt, and wishing to be dead.
[d]This cutoff is recommended for geriatric populations such as that employed by these investigators (see Kitchell, Barnes, Veith, Okimoto, & Raskind, 1982).

Source: Adapted from Wortman & Silver, 1990.

three-quarters of the sample, depending on the individual study. Second, the data provide limited evidence for the firmly entrenched assumption that lack of distress shortly after a loss will ultimately result in delayed grief. In all studies, only a handful of respondents who did not become distressed initially showed distress at the later assessment point.[3] Of course, one possibility is that these individuals became distressed at some point in the future but that this distress did not occur around the time of the second assessment. It should be noted that in two of the studies (Lund et al., 1986; Zisook & Shuchter, 1986), bereaved respondents were interviewed at frequent intervals. In addition, in the investigation by Zisook and Shuchter (1986), the assessments continued over a 4-year period. In both of these studies, there were very few respondents who moved from low distress at Time 1 to high distress at any subsequent interview.

Across these various data sets, when possible, we have carefully examined the hypothesis that those who showed low distress at Time 1 were not really attached to their loved ones. The data provide no support for this view. For example, in our study of coping with loss of an infant to SIDS, parents who initially showed low distress did not differ from those who initially evidenced high distress on such indicators as whether they reported that the pregnancy had come at a good time, whether or not the pregnancy had been unplanned, or whether or not it had been difficult to accept. Furthermore, these groups did not differ in their positive evaluations of their babies while alive. Although a detailed discussion of these findings is beyond the scope of this chapter, our analyses have also failed to support the notion that low initial distress is indicative of denial. Finally, there is little evidence in these data to support the widely held assumption that those who do not exhibit distress initially will show subsequent health difficulties or symptoms (see Wortman & Silver, 1990).

At present, we are continuing our analyses of data from all five data sets in order to enhance our understanding of those respondents who fail to show a typical grief reaction to the loss of their loved one. For example, we are attempting to determine whether those who failed to show the normal pattern of grieving were faced with situations involving an extended illness and/or caretaking responsibilities for their spouse. If so, such individuals may have grieved for their loss prior to the death. Another possibility is that as individuals become older, they are more likely to anticipate the loss of their spouse and may not show grief because they have already worked through the implications of the loss. As Table 8.1 indicates, those studies with the largest concentration of older respondents were the ones where "absent" grief was most prevalent. It should be noted, however, that even in the case of our study of parents who lost an infant to SIDS, which involved an unexpected and untimely loss, a sizable minority of respondents did not respond initially with intense distress.

In sum, the available research provides converging evidence that a sizable minority of individuals fail to experience intense distress shortly after the loss of a loved one. Moreover, the available research provides no evidence that failure to experience this distress results in subsequent mental or physical health problems. In fact, it appears that those who show high initial distress are most likely to show subsequent distress (see Wortman & Silver, 1987; 1989). Conversely, those who do not react to the loss initially with distress appear to show the best long-term adjustment. In the study by Lund et al. (1986), for example, those widows and widowers who indicated that they felt confident, who were amazed at their strength, and who were proud of how well they were coping 1 month after the loss were least likely to have difficulties coping with their spouse's death 2 years later. Thus, the data suggest that absent grief is not necessarily problematic, and, at least as it has been assessed in the studies conducted to date, delayed grief appears to be far less common than had been suggested in the theoretical and clinical literature.

Is it necessary to work through the loss and break down attachments to the lost loved one?

As reviewed above, the theoretical literature on grief clearly suggests that those who show evidence of working through their loss in the weeks or months following it will be more effective in mastering the loss than will those who do not. We have been able to locate only two studies (Parkes & Weiss, 1983; Silver & Wortman, 1990) that have offered a test of this hypothesis. In each case, contrary to expectation, those who showed early evidence of working through the loss were those who ultimately had the most difficulty adjusting to it.

Although they did not assess working through the loss specifically, Parkes and Weiss (1983) conducted a study that provides data relevant to the concept. Coders rated recently bereaved men and women on the degree to which they evidenced yearning or pining for their deceased spouse during the first interview, which occurred 3 weeks after the loss. Parkes and Weiss divided their sample into a high-yearning group, comprising those respondents who appeared to yearn or pine constantly, frequently, or whenever inactive, and a low-yearning group, comprised of those who yearned never, seldom, or only when reminded of the loss. At the first interview, about one third of their respondents fell into the low-yearning group, and two thirds fell into the high-yearning group. In fact, high yearning was found to be predictive of a poor mental and physical health outcome 13 months after the loss. As Parkes and Weiss (1983) expressed, "We might suppose that people who avoid or repress grief are the most likely to become disturbed a year later, yet this is not the case" (p. 74). They wrote that a "high level of yearning was often an early indicator of a recovery process which was going badly" (p. 228). Interestingly, high initial yearning was associated with poor outcome even 2 to 4 years after the loss.

In our study on parents coping with loss of an infant to SIDS, we also examined the impact of early evidence of working through the loss on subsequent adjustment (Silver & Wortman, 1990; Wortman & Silver, 1987). *Working through* was defined as active attempts by the parent to make sense of and process the death, including searching for an answer to why the baby died, thinking of ways the death could have been avoided, and being preoccupied with thoughts about the loss. Results indicated that the more parents were working through the death at 3 weeks, the more distressed they were, as assessed on a standardized measure of symptomatology, 18 months following the loss. In addition, those subjects who showed the least evidence of emotional resolution 18 months after the death of their infant (measured by distress in thinking and talking about the baby, feeling bitterness about the loss, and being upset by reminders of the baby) were those most likely to be working through the loss shortly after the death.

According to clinical lore in the area of grief and loss, the major purpose of working through the loss is to break down attachments to the lost loved one. Given these beliefs, it is interesting to note that continued and persistent attachments to the lost object appear to be very common. Fully 8 weeks after the loss, Glick et al. (1974) found that more than one half of the widows they interviewed, and about one fifth of the widowers, reported believing that their spouse might actually return. A year after bereavement, 69% agreed with the statement "I try to behave in ways he [or she] would have wanted me to." After 2 to 4 years, this type of attachment was still very prevalent, especially when the loss was sudden. Eighty-three percent of people who had suddenly experienced the loss of their spouse continued to agree with the statement, as did almost half of those who had forewarning about the loss. Similarly, Parkes and Weiss (1983) report that 2 to 4 years after the loss, 61% of those who lost their spouse suddenly reported sensing the presence of the dead person occasionally or always, as did 20% of those who had had some forewarning of the death.

Contrary to the suggestion that such continued attachments may inhibit adjustment or be disruptive, evidence suggests that those who encounter loss seem to find them comforting (see Goin, Burgoyne, &

Table 8.2. *Cognitive resolution of SIDS parents over time*

	3 weeks	3 months	18 months
Unable to find any meaning	65%	74%	75%
Unable to answer "Why me?" or "Why my baby?"	81%	88%	86%

Source: Adapted from Wortman & Silver, 1987.

Goin, 1979). Drawing from their study of widows, Glick et al. (1974) have argued that such attachments are not necessarily incompatible with independent action. As they have indicated, "Often the widow's progress toward recovery was facilitated by inner conversations with her husband's presence" (p. 154). Although these authors maintain that widows knew their spouses were not there, the widows nonetheless found it comforting to be able to talk through a problem with the "feeling" that their spouse was there to listen.

In summary, there is relatively little empirical evidence relevant to the question of whether it is necessary to work through the loss and break down one's attachment to the lost loved one. Nonetheless, if behaviors such as yearning for the deceased or being preoccupied with thoughts about the loss are conceptualized as working through, the assumption that working through is necessarily adaptive is challenged by available research. Like early evidence of intense distress, early signs of intense efforts to work through the loss may portend subsequent difficulties. Available data also suggest that behaviors indicative of attachment are surprisingly common and do not necessarily appear to be detrimental.

Are individuals typically able to achieve a state of resolution and recover their earlier level of functioning following loss?

Theories of grief and loss indicate that an important part of successful mastery of the loss involves achieving a state of resolution, or coming to terms with the loss, and recovering, or returning to a normal level of functioning. In one of the first studies we conducted on loss – the study of the loss of an infant to SIDS – we obtained data that were inconsistent with this view (Wortman & Silver, 1987). Parents were interviewed at three points in time during the first 18 months following the death of their infants: at 3 weeks, 3 months, and 18 months after the loss. Table 8.2 illustrates that at all three of the time points we studied, the vast majority of respondents were unable to find any meaning in their baby's death and were unable to answer the question "Why me?" or "Why my baby?" Thus, in our sample, only a small minority appears to have been able to achieve a state of resolution regarding the loss. A particularly intriguing feature of our data on coping with SIDS loss is that we found little evidence that resolution increases over time. Indeed, we found a significant decrease in the number of individuals who were able to find meaning in their babies' deaths between the first and second interviews. Regarding recovery and return to a normal level of functioning by 18 months after the loss, approximately 30% of the respondents in this sample were still experiencing intense distress (see Table 8.1).

Similar findings on lack of recovery among a significant minority of respondents have emerged in studies focusing on the loss of a spouse (see Osterweis et al., 1984; W. Stroebe & M. Stroebe, 1987, for reviews). Although symptoms appear to decline with time, many investigators have reported that a significant percentage of the bereaved continue to show marked symptoms 1 or 2 years after the loss. For example, Vachon and her associates found that 38% of the bereaved widows they studied were experiencing a high level of distress after 1 year. At the end of 2 years, 26% of the women were still classified as exhibiting high distress (Vachon, Rogers, et al., 1982; Vachon, Sheldon, et al., 1982). In a longitudinal study of bereaved widows and widowers conducted by Parkes and his associates (Parkes & Weiss, 1983), over 40% of the sample were rated by trained interviewers as showing moderate to severe anxiety 2 to 4 years after their loss. Feelings of depression, as well as problems in functioning, were also quite common at the 2- to 4-year interview. Such difficulties were particularly likely among respondents who had lost their spouse suddenly and with little forewarning. Parkes and Weiss reported that 72% of individuals whose spouses died without warning were moderately to severely anxious at the 2- to 4-year interview; 67% were moderately to severely upset or disturbed, and 44% agreed with the statement "Deep down, I wouldn't care if I died tomorrow," suggesting serious depression. In addition, 72% of those respondents with little forewarning prior to the death displayed difficulties in functioning as a spouse, parent, or worker. Among these respondents, there was also evidence to suggest lack of resolution of the loss, particularly if it was sudden. Sixty-one percent of the respondents who had suddenly lost their spouse and 29% of those who had forewarning were still asking why the event had happened as long as 2 to 4 years later. Almost half of the sample who had suddenly lost a spouse agreed with the statement "It's not real; I feel that I'll wake up and it won't be true," and even 15% of the individuals with forewarning agreed with this statement at the 2- to 4-year followup interview.

A few studies have examined individuals beyond the 2- to 4-year period following the loss of a spouse and have found evidence that a sizable percentage of individuals fail to recover from the loss. In a longitudinal investigation, Zisook and Shuchter (1986) assessed widows and widowers from 3 to 4 weeks after their loss to 4 years later, using interviews and questionnaires at 11 points in time. Even at the 4-year assessment, at least 20% of the bereaved rated their own adjustment to the loss as "fair to poor," and only 44% assessed it as "excellent" (see also Lund et al., 1986, for comparable findings).

In a case-control study on the long-term effects of losing a spouse or child in a motor vehicle crash (Lehman et al., 1987), we also found evidence that a sizable percentage of respondents were unable to resolve the loss or resume normal functioning. In this study, interviews were conducted with individuals who had lost a spouse or child in a motor vehicle accident 4 to 7 years previously. Bereaved respondents were matched with a control group of nonbereaved individuals on a case-by-case basis on sex, age, income, education, and number and ages of children. To further ensure that individuals in the bereaved sample would be comparable to those in the control sample except for having experienced the loss, the study was limited to people whose deceased spouses or children were "innocent victims" (i.e., occupants of automobiles in multiple-vehicle crashes in which the driver of the motor vehicle – whether the victim or someone else – was not at fault). Significant differences emerged between bereaved and control respondents on a variety of different indicators of effective coping and adjustment, including depression and other psychiatric symptoms, social functioning, and quality of life. Moreover, bereavement was associated with an increased mortality rate, a decline in financial status, and (in the parent study) a higher divorce rate. Finally, the data suggested that most respondents had not achieved a state of cognitive or emotional resolution regarding the loss. Almost half of the sample had reviewed events leading up to the accident in the month prior to the interview. A majority of the respondents were unable to find any meaning in the loss, had had painful memories of their spouse or child during the past month, and had had thoughts during the month prior to the interview that the death was unfair.

Finally, in a study we conducted of 45 senior citizens who had encountered a variety of losses over the course of their lives, we found that a considerable proportion of the sample reported ongoing cognitive and emotional involvement in the loss events, on average 23 years later (Tait & Silver, 1989, 1990). Decades after the occurrence of the event, more than half the respondents reported continuing to ruminate about their most negative life event, and almost 40% reported continuing to search for meaning in the outcome at least sometimes. Moreover, time did not moderate these effects.

On the basis of the foregoing research, what can be concluded about effective mastery of bereavement and widowhood? The available evidence we have reviewed suggests that prevailing notions of effective mastery of such an event may need to be reconsidered. Theories of grief and mourning, as well as clinical and cultural lore, maintain that virtually all individuals who experience the death of a significant person should go through the grief process, beginning with a phase of intense distress and followed by efforts to work through the loss. Ultimately, resolution and recovery are expected to be achieved over time as the bereaved comes to terms with the loss. Our review of available empirical work suggests that in contrast to this view, there is considerable variability in response to the loss of one's spouse. The data described above suggest that a substantial proportion of respondents do not experience intense distress following the loss. Similarly, some individuals appear to recover from the loss without working through what has happened. Moreover, at least with certain types of losses, some individuals are unable to resolve the loss and continue to remain distressed much longer than might have been expected. We believe that, taken together, these findings raise some challenging questions regarding effective mastery of bereavement.

Extending current conceptions of the grieving process

Traditional theories of grief and loss are of limited value in accounting for the variability in response to loss that we have documented. In our judgment, theoretical advancement in this area requires that attention be devoted to identifying factors that may account for this diverse pattern of findings. Moreover, the analysis offered above suggests that we may need to take a broader view of what it means to successfully master the loss of one's spouse.

Mediating factors that may promote or impede successful mastery of bereavement

Now that it is becoming clear that there is considerable variability in response to major losses, there is increasing interest in identifying those mediating factors that may promote or impede successful mastery of bereavement (Kessler, Price, & Wortman, 1985; Sanders, 1988; Silver & Wortman, 1980). Without such mediators, general theoretical models of the grieving process have limited utility in predicting reactions to conjugal loss. In recent years, a number of factors have been identified in the literature, including the nature of the relationship with the deceased, circumstances surrounding the loss, the presence of concomitant stressors, and the availability of social support.

The two relationship qualities that have been most carefully addressed in the literature on loss are ambivalence and dependence. Psychologists have generally assumed that relationships characterized by ambivalence or dependence have their roots in the early experiences of childhood. For example, Bowlby (1980) has maintained that for a variety of reasons some children come to feel insecure about the extent to which they can expect nurturance or protection from parents. As a result of these insecurities, they develop "working models" of themselves and others that influence their behavior in later relationships. Individuals who are predisposed to ambivalent relationships are primed to feel disappointment, betrayal, or abandonment by their loved ones and typically react to disappointments with intense hostility. For this reason, marriages in which one partner is ambivalent are generally characterized by considerable marital conflict (Bowlby, 1980). In fact, empirical support has been obtained for the hypothesis that those involved in ambivalent relationships will experience more long-term difficulties with bereavement than will those who do not (Parkes & Weiss, 1983).

Similarly, it has been suggested that as a result of anxiety concerning separation from one's parents, some children develop a tendency to form "clinging" relationships. Supposedly, such individuals carry this tendency into adulthood, in which they continue to react to real or threatened separation with fear or distress (Bowlby, 1980). Raphael (1983) has noted that such relationships are usually of the symbiotic kind and are reflected in such comments as "he was like a father to me." Parkes and Weiss (1983) reported that those spouses who had been involved in highly dependent relationships were more likely to have difficulties in coming to terms with their loss over time. Such individuals were also likely to experience intense yearning for the bereaved person, as well as feelings of helplessness and indecisiveness shortly after the death.

A second predictor of long-term difficulty following loss that has received considerable attention is the circumstances surrounding the loss. Although the evidence is not entirely consistent (see Osterweis et al., 1984, and Sanders, 1988, for reviews), several studies have suggested that sudden, unexpected, and untimely deaths, especially deaths of the young, are more likely to be associated with subsequent distress (see Lehman et al., 1987; Parkes, 1975; Parkes & Weiss, 1983). As Parkes and Weiss (1983) have written, such losses may have their impact through their "transformation of the world into a frightening place, a place in which disaster cannot be predicted and accustomed ways of thinking and behaving have proven unreliable and out of keeping with the actual world" (p. 245).

A third factor that has been mentioned consistently as likely to intensify distress following loss is the presence of concurrent crises (see Sanders, 1988, and Silver & Wortman, 1980, for reviews). In some cases, these crises may represent problems that existed at the time of the loss, such as chronic health ailments. In other cases, such problems may stem directly from the loss itself – for example, a widow may have to move out of her home as a result of financial strain that accompanies her husband's death. In two different studies, researchers have found a presence of other crises to be predictive of poor outcome among the bereaved (Parkes, 1975; Vachon, Rogers, et al., 1982).

Finally among people who are bereaved or have physical disabilities, the lack of available social support may also hinder the recovery process (see Osterweis et al., 1984; W. Stroebe & M. Stroebe, 1987; Vachon & Stylianos, 1988, for reviews). Clayton, Halikas, and Maurice (1972) have reported that subjects who were depressed at 1 month after the death of their spouse had significantly fewer children in the geographical area whom they considered close and available to render support (see also Bornstein et al., 1973; Dimond, Lund, & Caserta, 1987, for comparable results over time). In several studies, researchers have provided evidence that those who express feelings of lack of support, such as "nobody understands or cares," or feel that there is no one available to talk to or lean on shortly after their spouse's death are more likely to report subsequent problems (see Maddison & Walker, 1967; Vachon, Rogers, et al., 1982).

In our judgment, obtaining information concerning these risk factors is critical in assessing the extent to which an individual has successfully mastered a loss. Long-term difficulties in coming to terms with loss have generally been assumed to be indicative of coping failure on the part of the individual. Yet, such difficulties may be the norm in cases where the loss was sudden and unexpected, where it was accompanied by concomitant stressors, and among individuals who lack coping resources (e.g., children who live nearby and who are supportive).

To date, most of the research on factors that might mediate response to loss has tended to focus on those factors that impede recovery from the loss of a spouse. Yet one of the most intriguing findings to emerge from our review of the empirical literature is that many individuals never appear to become intensely distressed following the loss of a loved one. As noted earlier, such findings are typically regarded to be indicative of insufficient attachment or are expected to lead eventually to delayed grief. If future studies produce findings consistent with those reported here, however, it is important to acknowledge the possibility that some people may come through the bereavement process relatively unscathed. As psychologist Norman Garmezy (1982) has indicated, "... our mental health practitioners and researchers are predisposed by interest, investment, and training in seeing deviance, psychopathology, and weakness wherever they look" (p. xvii). By assuming latent pathology among those who fail to show intense distress following a loss, attention appears to have been deflected away from identifying strengths that may protect these people from distress (Wortman & Silver, 1989).

On the basis of our own research, we do not believe that those risk factors that have been most extensively studied, such as the presence of concomitant stressors or the availability of social support, will be highly influential in identifying individuals who appear to emerge unscathed from a major loss. Taken together, our work suggests that some people may have something in place beforehand – perhaps a religious orientation or outlook on life, or a personality predisposition – that enables them to cope with their experience almost immediately (Wortman & Silver, 1989). In fact, there has been increasing interest in philosophical perspectives or assumptions about the world and the role they may play in the coping process (Janoff-Bulman, 1985; Janoff-Bulman & Frieze, 1983; Wortman, 1983). For example, a person who holds a firm belief that all things are part of God's larger plan may show less distress following the loss of a spouse than a person who does not hold this particular belief. Similarly, individuals who have the perspective that bad things can happen at any time and that suffering is part of life may find it easier to cope with loss than those individuals who believe that if they work hard and are good people, they will be protected from misfortune (cf. Janoff-Bulman & Frieze, 1983). In our judgment, religious or philosophical orientations that might lead individuals to incorporate the loss into their view of the world, and hence be protected from distress, are in need of considerably more research.

Defining successful mastery of widowhood: The importance of a life-course perspective

In our judgment, current conceptions of successful mastery of widowhood could be enriched considerably by applying a life-course perspective to conjugal loss. Hultsch and Plemons (1979) have maintained that *when* an event occurs in the life cycle is perhaps as important as whether it occurs at all. Neugarten (1968) has introduced the concept of "on-time" and "off-time" to describe the occurrence of major events at various points in the life course. According to Neugarten (1968), individuals pass through a succession of major life transitions as they move from birth to death, including school, marriage, first job, parenthood, retirement, and widowhood. She maintains that there is a socially prescribed timetable for the ordering of most life transitions and that most adults hold a set of anticipations of the normal, expectable life cycle. Therefore, events are particularly likely to upset the sequence and rhythm of the life cycle, and hence pose a greater coping challenge, if they occur off-time rather than on-time (see also Brim, 1980). We will now attempt to illustrate how every aspect of the bereavement experience is influenced by the point in the life cycle at which the loss occurs, including the nature of what is lost, the tasks that need to be mastered following the loss, the appraisal or subjective meaning ascribed to the loss, and the resources available to cope with it.

In order to understand a person's reaction to conjugal bereavement, it is important to clarify what is lost. As a number of writers have emphasized, the nature of the loss is highly dependent on the particular roles normally performed by the spouse. In the individual case, losses that may or may not be experienced include the loss of companionship, emotional support, sexual intimacy, financial support, social status, and assistance with household tasks and childcare (Lieberman, 1975; Parkes, 1972). Clearly, the nature of the losses that are experienced is likely to vary across the life cycle. A young widow may be far more likely to endure losses of support and assistance than an elderly widow who was previously caring for her chronically ill husband. On the other hand, an elderly widow who has been married to her husband for 50 years may have a stronger and deeper attachment to her spouse than a younger widow. As a rule, elderly widows and widowers may also be more dependent on their spouses for companionship and assistance with the tasks of daily living, particularly if they are ill themselves.

Similarly, the tasks to be mastered following the loss of one's spouse are likely to be determined by the timing of the event with respect to the life cycle. For example, consider the tasks likely to be faced by a woman with young children whose husband was the primary source of income for the family. Tasks confronting this woman may include seeking additional training and employment, while managing on her own all household and parental responsibilities that were formerly shared by her husband. The loss of her husband is likely to leave her with the problem of too many roles. In contrast, an elderly woman may have experienced many role losses prior to the death of her spouse. If the woman's children are grown and she is retired, nurturing and caring for her husband may be the only meaningful role that she is performing. Thus, the major coping task facing such a woman may be dealing with the absence of social roles. Rosow (1973) has maintained that the systematic role losses experienced during old age take a heavy toll. He has suggested that people are dependent on their social roles for self-esteem and feelings of competence. According to Rosow, "role loss deprives them of their very social identity ... with a broad horizon of leisure and few obligations, many old people feel oppressively useless and futile" (p. 467).

As the above discussion illustrates, the objective situation facing a bereaved person is likely to be highly dependent on the point in the life cycle in which the loss occurs. In addition, the timing of the loss is likely to influence the person's subjective appraisal of it (Hultsch & Plemons, 1979). Neugarten (1968) has maintained that when the loss of a spouse occurs at the usual time in the life cycle, the event is "rehearsed, the 'grief work' completed, the reconciliation accomplished without shattering the sense of continuity of the life cycle" (p. 86). Similarly, Brim and Ryff (1980) have suggested that if individuals expect to be confronted with a given loss within a particular time frame, they have the opportunity to anticipate and plan for the challenges that lie ahead. If the loss has a high probability of occurrence (as widowhood does), they also have the opportunity to interact with and learn from others who have faced this event.

In a previous section of this chapter, we maintained that reactions to the loss of a spouse are likely to be influenced by the circumstances surrounding the loss. For the most part, research evidence has suggested that when a loss is sudden and unexpected, it may have a more debilitating effect. On the basis of the above discussion, however, it seems clear that the impact of such factors may be highly dependent on whether the event occurs on-time or off-time. Because of the greater preparedness for widowhood, as well as the anticipatory socialization that may occur among the elderly, older people may be less debilitated by a sudden loss. Younger widows may particularly benefit from forewarning, because it would provide an opportunity for them to prepare themselves for the loss (Ball, 1977). Of course, forewarning is typically present only in those cases in which the spouse dies after a period of illness. Caring for a chronically ill spouse may be particularly taxing for elderly widows, who may lack in coping resources themselves. Perhaps for this reason, forewarning has been shown to have no effect or to hinder subsequent adjustment among the elderly bereaved (see Gallagher et al., 1981/1982, for a review).

How successfully a person is able to master the loss of a spouse is also likely to be dependent on the coping resources available to the individual. Several resources have been studied in the coping literature, including health status, cognitive abilities, financial reserves, and social support.

There seems to be little doubt that these and other coping resources vary across the life cycle. While coping with the loss of their spouse, the elderly bereaved may also be coping simultaneously with impaired health, lowered physical stamina, and perhaps with the cognitive impairments that may be associated with aging. The importance of such resources has been illustrated in a study of the elderly conducted by Lieberman (1975). In this study, a multivariate analysis of several cognitive and physical characteristics accounted for 73% of the variance in predicting adaptation to altered living arrangements.

Generally speaking, socioeconomic status and income level often decline with advancing age. These resources can play an important role in coping with the loss of a spouse, because they allow for greater freedom in terms of manipulating one's environment following the loss (Hultsch & Plemons, 1979). Those with more economic resources, for example, can choose the living arrangement that they prefer following the loss and can purchase some of the services that may have been performed by the spouse, such as household maintenance.

One of the coping resources that has received the most attention in bereavement research is social support (see Kessler et al., 1985; Wortman & Silver, 1987, for a review). The nature and types of support available following the loss of a spouse are also likely to be strongly influenced by the timing of the event in the life course. As noted earlier, children may be more of a responsibility if the loss occurs off-time but may be an important source of support for the elderly widow or widower. Although the evidence is not entirely consistent, there is some reason to believe that younger individuals typically have a more extensive social network than most elderly individuals. Compared with younger individuals, the elderly tend to belong to fewer social groups, have fewer friends, and visit with them less (Rosow, 1973).

In several papers, we have suggested that those who have been through the experience may be in a particularly good position to provide support for a person who is going through a life crisis (see, e.g., Silver & Wortman, 1980). Such individuals can serve as role models regarding how to cope with the crisis and can offer concrete suggestions for dealing with specific problems. A problem facing the young widow or widower is that few opportunities may be available for interaction with other bereaved individuals (Brim & Ryff, 1980). In contrast, the elderly bereaved have many opportunities to interact with other bereaved individuals, both before and following the death of a spouse.

Although many coping resources decline with age, one resource that is likely to increase with age is accumulated knowledge. Hultsch and Plemons (1979) have suggested that accumulated knowledge can provide the individual with a broader perspective within which to evaluate a given life event. Along similar lines, Baltes and his associates have maintained that as life unfolds and more experiences take place, individuals accumulate more and more wisdom-related knowledge, which they define as exercising good judgment about important but uncertain matters of life (see, e.g., Smith, Dixon, & Baltes, 1989). Such wisdom-related knowledge may facilitate resolution of the tasks facing the bereaved.

Of course, the resources available to an individual at any particular point in time are dependent upon the stressors, in addition to the loss of a spouse, that have recently been encountered. Several studies have illustrated that the nature and timing of acute and chronic stressors differ across the life span (e.g., Lowenthal, Thurnher, & Chiriboga, 1975). As noted earlier, elderly individuals are more likely to be struggling with chronic health and financial problems at the time of their spouse's death than are younger bereaved. The elderly bereaved are also more likely to have experienced previous loss events (Rosow, 1973). At this point, however, little is known about the conditions under which experience with prior losses facilitates mastery of conjugal bereavement and the conditions under which such experiences deplete coping reserves and hence make successful mastery less likely.

Assessing successful mastery of widowhood: The importance of positive change

In the prevailing view of the grieving process, successful mastery of bereavement is often equated with recovery, or a return to homeostasis. A person is said to have recovered if, after a year or so, he or she is not showing continuing signs of psychological distress and has returned to normal functioning. As Riegel (1975) has expressed it, the notion of homeostasis or equilibrium as a desirable goal "has thoroughly penetrated the thinking of behavioral and social scientists" (p. 100).

In our view, conceptual and empirical work on bereavement would benefit from a broader view of what constitutes successful mastery. We would suggest that investigators add to their battery an assessment of growth, or the heightened ability to operate in a new set of circumstances (Lieberman, 1975). In addition to grieving the loss of her spouse, a widow must learn a variety of new skills, which may or may not include managing financial affairs, getting around town on her own, arranging for household maintenance and car repairs, and coping with the job market. Experiences that foster the development of such skills are likely to result in positive changes, such as enhanced feelings of self-esteem. Hence, in assessing effective mastery or competence following the loss, it may also be worthwhile to assess these and other skills that may be acquired, as well as the personal changes that might accompany the development of such skills (e.g., greater confidence, autonomy, or independence).

Thus far, the few bereavement researchers who have assessed constructs relevant to personal growth and change have found that such changes do indeed occur. For example, Lopata (1973) found that a majority of the widows she studied indicated that they had changed as a result of widowhood. Of these, 63% judged themselves to be more competent and independent, and another 10% regarded themselves as freer and more active individuals. Only 18% viewed their change in entirely negative terms. Similar findings have been reported by Thomas, DiGuilio, and Sheehan (1988).

Ongoing research efforts

Taken together, the evidence considered in this chapter suggests that in order to advance our understanding of successful mastery of bereavement, three issues must be addressed. First, more information is needed regarding factors that may place individuals at risk following bereavement, including gender, race, socioeconomic status, and age. Because most previous studies have focused on small samples of middle-aged white women, little is known about how sociodemographic factors influence the grieving process. Moreover, with few exceptions (e.g., Owen, Fulton, & Markusen, 1982), there is a dearth of studies that have examined the impact of bereavement at various points across the life span. A second issue involves clarifying our understanding of individuals who exhibit less distress than might be expected following conjugal loss, and who continue to function well at subsequent intervals. It is important to identify those variables or resources that individuals have in place prior to a loss that may allow them to emerge relatively unscathed. A third issue concerns identifying the long-term effects of conjugal bereavement and explicating the mechanisms linking bereavement to subsequent physical and mental health problems.

Over the past few years, we have had the opportunity to become involved in a large-scale national study that provides a unique opportunity to address the aforementioned questions. For this study, respondents were drawn from a national sample of 3,617 U.S. adults who were interviewed in 1986 and who were reinterviewed in 1989 as part of a large-scale study of productive activities across the life span called the Americans' Changing Lives study. This project is being conducted in collaboration with an interdisciplinary team of researchers including

James House and Ronald Kessler, sociologists; James Morgan, an economist; and Robert Kahn and Toni Antonucci, psychologists; among others. Personal interviews were conducted with adults from age 25 to 92 in 70 areas around the United States. In order to facilitate the study of people of different ages and races, blacks and elderly individuals (people over the age of 60) were oversampled. The interviews focused on respondents' experiences in various life roles, including work, marriage, and parenting; their leisure or voluntary productive activities; their stressful life experiences; and information about various coping resources such as personality, self-esteem, and social support. Information about physical and mental health and functioning was also obtained from all respondents. Ronald Kessler, James House, and Camille Wortman are collaborating on a large-scale national study of bereavement (National Widowhood Study) that is being conducted in conjunction with the Americans' Changing Lives study. All respondents who were widowed (or previously widowed and remarried) at the time of the first interview were questioned about the circumstances surrounding the loss, their thoughts and feelings about the loss (e.g., the frequency and intrusiveness of memories), and the extent of acceptance and recovery from the loss. At the Wave I interview, our bereaved sample included approximately 800 respondents who had lost a spouse between 1 and 66 years previously. We are currently in the process of analyzing the Wave I widowhood data from this project. Although a full account of our findings is beyond the scope of this chapter, we have found evidence for long-term effects of the loss of one's spouse (see Wortman, Kessler, Bolger, & House, 1990). Respondents who lost a spouse were compared with nonbereaved controls who were similar on a number of dimensions but who had not lost a spouse. It took bereaved respondents in our study approximately one decade to approach control respondents' scores on life satisfaction, and over two decades to approach their scores on depression. In addition, we asked respondents several questions about their current thoughts and memories regarding their spouse. Painful memories were found to decline over time, although it took several decades for such memories to reach their lowest level. Finally, several questions were included to assess cognitive resolution from the loss, such as whether the respondent had been able to find any meaning in the loss, or whether he or she regarded the loss as senseless and unfair. Interestingly, such questions showed no time effects whatsoever. Individuals who lost their spouse more than six decades earlier were no more likely to have generated a reason for what happened than individuals who lost their spouse during the past year.

At first glance, these findings may appear to be inconsistent with the longitudinal studies reported earlier, which suggest that a large percentage of people do not become depressed following the loss of a loved one. However, it is important to note that even though it took several years for respondents in the National Widowhood Study, as a group, to recover from the loss of their spouse, there is considerable variability within this sample. Some respondents appeared to be recovered shortly after their loss, whereas others showed enduring difficulties. A major goal of subsequent analyses will be to examine factors that may influence the amount of time it takes to recover. An advantage of a large cross-sectional design like this one is that it enables the investigator to examine recovery as a function of such variables as race, gender, age, and the circumstances surrounding the death. Such analyses are currently in progress, and preliminary results are intriguing. For example, Bolger, Wortman, and Kessler (1988) have found that younger individuals are more devastated by the loss of their spouse than older individuals, but older respondents take more time to recover from the loss. Various mechanisms that may underlie this effect are currently being explored. We are also conducting a systematic comparison of sudden, unexpected losses with losses that occur with greater forewarning.

In summary, this synthetic cohort analysis provides compelling evidence for long-term effects of loss, as well as evidence suggesting that the process of resolution from a loss may operate differently than we had previously thought. Taken together, the findings obtained thus far suggest that longitudinal studies following respondents beyond the first few years after the loss would be justified.

Although a large, representative cross-sectional study of bereavement can help to identify those groups of bereaved individuals who are particularly at risk for problems and can provide preliminary evidence of enduring difficulties, such a design fails to clarify our understanding of individuals who show little distress following the loss of their spouse. Nonetheless, our earlier review (see Table 8.1) showed that by 1 month following the loss, there is already marked variability in response to the loss of a loved one, with some individuals reacting with intense distress and others less so. As noted, these early reactions appear to be highly predictive of long-term adjustment. Clearly, in studies beginning after the loss event, it is impossible to determine the antecedents of initial adjustment. Moreover, it is difficult to determine whether variables assessed after the event, such as respondents' mental health or social networks, have been altered by the loss. Because of such interpretive difficulties, it has been suggested that the logical next step in advancing our understanding of the relation between stressful life events and health outcomes is a prospective study, which would assess relevant risk factors and potential confounding variables (e.g., initial health status) prior to the stressor. In fact, a major conclusion drawn in the recent report on bereavement completed by the Institute of Medicine is that "prospective longitudinal studies that begin before and run for several years after bereavement are needed" (Osterweis et al., 1984, p. 11).

At present, we are involved in two prospective studies that we hope will help to clarify the issues discussed in this chapter. The first study builds on the National Widowhood Study (Figure 8.1). We noted that, as part of a large-scale study of stress and coping across the life span, we conducted interviews with several thousand individuals in 1986 and reinterviewed these respondents in 1989. Between the first and second interviews, approximately 75 of the respondents became widowed. Pre-loss information concerning risk factors and moderating variables is available from the Wave I interview. At the Wave II interview, those respondents who lost a spouse were questioned about their reactions to the loss. They also provided information about their current health and functioning.

Because of the importance of obtaining a prospective assessment of relevant risk factors, the project was designed to include a larger, more intensively focused prospective study in the Detroit, Michigan, area (see Figure 8.2). In 1987, baseline information was collected on 1,532 respondents who were at risk for bereavement (couples where the spouse is 65 years or older). The baseline interview provided a careful assessment, prior to the loss, of potential risk factors, confounding variables, and coping resources such as social support. Michigan death records are being monitored to determine when deaths occur among this sample. It is projected that approximately 200 respondents will become bereaved over the next 3 years. These respondents will be contacted and invited to participate in a study of conjugal bereavement. If they agree, they will be interviewed at 6 to 8 months, 18 months, 37 months, and 61 months after the loss. A control group of married respondents matched on age, sex, race, age of (deceased) spouse, and spouse's prior physical health will be selected from those who participated in the baseline interview and interviewed at parallel time points to provide comparison data about functioning. In addition, a separate interview is being conducted with a subset of our respondents to collect biomedical, physical, and cognitive-functioning data. Such information, including blood and urine samples, will be obtained from all baseline respondents who are age 70 or older and from all respondents who become bereaved, as well as from matched controls. Thus, the study represents an opportunity to examine the relation between biomedical and psychosocial indicators of functioning among a representative sample of individuals who experience the loss of their spouse. We hope the results will contribute to our knowledge of resilience or vulnerability in the face of a major loss.

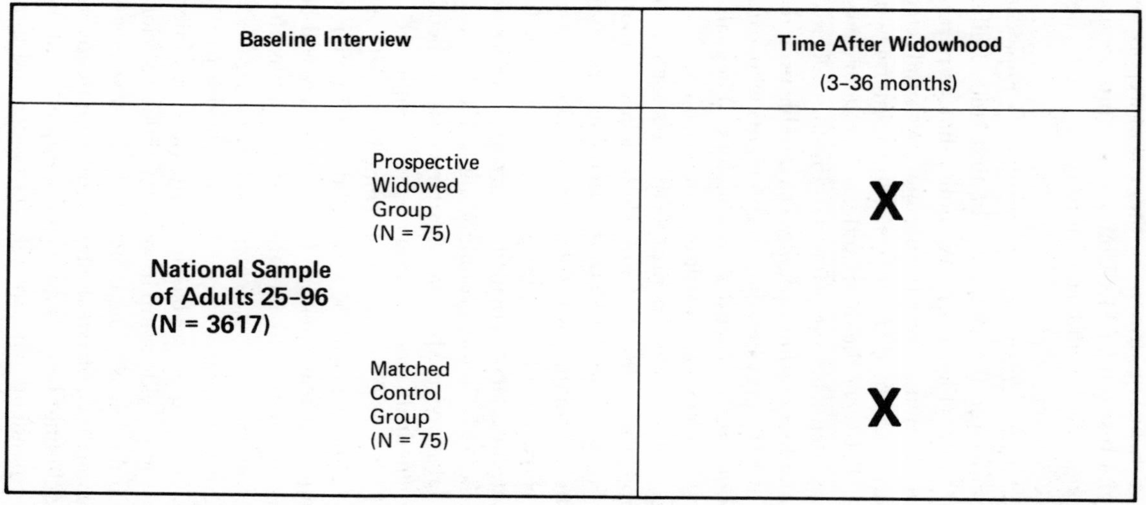

Figure 8.1. Study I: National prospective longitudinal study on bereavement.

Baseline Interview		Time After Widowhood			
		6–8 mo.	18 mo.	37 mo.	61 mo.
Detroit Sample of Older Couples (N = 1532)	Prospective Widowed Group (N = 200)	X	X	X	X
	Matched Control Group (N = 200)		X	X	X

Figure 8.2. Study II: Detroit prospective longitudinal study on bereavement.

Future research directions

The data reviewed earlier suggest that across several studies, a substantial proportion of respondents do not experience intense distress following the loss of a loved one. There is little evidence from these studies that such individuals develop subsequent problems. However, these studies were not designed to explore the grief process as a function of respondents' initial levels of distress. Thus, they leave many questions unanswered about individuals who appear to be well adjusted following a loss. For example, do such individuals experience classic signs of grief and mourning despite their lack of distress? Are they preoccupied with thoughts about the lost loved one? Do such individuals devote a lot of energy to avoiding reminders of the loss, or are they able to encounter reminders with equanimity? Is there any evidence to suggest that such individuals have not yet accepted the reality of the loss, and this is why they show little distress? At present, we are examining these and other questions about the failure to exhibit early distress among respondents in our study of coping with SIDS loss. To date, our analyses suggest that individuals who fail to experience distress following the loss are not preoccupied with thoughts about the loss, nor do they avoid reminders of the baby (see Silver & Wortman, 1990).

In subsequent studies, it will be important to employ research designs that go beyond the self-report methodology that is used almost exclusively in current research in this area. Individuals who indicate that they are not distressed shortly after a loss may also be unwilling to admit subsequent problems in other areas of their lives. An important direction for subsequent work would be to supplement self-reports of symptomatology with more objective indicators of problems, such as measures of behavioral and physiological functioning (e.g., from health records or from observational ratings made by members of the individual's social networks).

If results obtained from further studies are consistent with the results reviewed in this chapter, it will be important to identify those strengths or coping resources that may protect some people from distress following loss. At present, most of the work on coping resources has focused on such variables as socioeconomic status, financial resources, intelligence, self-esteem, premorbid coping style, and social support (see Kessler et al., 1985, for a review). We believe that an individual's religious orientation, or view of the world, may be particularly likely to serve a protective function against the initial, potentially devastating effects of conjugal bereavement. Prospective research designs, which permit such resources to be identified prior to the crisis, afford the opportunity to assess their protective value. In considering the role of coping resources in the effective mastery of widowhood, it should be kept in mind that those resources that may lessen the initial impact of the loss may be quite different from those resources that predict recovery among those who are initially distressed.

In predicting what personal qualities are likely to serve as a coping resource, past research suggests that we should think expansively. Previous research has found that qualities seeming to be quite negative can often facilitate adaptation to a crisis. For example, Lieberman (1975) has reported that those elderly individuals who were most aggressive, irritating, narcissistic, and demanding were those most likely to survive a crisis involving relocation. Those who were liked by the staff – who were not troublemakers and who were easy to relate to – fared less well. Similarly, Lowenthal, Thurnher, and Chiriboga (1975) report that lifelong social isolation, which is generally considered a major indicator of maladaptation, is not necessarily associated with poor adjustment in later life. Apparently, the lifelong social isolate does not suffer as much from age-linked social losses, because he or she has never had social ties. Whether this finding has a parallel among married couples remains to be seen. Similarly, these investigators report that among the older age-groups that they studied, resources such as insight, perspective, and competence do not necessarily contribute to a sense of well-being. Those with many resources were even more unhappy than those with few resources and few deficits. The authors speculate that those who have many resources may become increasingly frustrated in their attempts to realize their maximum potential during old age. Again, it is unclear whether this finding has a parallel among elderly who are coping with the loss of their spouse.

In studying effective mastery of conjugal bereavement, we believe that a question of major importance concerns how coping skills, resources, and personal qualities are affected by the loss of a spouse. Although some resources may be diminished by such a loss, there is every reason to expect that others may be enhanced. If so, the individual may show considerable personal growth as a result of the crisis. Of course, there are many important questions regarding such positive change, or personal growth, that must be addressed, including how common such changes are, how long it takes before a change is achieved, and whether a person must go through a period of initial distress in order to experience growth. Are respondents who show little initial distress following the loss of their spouse less likely to experience personal growth than those who struggle with intense depression and anxiety?

If a person's coping resources are indeed altered by life crises such as the loss of a loved one, then successful mastery of conjugal bereavement may be influenced by experience with prior crises or with concomitant stressors. In almost all cases, conjugal bereavement is likely to be experienced against the backdrop of other life stressors. As noted above, the elderly may be particularly likely to experience other losses prior to the loss of their spouse (Rosow, 1973). A final research question of central importance concerns the cumulative effects of such stressors. Some investigators have suggested that experiencing prior losses may bolster a person's ability to cope with later losses. For example, Hamburg and Adams (1967) contend that an individual will develop new coping strategies as a response to life events that are intensely stressful. They have maintained that if effective, these strategies become available for use in future crises and may augment the individual's problem-solving capacity. However, others have argued that losses may be cumulative in their effects (e.g, Engel, 1964). Negative effects may be especially likely if the prior crisis has not been satisfactorily resolved (Caplan, 1964; Haan, 1977). In fact, Haan (1977) has suggested that a crisis may trigger "ominous meaning" or associations for people because of past unresolved conflicts. More research is necessary to determine whether experience with prior life crises enhances or diminishes a person's ability to cope with conjugal bereavement, and whether the effect depends on whether the prior crisis also involved loss, as opposed to a different type of stressor.

It is also unclear whether an individual's reaction to the loss of a spouse is influenced by other stressors present at the time of the loss, such as limited financial resources or chronic health problems. Such resources may "use up" one's coping reserves and leave one especially vulnerable for adjustment problems following widowhood. Of course, this would not be the case if the chronic stressor involved the spouse. Wheaton (1988) has advanced the provocative argument that in some cases what appears to be a stressful life event marks the end of a chronic stressor. This would be the case, for example, for a person involved in a bad marriage or for someone who was married to a spouse who was extremely ill and who required constant care. In such cases, the loss of the spouse spells the end of the chronic stress involved.

Concluding comments

In conclusion, we have drawn from our own program of research, as well as from the work of others, to critically evaluate prevailing views regarding what constitutes successful mastery of bereavement. Because individuals are increasingly confronted with the loss of loved ones as they age, it is crucial to consider the possibility that prevailing views of adjustment to loss may be too narrow. In fact, a close look at available empirical findings suggests that we need to remain open-minded about what constitutes successful mastery of the bereavement experience. As Zisook and Shuchter (1986) have written, at the present time "there is no prescription for how to grieve properly ... and no research-validated guideposts for what is normal vs. deviant mourning .... We are *just beginning* to realize the full range of what may be considered 'normal' grieving" (p. 288, italics added). It is important that this variability be recognized in subsequent theorizing and research on mastery of bereavement across the life span.

NOTES

Research and preparation of this chapter were supported by U.S. Public Health Services grant MCJ-260470 and by National Institute of Aging Program project grant A605561 to both authors.

1 In this chapter, we have chosen to focus on the classic psychoanalytic model, on Bowlby's (1980) attachment model, and on stage models of emotional reaction to loss, because we believe that these approaches have been the most influential in shaping people's assumptions about coping with loss. Of course, many other types of models have been applied to the study of bereavement, including crisis models, illness and disease models, and the stress and coping approach (for reviews, see Kessler, Price, & Wortman, 1985; Osterweis et al., 1984; Raphael, 1983; W. Stroebe & M. Stroebe, 1987).

2 For the purposes of this discussion, it may be useful to distinguish between the concepts of depression, grief, and mourning. In Freud's classic paper on the subject, "Mourning and Melancholia" (1917/1957), he drew a distinction between the feelings associated with mourning, a process initiated by the loss of a loved one, and melancholia or depression. Freud maintained that both conditions were characterized by the cessation of interest in the outside world, loss of the capacity to love, inhibition of activity, and profoundly painful feelings of dejection. He suggested, however, that melancholia or depression is characterized by an impoverished ego, or low feelings of self-regard, whereas mourning is not. Throughout his writings, Freud used the term *mourning* to refer to the internal psychological process through which one breaks down attachments to the loved one and becomes free to form new relationships.

   For the most part, contemporary researchers have attributed a somewhat different meaning to these terms than that ascribed by Freud (see Osterweis et al., 1984, p. 10). Unfortunately, there has been little consensus in the way the terms *mourning, grieving,* and *depression* are utilized. *Mourning* is sometimes used to refer to the intrapsychic process through which individuals work through their distress following the loss of a loved one and sometimes used to refer to the social or public expression of grief. *Grief* is sometimes utilized to refer to the feelings of mental anguish that occur when a loved one is lost. Other researchers have utilized the term *grieving* to refer to the process of working through or mourning the loss of a loved one – pining for the loved one, reviewing thoughts and memories, perhaps crying. Some investigators have utilized the terms *grief* and *depression* synonymously; others have utilized *grieving* to refer to the expression of sad feelings – "getting the feelings out" – through sharing them with others or through crying. Conceptual confusion about the meaning of these terms has made it difficult to interpret research findings in the area. In this paper, we use the terms *mourning* and *grieving* synonymously, to refer to the intrapsychic process of experiencing painful feelings associated with the loss, preoccupation with thoughts of the lost loved one, and perhaps crying.

3 The only evidence for delayed grief that we have been able to uncover comes from a study by Parkes and Weiss (1983). These investigators found that widows who reported having had marriages characterized by high conflict displayed little or no emotional distress in the weeks following their loss. However, at the 13-month and 2- to 4-year followup interviews, these widows were evidencing greater difficulties than those women whose marriages were characterized by low conflict.

REFERENCES

Ball, J. F. (1976–1977). Cluster analysis. In D. R. Heise (Ed.), *Sociological methodology*. San Francisco, CA: Jossey-Bass.

Ball, J. F. (1977). Widows' grief: The impact of age and mode of death. *Omega, 7,* 307–333.

Bock, E. W., & Webber, I. L. (1972). Suicide among the elderly: Isolating widowhood and mitigating alternatives. *Journal of Marriage and the Family, 34,* 24–31.

Bolger, N., Wortman, C. B., & Kessler, R. (1988, August). Temporal and situational factors in adjustment to widowhood. In R. Janoff-Bulman (Chair), *Personal and situational sources of variation in adjustment to loss*. Symposium conducted at the meeting of the American Psychological Association, Atlanta, GA.

Bornstein, P. E., Clayton, P. J., Halikas, J. A., Maurice, W. L., & Robins, E. (1973). The depression of widowhood after thirteen months. *British Journal of Psychiatry, 122,* 561–566.

Bowlby, J. (1961). Processes of mourning. *International Journal of Psychoanalysis, 42,* 317–340.

Bowlby, J. (1973). *Attachment and loss: Vol. 2. Separation: Anxiety and anger.* New York: Basic Books.

Bowlby, J. (1980). *Attachment and loss: Vol. 3. Loss: Sadness and depression.* New York: Basic Books.

Brim, O. G., Jr. (1980). Types of life events. *Journal of Social Issues, 36* (1), 148–157.

Brim, O. G., Jr., & Ryff, C. D. (1980). On the properties of life events. In P. B. Baltes & O. G. Brim, Jr. (Eds.), *Life-span development and behavior*, Vol. 3. New York: Academic Press.

Brown, J. T., & Stoudemire, G. A. (1983). Normal and pathological grief. *Journal of the American Medical Association, 250,* 378–382.

Caplan, G. (1964). *Principles of preventative psychiatry.* New York: Basic Books.

Carey, R. G. (1977). The widowed: A year later. *Journal of Counseling Psychology, 24,* 125–131.

Carter, H., & Glick, P. (1976). *Marriage and divorce: A social and economic study.* Cambridge, MA: Harvard University Press.

Clayton, P. J. (1979). The sequelae and nonsequelae of conjugal bereavement. *American Journal of Psychiatry, 136,* 1530–1534.

Clayton, P. J., Halikas, J. A., & Maurice, W. L. (1972). The depression of widowhood. *British Journal of Psychiatry, 120,* 71–78.

Craig, Y. (1977). The bereavement of parents and their search for meaning. *British Journal of Social Work, 7,* 41–54.

Deutsch, H. (1937). Absençe of grief. *Psychoanalytic Quarterly, 6,* 12–22.

Dimond, M. F., Lund, D. A., & Caserta, M. S. (1987). The role of social support in the first two years of bereavement in an elderly sample. *Gerontologist, 27,* 599–604.

Donovon, M. I., & Girton, S. E. (1984). *Cancer care nursing.* Norwalk, CT: Appleton-Century-Crofts.

Doyle, P. (1980). *Grief counseling and sudden death: A manual and guide.* Springfield, IL.: Charles C. Thomas.

Engel, G. L. (1964). Grief and grieving. *American Journal of Nursing, 64,* 93–98.

Feighner, J. P., Robins, E., Guze, S. B., Woodruff, R. A., Jr., Winokur, G., & Munoz, R. (1972). Diagnostic criteria for use in psychiatric research. *Archives of General Psychiatry, 26,* 57–63.

Freud, S. (1957). Mourning and melancholia. In J. Strachey (Ed. and Trans.), *The standard edition of the complete original works of Sigmund Freud* (Vol. 14, pp. 152–170). London: Hogarth Press. (Original work published 1917)

Gallagher, D. E., Thompson, L. W., & Peterson, J. A. (1981/1982). Psychosocial factors affecting adaptation to bereavement in the elderly. *International Journal of Aging and Human Development, 14,* 79–85.

Garmezy, N. (1982). Foreword. In E. E. Werner & R. S. Smith (Eds.), *Vulnerable but invincible* (pp. xiii–xix). New York: McGraw-Hill.

Glick, I. O., Weiss, R. S., & Parkes, C. M. (1974). *The first year of bereavement.* New York: John Wiley and Sons.

Goin, M. K., Burgoyne, R. W., & Goin, M. J. (1979). Timeless attachment to a dead relative. *American Journal of Psychiatry, 136,* 988–989.

Gove, W. R. (1972). Sex, marital status, and suicide. *Journal of Marriage and the Family, 34,* 24–31.

Haan, N. (1977). *Coping and defending: Processes of self-environment organization.* New York: Academic Press.

Hamburg, D. A., & Adams, J. E. (1967). A perspective on coping behavior: Seeking and utilizing information in major transitions. *Archives of General Psychiatry, 17,* 277–284.

Heyman, D., & Gianturco, D. (1973). Long term adaptation by the elderly to bereavement. *Journal of Gerontology, 28,* 359–362.

Horowitz, M. J. (1976). *Stress response syndromes.* New York: Aronson.

Horowitz, M. J. (1985). Disasters and psychological responses to stress. *Psychiatric Annals, 15,* 161–167.

Hultsch, D. F., & Plemons, J. K. (1979). Life events and life-span development. In P. B. Baltes & O. G. Brim, Jr. (Eds.), *Life-span development and behavior* (Vol. 2, pp. 1–35). New York: Academic Press.

Janoff-Bulman, R. (1985). The aftermath of victimization: Rebuilding shattered assumptions. In C. R. Figley (Ed.), *Trauma and its wake: The study and treatment of Post-Traumatic Stress Disorder* (pp. 15–35). New York: Brunner/Mazel.

Janoff-Bulman, R., & Frieze, I. H. (1983). A theoretical perspective for under-standing reactions to victimization. *Journal of Social Issues, 39*(2), 1–17.

Jette, S. H. (1983). Nursing the person with loss. In J. Lindbergh, M. Hunter, & A. Kruszewski (Eds.), *Introduction to person-centered nursing* (pp. 641–657). Philadelphia: Lippincott.

Kessler, R. C., Price, R. H., & Wortman, C. B. (1985). Social factors in psychopathology: Stress, social support, and coping processes. *Annual Review of Psychology, 36*, 531–572.

Kitchell, M. A., Barnes, R. F., Veith, R. C., Okimoto, J. T., & Raskind, M. A. (1982). Screening for depression in hospitalized geriatric medical patients. *Journal of the American Geriatrics Society, 30*, 174–177.

Klinger, E. (1975). Consequences of commitment to and disengagement from incentives. *Psychological Review, 82*, 1–25.

Klinger, E. (1977). *Meaning and void: Inner experience and the incentives in people's lives.* Minneapolis: University of Minnesota Press.

Kubler-Ross, E. (1969). *On death and dying.* New York: Macmillan.

Lehman, D. R., Wortman, C. B., & Williams, A. F. (1987). Long-term effects of losing a spouse or child in a motor vehicle crash. *Journal of Personality and Social Psychology, 52*, 218–231.

Lieberman, M. A. (1975). Adaptive processes in late life. In N. Datan & L. H. Ginsberg (Eds.), *Life-span developmental psychology: Normative life crises.* New York: Academic Press.

Lopata, H. Z. (1973). Self-identity in marriage and widowhood. *Sociological Quarterly, 14*, 407–418.

Lowenthal, M. F., Thurnher, M., & Chiriboga, D. (1975). *Four stages of life.* San Francisco, CA: Jossey-Bass.

Lund, D. A., Dimond, M. F., Caserta, M. S., Johnson, R. J., Poulton, J. L., & Connelly, J. R. (1986). Identifying elderly with coping difficulties after two years of bereavement. *Omega, 16*, 213–224.

MacMahon, B., & Pugh, J. (1965). Suicide in the widowed. *American Journal of Epidemiology, 81*, 23–31.

Maddison, D. C., & Viola, A. (1968). The health of widows in the year following bereavement. *Journal of Psychosomatic Research, 12*, 297–306.

Maddison, D., & Walker, W. L. (1967). Factors affecting the outcome of conjugal bereavement. *British Journal of Psychiatry, 113*, 1057–1067.

Marris, P. (1958). *Widows and their families.* London: Routledge and Kegan Paul.

Miles, M. S., & Crandall, E. K. (1983). The search for meaning and its potential for affecting growth in bereaved parents. *Health Values: Achieving High Level Wellness, 7*, 19–23.

Moos, R. H., & Schaefer, J. A. (1986). Life transitions and crises: A conceptual overview. In R. H. Moos (Ed.), *Coping with life crises: An integrated approach* (pp. 3–28). New York: Plenum Press.

Neugarten, B. L. (1968). Adult personality: Toward a psychology of the life cycle. In B. L. Neugarten (Ed.), *Middle age and aging.* Chicago: University of Chicago Press.

Osterweis, M., Solomon, F., & Green, M. (Eds.). (1984). *Bereavement: Reactions, consequences, and care.* Washington, DC: National Academy Press.

Owen, G., Fulton, R., & Markusen, E. (1982). Death at a distance: A study of family survivors. *Omega, 13*, 191–225.

Palmore, E., Cleveland, W. P., Nowlin, J. B., Ramm, D., & Siegler, I. C. (1979). Stress and adaptation in later life. *Journal of Gerontology, 34,* 841–851.

Parkes, C. M. (1964). The effects of bereavement on physical and mental health – A study of the medical records of widows. *British Medical Journal, 2,* 274–279.

Parkes, C. M. (1972). Components of the reaction to loss of a limb, spouse or home. *Journal of Psychosomatic Research, 16,* 343–349.

Parkes, C. M. (1975). Unexpected and untimely bereavement: A statistical study of young Boston widows and widowers. In B. Schoenberg, I. Gerber, A. Wiener, A. H. Kutscher, D. Peretz, & A. C. Carr (Eds.), *Bereavement: Its psychosocial aspects* (pp. 119–138). New York: Columbia University Press.

Parkes, C. M., & Brown, R. (1972). Health after bereavement: A controlled study of young Boston widows and widowers. *Psychosomatic Medicine, 34,* 449–461.

Parkes, C. M., & Weiss, R. S. (1983). *Recovery from bereavement.* New York: Basic Books.

Rando, T. A. (1984). *Grief, dying and death: Clinical interventions for caregivers.* Champaign, IL: Research Press.

Raphael, B. (1983). *The anatomy of bereavement.* New York: Basic Books.

Riegel, K. F. (1975). Adult life crises: A dialectic interpretation of development. In N. Datan & L. H. Ginsberg (Eds.), *Life-span developmental psychology: Normative life crises.* New York: Academic Press.

Rosow, I. (1973). The social context of the aging self. *Gerontologist, 13,* 82–87.

Rubin, S. S. (1982). Persisting effects of loss: A model of mourning. In C. D. Spielberger, I. G. Sarason, & N. A. Milgram (Eds.), *Stress and anxiety* (Vol. 8, pp. 275–282). Washington, DC: Hemisphere Publishing.

Rubin, S. S. (1985). The resolution of bereavement: A clinical focus on the relationship to the deceased. *Psychotherapy, 22,* 231–235.

Sanders, C. M. (1988). Risk factors in bereavement outcome. *Journal of Social Issues, 44*(3), 97–111.

Shuchter, S. R. (1986). *Dimensions of grief: Adjusting to the death of a spouse.* San Francisco: Jossey-Bass.

Siller, J. (1969). Psychological situation of the disabled with spinal cord injuries. *Rehabilitation Literature, 30,* 290–296.

Silver, R. C., & Wortman, C. B. (1980). Coping with undesirable life events. In J. Garber & M. E. P. Seligman (Eds.), *Human helplessness: Theory and applications* (pp. 279–340). New York: Academic Press.

Silver, R. C., & Wortman, C. B. (1990). *Is "processing" a loss necessary for adjustment? A study of parental reactions to the death of an infant.* Unpublished manuscript, University of California, Irvine.

Smith, J., Dixon, R. A., & Baltes, P. B. (1989). Expertise in life planning: A new research approach to investigating aspects of wisdom. In M. L. Commons, J. D. Sinnott, F. A. Richards, & C. Arman (Eds.), *Adult development: Vol. 1. Comparisons and applications of developmental models* (pp. 307–331). New York: Praeger.

Stroebe, M., & Stroebe, W. (1983). Who suffers more? Sex differences in health risks of the widowed. *Psychological Bulletin, 93,* 297–301.

Stroebe, W., & Stroebe, M. S. (1987). *Bereavement and health: The psychological and physical consequences of partner loss.* New York: Cambridge University Press.

Tait, R., & Silver, R. C. (1989). Coming to terms with major negative life events.

In J. S. Uleman & J. A. Bargh (Eds.), *Unintended thought* (pp. 351–382). New York: Guilford.

Tait, R., & Silver, R. C. (1990). *The long-term psychological impact of major negative life events.* Manuscript submitted for publication.

Thomas, L. E., DiGiulio, R. C., & Sheehan, N. W. (1988). Identity loss and psychological crisis in widowhood: A re-evaluation. *International Journal of Aging and Human Development, 26,* 225–239.

Vachon, M. L. S. (1976). Grief and bereavement following the death of a spouse. *Canadian Psychiatric Association Journal, 21,* 35–43.

Vachon, M. L. S., Rogers, J., Lyall, W. A. L., Lancee, W. J., Sheldon, A. R., & Freeman, S. J. J. (1982). Predictors and correlates of adaptation to conjugal bereavement. *American Journal of Psychiatry, 139,* 998–1002.

Vachon, M. L. S., Sheldon, A. R., Lancee, W. J., Lyall, W. A. L., Rogers, J., & Freeman, S. J. J. (1982). Correlates of enduring stress patterns following bereavement: Social network, life situation, and personality. *Psychological Medicine, 12,* 783–788.

Vachon, M. L. S., & Stylianos, S. K. (1988). The role of social support in bereavement. *Journal of Social Issues, 44*(3), 175–190.

Wheaton, B. (1988, August). *When more stress is stress relief: Life events as the resolution of ongoing stress.* Paper presented at the Society for the Study of Social Problems Meetings, Atlanta, GA.

Wortman, C. B. (1983). Coping with victimization: Conclusions and implications for future research. *Journal of Social Issues, 39*(2), 197–223.

Wortman, C. B., Kessler, R. C., Bolger, N., & House, J. (1990). *Recovery and resolution following loss of a spouse.* Unpublished manuscript, University of Michigan.

Wortman, C. B., & Silver, R. C. (1987). Coping with irrevocable loss. In G. R. VandenBos & B. K. Bryant (Eds.), *Cataclysms, crises, and catastrophes: Psychology in action (Master Lecture Series, Vol. 6,* pp. 189–235). Washington, DC: American Psychological Association.

Wortman, C. B., & Silver, R. C. (1989). The myths of coping with loss. *Journal of Clinical and Consulting Psychology, 57,* 349–357.

Wortman, C. B., & Silver, R. C. (1990). *Coping with the loss of a loved one: The grieving process re-examined.* Unpublished manuscript, State University of New York, Stony Brook.

Zisook, S., & Shuchter, S. R. (1986). The first four years of widowhood. *Psychiatric Annals, 15,* 288–294.

Zung, W. W. K. (1965). A self-rating depression scale. *Archives of General Psychology, 13,* 508–516.

9 The Bonn Longitudinal Study of Aging: Coping, life adjustment, and life satisfaction

GEORG RUDINGER AND HANS THOMAE

The Bonn Longitudinal Study of Aging

The Bonn Longitudinal Study of Aging (BOLSA) was started in 1965 with a sample of 222 women and men born between 1890 and 1895 and between 1900 and 1905. The majority of the subjects (97%) lived in their own households in different parts of West Germany. Average length of education was 11.2 years, slightly above the average education of the German population, lower-middle-class status prevailing. In agreement with the planners of the Berkeley, Baltimore (Shock, 1984), and Duke longitudinal studies (Busse & Maddox, 1986), our design did not focus on testing specific hypotheses. Rather, we tried to assess the psychological, social, and physical situation of our subjects at each measurement point as comprehensively as possible. Each measurement session lasted 5 days; during this period, three semistructured interviews were conducted, each of which focused on different aspects of our subjects' lives. At the first interview, the current situation in all of its social, psychological, and physical aspects was emphasized, whereas the second and third interviews were directed toward the past and the future. Furthermore, subjects underwent a series of cognitive, psychomotor, and personality tests and were examined by a specialist for internal medicine. Data were collected between 1965 and 1984 in eight steps: first measurement in 1965/66, second in 1966/67, third in 1967/68, fourth in 1969/70, fifth in 1972/73, sixth in 1976/77, seventh in 1980/81, and eighth in 1983/84.

General hypothesis and global strategy of the BOLSA

The design of the study was influenced by the second author's experience, gained as psychological director of the German Longitudinal Study of

Children (Coerper, Hagen, & Thomae, 1954; Hagen & Thomae, 1962), from longitudinal studies on middle-aged white-collar employees (Lehr & Thomae, 1958), and from a cross-sectional study of men and women born between 1885 and 1930 (Lehr & Thomae, 1965; Lehr, 1969).

These studies led to the formation of a more global hypothesis for this longitudinal study, based also on the assumption that *aging* is an extremely complex process that differs under various biological, social, biographical, and person-specific conditions. The history of the great longitudinal studies, which began in the United States in the late twenties or early thirties of this century, shows that some of the most valuable results of these studies emerged from hypotheses or theories that became relevant several years after the studies had been initiated.

On the other hand, the realization of each study is affected by organizational and financial restrictions. Because we included a fairly extensive psychological testing program, we had to limit the medical program for financial as well as psychological reasons. However, a specialist for internal medicine examined each subject's general health at each measurement point. In 1972 and 1980, all subjects underwent a clinical checkup in a hospital.

We also had to limit the assessment of learning and social conditions preceding transition into old age: These two aspects could be assessed only by interviewing the subjects themselves. Therefore, our findings reflect the self-reported socialization history rather than the "real" one. The decision to dedicate the major part of the week to interviews can be justified by theoretical considerations formulated in terms of a "cognitive theory of personality" (Thomae, 1968) and of aging (Thomae, 1970). This theory places special emphasis on the influence of the situation as perceived by the individual. Because our subjects were quite motivated and very cooperative, their responses in the interviews may legitimately be regarded as rather valid cues to their perception of present, past, and future life situations. On the other hand, we applied intelligence and personality tests to get as much objective information as possible on their psychological situation. Because cognitive and motivational aspects of behavior are interrelated in a very complex manner, we decided to introduce as many variables as possible, in order to be able to identify different patterns of aging as well as the cognitive, motivational, social, and biological correlates of these patterns.

The BOLSA sample

The basic intention in planning BOLSA was to draw a random sample of the population from the western part of the West German Ruhr area, including Bonn and suburbs, Frankfurt, Mannheim, and Heidelberg. However, like most of the previous researchers, we faced many difficulties in doing so. Sampling procedures for a 2-hour interview are completely different from those for a complex psychological and medical examination that requires attendance at a university institute for a whole week. Therefore, we had to complete our random sample with referrals from churches, doctors, voluntary organizations, and industrial plants, to whom we explained our aims and plans. We required that each participant be in good health and live in his or her own household. The subjects we included had to be able to travel to Bonn by train and to stay in small hotels near the department of psychology; those living in the Bonn area were expected to reach the institute every day using public transportation. Another selection criterion was lower-middle-class or middle-middle-class status. We also tried to equate the sample for religious background and place of birth (West Germany versus former German provinces that now belong to Russia, Poland, and Czechoslovakia). A detailed description of the original sample can be found in Rudinger and Schmitz-Scherzer (1976).

Cohorts. A major decision concerned the age cohorts. The design included four groups of men and women of lower-middle-class status: (1) men born between 1900 and 1905, (2) women born between 1900 and 1905, (3) men born between 1890 and 1895, and (4) women born between 1890 and 1895. This design made it possible to compare longitudinal and cross-sectional findings. The two cohorts did not differ regarding socioeconomic status (SES), and health differences were confined to the group of older women at the beginning of the study. However, the biographies of the older cohort during childhood, adolescence, and young adulthood were characterized by the experience of peace and security, although subjects very often reported great economic hardship and few opportunities for better education or occupational training. The older men's period of adulthood was influenced by military service during World War I, whereas the older women very often either had lost a husband or fiancé in this war or had been separated from a husband for years. Very often subjects reported great economic difficulties and even starvation during this period. Only very few of the "younger" men were soldiers in World War I (during the last years). Most of them were adolescents during the war and had to work quite hard to help support their families. Both groups remembered in the same intense and negative manner the time around 1930, when there was widespread unemployment in Germany. Most of the younger men were in the German army in World War II, and most of them reported their experiences as prisoners of war.

Attrition. The original sample in 1965/66 included 222 persons, divided into the two cohorts 1900–1905 and 1890–1895. The younger cohort consisted of 114 persons and the older of 108. Of the 114 younger subjects, 55 were women and 59 men; in the older cohort, there were 49 women and 59 men. In every gerontological longitudinal study, the sample is inevitably subject to attrition processes. In BOLSA, this attrition process reduced the sample from the first to the eighth measurement point in the following way: first measurement in 1965/66, $N = 222$; second in 1966/67, $N = 202$; third in 1967/68, $N = 184$; fourth in 1969/70, $N = 146$; fifth in 1972/73, $N = 121$; sixth in 1976/77, $N = 81$; seventh in 1980/81, $N = 48$; eighth in 1983/84, $N = 34$. At the last measurement point, the sample had dropped to 25 women and 9 men. Attrition was due to death or poor health in about 95% of the cases. There were no dropouts due to lack of motivation. In the following analyses, we refer mainly to the reduced sample of the sixth measurement point (1976/77, $N = 81$). The chronological age of this subsample ranged from 70 to 85 years in 1976/77.

Survival, selection, and "successful" aging. Considering the deprivation, stress, and personal loss experienced and reported by most of our subjects, they may be regarded as the survivors of serious strains even at the beginning of our study in 1965. The men in particular were survivors in the true sense of the word. According to census data of the Federal Republic of Germany (FRG) in 1961, 1890–1895 cohorts consisted of about 1 million men and 1.658 million women; the 1900–1905 cohorts included 2.076 million men and about 2.5 million women. These sex differences in survivorship are only partially explained by the two world wars. Estimations of survival rates for these cohorts pointed to a decreasing life expectancy for men compared with a slowly increasing life expectancy for women (Schwarz, 1974). This difference, according to some authors, is because men's occupations entail more severe stress and other conditions conducive to coronary vascular disease in middle age. However, female life expectancy is not getting any lower, even now that the number of women in similar stressful work situations is steadily increasing.

Against this background, our subjects might be defined as a biological "elite," even if they have by no means attained the status of centenarians. Especially those who participated in the study at all points of measurement from 1965 to 1983 may be regarded as "successfully" aged people per se. Inasmuch as this pattern of successful aging is defined by the ability to lead a fairly independent life, it certainly is more representative of the aged population than the picture drawn by studies using social welfare samples. Of all persons living in the FRG aged 65 or above, approximately 96%–97% live in their own households. In our original sample (in 1965/66), 3%–4% of the men and women were living in a home for the aged. Unfortunately, the image of the sickly, helpless, or at least dependent old person has been reinforced many times by overgeneralization from experiences with physically or mentally impaired patients. Even if the BOLSA sample is defined as an elite group (although subjects belong mainly to lower SES), which of course restricts generalizability of findings to the entire population, inferences from samples of this kind can help to revise the stereotypes that have emerged from overgeneralized experiences with physically and/or economically highly dependent persons. A major task of the BOLSA is to uncover different patterns of aging and to elaborate ways of evaluating, predicting, and controlling them. Therefore, the image of aging we should like to reinforce is neither optimistic nor pessimistic; it is realistic in the sense that it tries to outline and differentiate the highly complex process of aging.

Successful aging and life satisfaction

The concept *successful aging* in its original meaning implies life satisfaction as the most salient indicator (Havighurst, 1961; Williams & Wirths, 1965). According to the widely accepted early conceptualization (see Adams, 1971), life satisfaction is related to the main goal of life in old age: maintaining and/or restoring psychological well-being in a situation implying many biological, social, and psychological crises and risks (see, e.g., Kuypers & Bengtson, 1973).

Correlates, conditions, and prediction of life satisfaction

In a condensed, but comprehensive paper about correlates of life satisfaction, Adams (1971) splits these correlates into major (but not independent) areas for clarity of presentation, namely, biological, psychological, and sociological. Subsequent reviews (such as Larson, 1978) as well as the introductory contributions by Fries, Baltes and Baltes, and Featherman, Smith, and Peterson (this volume) follow this tripartite taxonomy. The following brief summary of recent approaches and findings in the area of life satisfaction and well-being in old age is given to clarify the BOLSA approach in the study of life satisfaction.

Biological correlates. Age and health were the predominant biological characteristics that were considered very extensively during the planning and realization of the BOLSA. Because age as a correlate of satisfaction (as indicator of successful aging) turns out to be slightly circular, we focused on health. Also, recent studies point consistently in the following direction: Dissatisfaction depends not only on objective health assessed by a physician but also on physical disability and loss of physical mobility, combined with the self-perception of poor health. One frequent explanation is that poor health generally restricts possible social contacts (e.g., Medley, 1976; Whitbourne, 1987) and that this reduction has an adverse effect on life satisfaction. This interpretation is plausible, but it is, of course, not the only one. It might be the dependence on others (i.e., loss of independence), the pain caused by illness, the realization of a limited life span, or disappointment with the lack of mobility that results in dissatisfaction.

Sociological correlates. Sociological correlates can be divided into personal characteristics, roles and role changes, and social relations and activities. Research on roles and role changes and social relations and activities points to a positive relationship between intensity and frequency of social contact and satisfaction, particularly within the family system (marriage, familial roles and activities). Continuity and stability of social network and support are decisive factors, for example, being single or married as opposed to widowed, divorced, or separated (Larson, 1978). Salient "personal characteristics" affecting satisfaction are SES indices, such as income, home ownership, education.

Social networks. Ward (1985) offers a research guide and discusses the processes by which informal social networks (such as family, friends, neighbors, kin, and children) are assumed to affect the well-being and quality of life of older people. In order to understand this contribution of informal social support to the quality of life, one has to differentiate sources and types of social networks: for example, immediate kin (parents, children, etc.) from more distant kin (aunts and uncles, etc.), neighbor friends versus non-neighbor friends, and structural and functional properties (e.g., member, proximity, reciprocity, or nature of contact: casual, intimate, supportive, etc.). On the other hand, one also has to pay attention to the dimensionality of the "criterion," for example, satisfaction or well-being. Social support by family members (spouse, children, etc.) may contribute to global life satisfaction, but it may also have relatively little bearing on whether the whole life is viewed as rewarding. Less global and more specific measures of well-being, such as emotions or symptoms of distress, may more adequately reflect the contribution of current social involvement and support. We will return to this problem of global versus specific measures of life satisfaction in the section on assessment and scales of life satisfaction.

Historical and social antecedents. Caspi and Elder's (1986) approach to life satisfaction in the later years explores personal resources as determinants of the choices and actions that shape the life course under various conditions. Their central thesis is that life appraisals in old age are shaped by past experience, which, in turn, is shaped by personal resources that augment, reduce, or buffer the effect of stressful events, including historical events that alter lives in unforeseen ways and social conditions that provide or curtail opportunities. Their theoretical model on successful aging stresses the importance of personal resources in early adulthood (intellectual ability and emotional health) and hardship experience (in their study, the Great Depression) as antecedent factors to successful aging. Social involvement in old age mediates between early personal resources and economic loss.

Psychological correlates. Essential "classical" psychological correlates of satisfaction are self-perception of age, self-esteem, self-concept, and perceptions of relative deprivation and contracting life space; recently, *personal control* turned out to be an important psychological dimension (see Baltes & Baltes, 1986). Klemmack and Roff (1984) examined the relationship between social and psychological factors (such as income, education, welfare status, race, perceived health) and subjective well-being in a cross-sectional sample of 595 Alabamians (55 years and older). Well-being was measured by a subset of Life Satisfaction Index (LSI) items (see Adams, 1969). In particular, fear of aging was assumed to be an intervening variable, mediating effects of education and perceived health on well-being. One of the major results of their descriptive multiple regression analysis is that fear of aging (as a subjective variable) is inversely related to current subjective well-being, independent of the psychological and social factors mentioned above. The authors point to similarities between fear of aging and "attitude toward future," as defined in BOLSA: Positive attitudes are associated with higher satisfaction concerning the current life situation (Lehr, 1967).

Unanswered questions

There is a certain agreement on some preconditions or at least correlates of life satisfaction, yet there are still a number of open interrelated questions.

Theoretical conceptualization. One set of questions refers to the theoretical conceptualization: Should life satisfaction be embedded in a theoretical context such as activity and/or disengagement theory (Hoyt, Kaiser,

Peters, & Babchuk, 1980)? Does it have to be connected with adjustment, restructuring, or homeostatic processes? Should it be defined in terms of interaction? Should it be conceptualized in terms of an action perspective (Brandstädter, 1984) or rather be considered as a trait?

The pioneers in research on life satisfaction in old age have been criticized for lack of theory (Ryff, 1986). An analysis of the contributions of Pollak (1948), Burgess, Cavan, Havighurst, and Goldhammer (1949), and Havighurst (1963) shows, however, that explicitly as well as implicitly, this research was guided by homeostatic principles. Life in old age was considered to imply several deficits in well-being concerning health, income, social contacts, or social status. Measures of life satisfaction, from this point of view, were measures of reestablished homeostasis or of adjustment (see also Hoyt & Creech, 1983). This method of assessing successful aging by measuring life satisfaction assumes that a successfully aging person is satisfied with his or her present and past life. Havighurst (1963) identified life satisfaction as the "inner subjective" aspect of successful aging and developed with his co-workers the LSI, which includes five components: zest versus apathy, resolution and fortitude, goodness of fit between desired and achieved goals, positive self-concept, and mood tone. These five suggested components were reduced to three by Hoyt and Creech (1983) and (through confirmatory factor analysis) by Liang (1984), namely, mood tone, zest, and congruence.

Since its early conceptualization, the theory of successful aging has undergone many transformations, modifications, specifications, and enlargements. It has sometimes been equated with more objective features such as survival (longevity) and health (lack of disability). In recent years, essential aspects already inherent in the original definition have been reemphasized from an interactional and contextual point of view: Successful aging is considered to be an effective adaptation process, labeled "selective optimization with compensation" (Baltes, 1987; Baltes & Baltes, 1986, and this volume). This interactional perspective takes into account the interplay between interindividual differences and intraindividual variability in the aging process, on the one hand, and the variety of (objective) life domains, (subjective) life spaces, environments, and ecologies, on the other (see also Lehr, 1985). A comprehensive theory of successful aging has to pay attention to all these components: the objective and the subjective "inner" facets, the adaptive and selective processes, and the interactional structure of the complex person–environment network.

Assessment of life satisfaction. Related to this discussion is another set of questions: Should life satisfaction be defined as a general (unidimen-

sional, traitlike) concept or as a domain-specific, interactional, or process-oriented multicomponent construct with conceptually different but
interrelated facets? We will return to this problem in the third part of this
section.

Medley (1976) investigated the problem of explaining the interrelationships of selected determinants of satisfaction with life as a whole, such
as satisfaction with the financial situation, health satisfaction, satisfaction
with standard of living, and satisfaction with family life. The data were
obtained from persons 65 years of age and older, representing a subsample
($N = 301$) taken from a larger national probability sample of people of
all ages. The results stress the importance of family life satisfaction for
satisfaction with life as a whole. The financial situation did not have a
significant, direct impact on life satisfaction; males, however, were indirectly but substantially influenced by the financial situation mediated
by expectations about standard of living. Satisfaction with standard of
living may be of greater importance for an individual's outlook on life than
his or her actual financial condition. This finding supports the notion that
subjective evaluation is a crucial determinant in the formation of an
individual's view of reality, as well as the fact (reported in a great number
of studies) that health is an essential component of life satisfaction.

Interactional orientation. The third set of questions focuses on the problem of
the interaction of social, historical, and psychological factors in the course
of successful adaptation and aging. Satisfaction may be directly linked
to biological, historical, sociological, and psychological variables, or indirectly mediated by differential life-styles, values, role relations, and
expectations. This approach goes beyond the search for correlates, because interactive or time-bound "causal" interconnections between preconditions of satisfaction are hypothesized, explored, and tested.

The methodological problem inherent in correlation studies or simple
regression ("prediction") studies can be illustrated with an example taken
from the Duke study (Palmore, 1979; Palmore & Kivett, 1977). The
significance of predictors of successful aging such as group activity,
physical activity, physical function abilities, and happiness is understood
to support the activity theory of aging (Havighurst, 1961). The activity
theory is unidirectional. It states that those who are more active are more
likely to be happy. But there is also evidence that those who are happy are
more likely to remain active. Even though this reciprocal relation can be
studied within a longitudinal context, it should be mentioned that neither
the Duke study nor the BOLSA have done this type of statistical analysis.
In the present paper we mainly confine ourselves (with one exception) to
the (cross-sectional) prediction type of research for a variety of domains

and a relatively large number of variables. These analyses should be considered a first attempt to cover a more extensive period of the life course of older subjects of the BOLSA.

Life satisfaction indices in the BOLSA

As outlined in the preceding paragraphs, the examination of the biographical and situational correlates of life satisfaction or well-being of old people is a central issue in research on successful aging. However, the difficulty in trying to assess subjective well-being or life satisfaction has resulted in a variety of concepts, definitions, and measurements (see Diener, 1984). The definitions of the concepts are semantically similar and the scales measuring them – such as satisfaction, happiness, morale, adjustment, and adaptation – are related empirically. In addition to these investigations into the conditions of life satisfaction, other studies are concerned with the construction, validation, and overall reexamination of satisfaction scale and well-being scales per se (for a review see Stock, Okun, & Benin, 1986). There is an increasing trend to study the construct validity of life-quality scales, life-satisfaction scales, and measures of well-being and morale by means of confirmatory factor analysis (e.g., Liang, Lawrence, & Bollen, 1986). This technique tests the theoretical presuppositions for multidimensionality of life satisfaction scales, such as the Philadelphia Geriatric Center Morale Scale (PGS) and the Life Satisfaction Index A (LSI-A).

For our purpose, it is not necessary to go into the details of this validation process. Instead, we will now turn to the issue of global versus domain-specific measures of life satisfaction. As "a cognitive assessment of progress toward desired goals," life satisfaction refers to life in general "from a long-term time perspective" (George, 1981, p. 351). This global and traitlike concept of life satisfaction, which is also inherent in most life satisfaction scales, is to be distinguished from domain-specific, concrete measures. The latter do not refer to life in general but to specific areas of life such as family life, health, income, housing, and so forth. Assessments of these specific aspects of life satisfaction are more likely to be affected by situational change, whereas "satisfaction with life in general" is related to rather basic and stable attitudes. We therefore expect domain-specific ratings across time to be less stable than global ratings of satisfaction.

At the beginning of the BOLSA in 1965, a German standardization of the LSI or of other satisfaction scales was not available. Thus, we had to rely on a set of global ratings such as the "positive/negative appraisal of the last year" (determined by the prevalence of pleasant or unpleasant experiences during the last year), on the one hand, and on more domain-specific ratings such as satisfaction with housing, income, family, or health, on the other hand. For example, satisfaction in the domain of the family was assessed by one global scale ("congruence between desired and achieved goals in the family") and several specific measures related to different roles in the family. The inclusion of extrafamilial roles and of satisfaction with housing was especially important. In choosing these domains, we were guided by Cantril's (1965) finding that the areas of income, family relationships, and health are the primary referents for the assessment of subjective well-being. The interview schedule and the rating scales were adapted from those applied in a cross-national study on adjustment to aging (Havighurst, Munnichs, Neugarten, & Thomae, 1969). The interview material was rated by the psychologists of the BOLSA research staff. Thus, the assessment of satisfaction as well as of "concerns" and responses to stress such as coping (see below) is not based on self-ratings of our older subjects but on ratings by the interviewing research psychologists.

Following the validation procedures for several life satisfaction scales (Adams, 1969; Carp & Carp, 1983; Liang, 1984, 1985; Liang & Bollen, 1983; Liang, Lawrence, & Bollen, 1986; Stock, Okun, & Benin, 1986), we tested both a unidimensional model for the BOLSA satisfaction indices and an a priori specified multicomponent model.[1] In the one-factor model, the ratings are assumed to represent only a single, underlying construct of general satisfaction, without any differentiation into components. The multicomponent model corresponds to a multifactor solution with correlated factors. It reflects the expectation that the measures of satisfaction in the BOLSA are indeed conceptually different but not necessarily statistically independent.

Because of the acceptable goodness of fit index (GFI) for the multicomponent model (GFI = .93) compared with the GFI for the one-factor model (GFI = .86), we opted for the multiple-factor solution (see Table 9.1 for the nontechnical description of the correspondence between ratings and factors). In terms of goodness of fit, a hierarchical factor model, which turned out to be quite appropriate in the recent analyses of various life satisfaction scales, did not differ substantially from the one-factor solution. The four main components out of the six factors are

- a factor comprehending fairly global ratings – mood tone,
- satisfaction with economic/ecological conditions,
- satisfaction with family roles, and
- satisfaction with extrafamilial roles.

In the analyses presented in the next section, we will concentrate on the facets of satisfaction as suggested by the multicomponent model.

Table 9.1. *Multicomponent model of the BOLSA rating scales of life satisfaction*

Factors	Ratings
Basic and General Feeling	• Attitude toward future • Mood as observed during 1-week session • Positive or negative appraisal of last year
Evaluation of Everyday Life With Respect to Economics and Ecological Conditions	• Satisfaction with housing • Positive or negative appraisal of daily activities • Congruence between desired and achieved goals in family • Satisfaction with private economic situation
Satisfaction With Family Roles	• Satisfaction with situation in parent role • Satisfaction with situation in grandparent role • Satisfaction with situation in spouse role
Satisfaction With Extrafamilial Social Roles and Activities	• Satisfaction with perceived change of work and rest • Satisfaction with situation in acquaintance role • Satisfaction with situation in kin role • Satisfaction with situation in citizen role • Satisfaction with situation as club member
Satisfaction With Friend Role	• Satisfaction with situation in friend role
Satisfaction With Neighbor Role	• Satisfaction with situation in neighbor role

Life satisfaction in different domains: Empirical results from the BOLSA

This section presents six path analyses with latent variables using concurrent data from the BOLSA. The models were developed according to a priori predictions based on the cognitive theory of aging and its very general postulates:

- Human behavior is dependent on the cognitive representation of a situation rather than on its objective quality.
- Perception and cognitive representation of a situation are influenced by the person's dominant concerns and expectations.
- Adjustment to aging is a function of the attained balance between the person's cognitive and motivational–emotional system.

The confirmatory strategy of testing models changed slightly to a more-or-less exploratory procedure in order to find a model whose fit was rather satisfactory. We did not test theoretically alternative (noncognitive) models. The majority of the analyses use data from the sixth assessment in 1976/77. Dependent variables include satisfaction with health, family life, the economic and ecological situation, and everyday life, as well as an evaluation of the present situation.

Health and satisfaction with health

From the earliest reviews of correlates and conditions of life satisfaction up to recent ones (Okun, 1986), health has been found to be one of the most powerful predictors of well-being in old age. Health as perceived by the person is considered even more predictive than the medically assessed health status (Okun, 1986).

Independent variables. In view of the evidence for the relationship between health and social status (e.g., Blume, Hauss, Kuhlmeyer, & Oberwittler, 1974), we used SES and income as one set of independent variables, indicating the theoretical concept "socioeconomic background." Another set of variables, including intelligence and education level, defines "competence." As measures for health we included both health rated "objectively" by our medical staff member and ratings of the subjective evaluation of health status. Objective health status is used as an independent variable.

Dependent variables. Because BOLSA does not include a scale "satisfaction with health," we substituted the ratings of "perceived need for help in daily life" and "perceived disability." Because the sample of survivors at the sixth measurement consists almost entirely of persons living independently in their own households, need for help refers to required assistance in special situations such as cleaning the windows, climbing stairs, or doing errands downtown. Perceived disability is in most cases related to difficulties in hearing, seeing, or moving. Of course, realizing that one "needs help" and that one is becoming "increasingly disabled" may well be a stressful and unfavorable experience. The reverse of satisfaction with health, labeled "perceived physical dependency" as defined by these ratings, is the dependent variable in our analysis.

Intervening variables. "Subjective health status" is described by a set of rating scales, such as "frequency and intensity of reported illness," "concern about health," "subjective evaluation of health status," and "appraisal of the last year." Events reported to affect the appraisal of the last year were exclusively health related. "Subjective health status" defined this way is considered to be a theoretical variable, mediating the influence of objective health on perceived physical dependency.

From the large set of possibilities to cope with health problems, we chose "achievement-related behavior," that is, the degree of active coping, and "adjustment to institutional aspects of the situation." In the context of health, this "adjustment" variable includes all efforts of the BOLSA subjects to make use of the services offered by the German health care system for the prevention and treatment of illness.

Finally, we also took into account a "cognitive" way of dealing with health problems, namely, "accepting the situation as it is." From a theoretical point of view, these variables are also assumed to mediate the influences of the "objective" independent variables (see Figure 9.1 for a list of variables and the specification of the model).

1976/77 Results (sixth measurement). The model outlined and presented in Figure 9.1 explains a great proportion of variance (45%) of perceived physical dependency ("dis/satisfaction with health"). In accordance with previous research (see Lehr, 1982), subjective health is the main explanatory factor (total direct and indirect effect: .63). In comparison, the total effect of objective health was much smaller (.29). None of the competence variables turned out to be relevant in predicting satisfaction with health.

1967/68 Results (third measurement). In this path analysis, the model developed and tested for the sixth assessment is applied to data from the longitudinal sample ($N = 81$) of the third assessment (1967/68). This analysis provides some quasi-longitudinal evidence and is an attempt to cross-validate the model from 1976/77. *Quasi-longitudinal* means that intraindividual changes in stress, coping, and satisfaction are not analyzed. The results are given in Figure 9.2.

Conclusion. The network of interrelations among competence, socioeconomic conditions, and objective health changes from 1967 to 1976. The strength of relations is decreasing; the components become independent. The objective health status changes for the worse, regardless of the social and psychological conditions. These conditions seem to lose their buffering function in old age. The independence of the subjective realm of competence and socioeconomic conditions in 1967 and 1976 might be explained by a selective attrition process, inevitably taking place in a longitudinal study and leading to increasing homogeneity of the sample. The social status stratification in the BOLSA sample, however, remained unchanged from the first to the seventh measurement, in 1980 (Lehr & Thomae, 1987). Therefore, attrition is probably not the explanation. Methodological distinction offers another possible interpretation: SES and intelligence (measured by WAIS) are "objective" assessments, that is, observed under stimulus-like conditions, as opposed to "subjective"

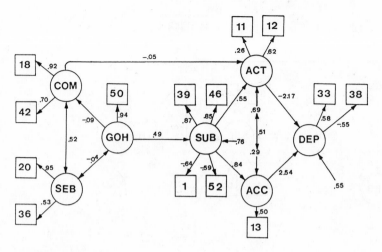

Goodness of fit index = .93

Latent variables	Observed variables
COM – competence:	18 – educational status
	42 – WAIS score
SEB – socioeconomic background:	20 – socioeconomic status (1 = low, 5 = high)
	36 – income
GOH – objective health status:	50 – general health status (from good to poor)
SUB – subjective health status:	39 – recent stressful events (regarding health)
	1 – positive/negative appraisal of last year
	46 – concern about health
	52 – subjective evaluation of health status
ACT – activity for improvement of health conditions:	11 – achievement-related behavior regarding health
	12 – adjustment to institutional aspects of situations
ACC – accepting the situation:	13 – accepting health situation
DEP – perceived physical dependency:	33 – need for help in everyday life
	38 – perceived disability (from high to low)

Figure 9.1. Domain "health": model for prediction of "physical dependency/helplessness" (sixth measurement, 1976/77). Standardized solution. Latent variables are shown within circles, and observed variables are shown within squares.

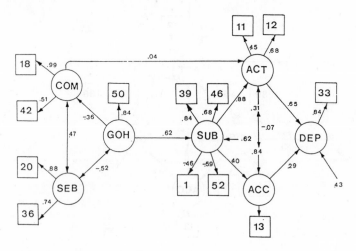

Goodness of fit index = .96

Latent variables	Observed variables
COM – competence:	18 – educational status
	42 – WAIS score
SEB – socioeconomic background:	20 – socioeconomic status (1 = low, 5 = high)
	36 – income
GOH – objective health status:	50 – general health status (from good to poor)
SUB – subjective health status:	39 – recent stressful events (regarding health)
	1 – positive/negative appraisal of last year
	46 – concern about health
	52 – subjective evaluation of health status
ACT – activity for improvement of health conditions:	11 – achievement-related behavior regarding health
	12 – adjustment to institutional aspects of situations
ACC – accepting the situation:	13 – accepting health situation
DEP – perceived physical dependency:	33 – need for help in everyday life

Figure 9.2. Domain "health": model for prediction of "physical dependency/helplessness" (third measurement, 1967/68). Standardized solution.

assessments. It is in complete agreement with cognitive theories of aging that concepts of this "objective" type do not contribute to the explanation of "subjective" dis/satisfaction with health. However, the close connection between dis/satisfaction with health and cognitive representations of different aspects of the personal health condition coincides with cognitive theories of behavior. According to these theories, the regulation and selection of responses to stressful situations are guided by the cognitive representation of a situation rather than by the objective quality of the situation.

The striking difference between the two models can be found in the domain of coping strategies and their effect on physical dependency. In 1967 both strategies were associated with an increase of perceived disability, but 9 years later "activity" reduced and "acceptance" increased the feeling of dependency. Of course, it is premature to infer a systematic change in coping with health problems. Yet in 1976 our subjects (average age, 77 years) probably had adopted effective ways of adjusting to their health problems, whereas in 1967 (average age, 68 years) health problems led to a feeling of physical dependency.

Satisfaction with family life

Satisfaction with family life is considered one of the main conditions for well-being in old age (Atchley & Miller, 1980; Hagestad, 1986). However, there seems to be some interaction between social status, personality variables, intrafamilial interaction, extrafamilial activities, and life satisfaction (Lehr, 1987).

Independent variables. One of the variables not analyzed sufficiently in previous studies is continuity versus discontinuity in family life. Because continuity in life conditions is regarded as a major determinant of well-being in old age, discontinuity in family life should have some adverse effects on satisfaction with life (see Palmore, 1981). To test this assumption, we defined a dis/continuity variable by dividing "family status" into two ordered categories: those always single or always married (continuity) versus widowed, divorced, and so forth (discontinuity). Another "independent" variable we selected was stressful events connected with family life, that is, a rating of the perceived stress in family life.

Dependent variable. The dependent variable is "congruence between desired and achieved goals in the family," as defined in the cross-national study on adjustment to retirement (Havighurst et al., 1969). This variable can be considered a more general indicator of satisfaction with family life.

Intervening variables. Three responses to stress – "adjustment to needs and habits of others," "identification with the aims and fates of children and grandchildren," and 'achievement-related behavior" – and some domain-specific ratings like satisfaction with the roles of parent, grandparent, and spouse were introduced as indicators of a set of three intervening variables: "prosocial behavior," "achievement-related behavior," and "satisfaction with family roles." They are assumed to mediate the influences of "objective" conditions on global satisfaction (Figure 9.3).

Results. The network of theoretical paths explains 80% of the variance of "congruence between desired and achieved goals in the family," that is, of satisfaction with family life in general. As expected, stressful events in family life have a strong (direct) negative effect on congruence (−.67). However, the chain from stressful events to congruence mediated by behavioral responses is quite remarkable. Stress "leads" to prosocial behavior; prosocial behavior has a (direct) positive effect on satisfaction and "leads" to achievement-related behavior, which in turn has a positive effect on satisfaction with family life and an (indirect) effect on general congruence. In other words, "coping" leads to general satisfaction, and stressful events per se have a negative influence on the global satisfaction with family life. Discontinuity has direct and indirect negative effects on "congruence" as an indicator of global satisfaction. As expected, discontinuity turns out to be a relevant variable; the Duke Longitudinal Studies have used it with similar effects.

Conclusion. If only stress (conceptualized as environmental input) and behavioral outcomes were taken into account, low satisfaction would be the inevitable result of this unfavorable situation. However, if personality variables (conceptualized in terms of different ways of coping) are included in the model, the active part of the individual's contribution to her or his own well-being can be traced. It should be emphasized, however, that these personality variables are action-oriented rather than trait-oriented. They refer to specific patterns of behavior rather than to global personality dispositions.

Satisfaction with the economic and ecological situation

The importance of socioeconomic correlates of global life satisfaction has been underlined in many studies (e.g., Adams, 1971; Palmore, 1981). The economic and ecological situation as a material domain is important for subjective well-being. These relationships, however, could not be confirmed consistently across different studies (Okun, 1986). The ecological

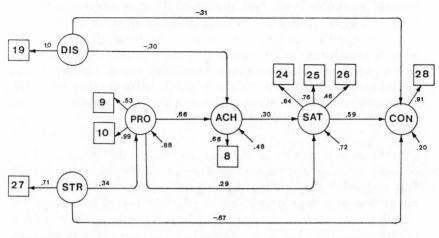

Goodness of fit index = .93

Latent variables	*Observed variables*

DIS – discontinuity:

19 – discontinuity in family life over the life course (1 = married or single during the whole life, 2 = widowed, divorced, etc.)

STR – stressful events:

27 – stressful events connected with family life

PRO – prosocial behavior:

9 – identification with aims and fates of family members

10 – adjustment to the needs and habits of family members

ACH – achievement-related behavior:

8 – achievement-related behavior research regarding family affairs

SAT – satisfaction with family roles:

24 –
25 – satisfaction with { parent / grandparent / spouse } role
26 –

CON – congruence:

28 – congruence between desired and achieved goals in the family

Figure 9.3. Domain "family": model for prediction of "congruence between desired and achieved goals in the family" (sixth measurement, 1976/77). Standardized solution.

variable studied most has been that of rural–urban differences. Results point to a higher degree of well-being in urban areas.

The main environment for aged people is the home; thus, satisfaction with the situation in this area should be a major component of well-being. In the longitudinal analyses of these satisfaction scores, Thomae (1983a, 1983b) found a large number of significant correlations between satisfaction with housing and satisfaction with both intra- and extrafamilial roles, as well as with health variables.

Variables under study. Our model aims to analyze the influence of the economic situation and personal resources on satisfaction in this domain. It is assumed that stress due to housing and coping with stress determine satisfaction to a large degree. Stress might be caused by unfavorable circumstances, such as an apartment house without a lift or central heating where fuel has to be transported up several flights of stairs. Dissatisfaction with housing may also be due to conflicts within the neighborhood or to ecological deficits caused by a nearby highway. Satisfaction is assessed by ratings of "congruence between desired and achieved goals regarding the private economic situation" and "economic independence" (Figure 9.4).

Results. Objective economic conditions and the mediating subjective evaluations, such as satisfaction with housing, explain 66% of the variance of satisfaction with the economic and ecological situation. Although the perceived degree of stress due to housing has a negative effect on satisfaction with the economic and ecological situation, stress is connected with satisfaction in a positive way if mediated by active coping with housing problems.

The negative path from competence as defined by education and WAIS score to satisfaction with economic conditions is an unexpected result.

Conclusion. From the sources of perceived stress described above, it can be seen that the objective economic situation and satisfaction with housing are independent dimensions, as shown in our analysis. The results of Carp's (1975) study offer some explanation. She found that elderly people living in run-down quarters that were to be pulled down because of their poor condition were very satisfied with their housing situation. There seem to be defense mechanisms working toward a positive self-concept. They start operating given a critical discrepancy between objective quality of the housing situation and subjective evaluation of this situation. In

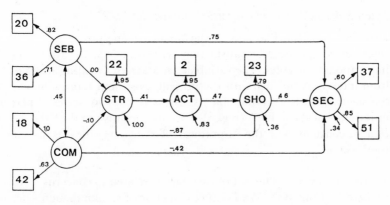

Goodness of fit index = .93

Latent variables	*Observed variables*
SEB – socioeconomic background:	20 – socioeconomic status (from low to high)
	36 – income
COM – competence:	18 – educational stress
	42 – WAIS score
STR – stress due to housing:	22 – stress due to housing
ACT – activity regarding housing:	2 – activities to reduce stress due to housing
SHO – satisfaction with housing:	23 – satisfaction with housing
SEC – satisfaction with economic/ ecological situation:	37 – economic independence
	51 – congruence between desired and achieved goals regarding the private economic situation

Figure 9.4. Domain "economic situation": model for prediction of "satisfaction with economic and ecological situation" (sixth measurement, 1976/77). Standardized solution.

our sample, perceived unchangeable housing conditions can be considered a major cause of this discrepancy.

This stabilizing mechanism does not seem to work in every situation. Thus, the negative relation between competence and satisfaction may be explained as follows: A higher education level and higher mental competence are associated with higher life goals in the economic domain. If these goals cannot be achieved because of adverse circumstances, there is a negative balance, namely, a discrepancy between expectations and outcome.

Extrafamilial activities and satisfaction with everyday life

Dependent variables. The aim of the following analysis is to predict two separate components of satisfaction with daily life by attitudinal and motivational variables. The variables are assessed by rating scales derived from interviews dealing with the present, past, and future life situation. Satisfaction with everyday life is assessed by two scales: "perceived uniformity of daily life" (regarded as the negative end of the satisfaction dimension) and the "appraisal of daily activities as pleasant or unpleasant."

Independent variables. One set of variables is related to concerns as conceptualized by Cantril (1965): Frequent mention of certain thoughts, feelings, or worries is taken as indicating concern. Among others, "concerns of maintenance, extension, and restrictions of range of social contacts" were assessed from the subjects' spontaneous remarks during three extensive interviews. Included in this group is another theme: memories and feelings our subjects expressed spontaneously about pleasant encounters or experiences in everyday life, like watching a bird or a squirrel, enjoying spring after a hard winter, and so forth. It is labeled "using chances."

Intervening variables. Another set of variables includes coping strategies such as "degree of coping with conflict and strain in extrafamilial roles" and "cultivating social contacts" in order to solve these problems. A final set is labeled "specific social activities" and includes things like paying visits, going on trips or tours, and having social engagements. The scale "perceived amount of favorable/pleasant as well as unfavorable/unpleasant events during the last year" also belongs to this set, because the events reported were mainly social activities. The variables are listed in Figure 9.5.

Results. The model delivers only a satisfactory prediction of "perceived uniformity of daily life" and does not predict "appraisal of daily activities as pleasant or unpleasant" at all. The fact that perceived uniformity is linked to the motivational concept "attitude toward social engagement" (which reflects concerns about social participation) suggests that cognitive representations of everyday life depend on emotions and motives. This influence is mediated, however, by the set of variables related to "extrafamilial social activities."

Conclusion. Concerns about maintenance or extension of social contacts initiate more social activities, which make everyday life less uniform. We

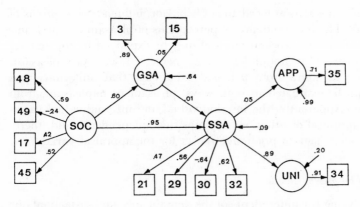

Goodness of fit = .95

Latent variables	Observed variables
SOC – attitude toward social engagement:	
	48 – desire to extend the range of social contacts
	41 – concern about restrictions of the range of social contacts
	17 – concern about maintaining the range of social contacts
	45 – using chances
GSA – general social activities:	3 – coping with conflict and strain in extra-familial roles
	15 – cultivating social contacts
SSA – specific social activities:	21 – perceived number of favorable as well as unfavorable events during the last year
	29 – making visits
	30 – social ventures
	32 – making trips
APP – positive/negative appraisal of daily activities:	35 – cognitive appraisal of daily activities (pleasant/unpleasant)
UNI – perceived uniformity of everyday life:	34 – perceived uniformity of daily life

Figure 9.5. Domain "extrafamilial social activities": model for prediction of "satisfaction with everyday life" (sixth measurement, 1976/77). Standardized solution.

see that motivations, as antecedents of behavior, influence perceptions of everyday life. The independence of perceptions of pleasantness and uniformity is contrary to expectations and may be explained by the activity theory implying that nonuniformity is perceived as more pleasant. However, we all know from personal experience that uniformity and variation can be evaluated in both ways, pleasant or unpleasant, from time to time. Apparently, the interindividual and intraindividual variation in the appraisal of situations explains this independence and, therefore, our model's lack of predictive power for the appraisal variable.

Evaluation of the present situation

Besides analyzing the antecedents of the domain-specific satisfaction, our final model tries to predict a more global satisfaction captured by "evaluation of the present situation,."

Dependent variables. Three variables were selected for the definition of global satisfaction: "desire for change in the personal life-style," "attitude toward one's own age," and "concern about general disappointment in life."

Independent variables. Two "independent" variables were introduced: The first related to the "appraisal of the recent past," and the second to "competence." The first was defined by the variables "amount of important events during the last year" and "amount of perceived stress experienced during the last year." Competence was operationalized by the intelligence test measures and educational level.

Intervening variables. Two mediating constructs were traced for each of these independent variables: "Perceived reduction and restriction of life space" and "quality of future time perspective" were connected with "appraisal of the recent past." The concepts "using the chances and possibilities left" and "satisfaction with everyay life" (defined by variables like "satisfaction with the change of work and rest in everyday life" and "perceived uniformity of life") are connected with "competence" and "appraisal." The variables are listed in Figure 9.6.

Results. In general, this model turns out to be one of the best in terms of prediction of the dependent variable. A relatively simple causal chain of the "first order" explains 70% of the variance concerning the evaluation of the present situation. As expected, positive appraisal of the recent past is associated with a low "concern about reduction of life space." Greater

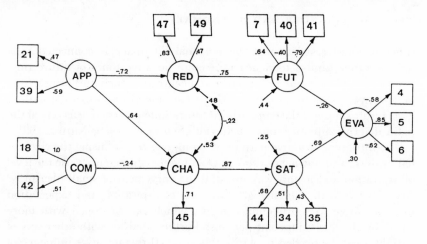

Goodness of fit index = .90

Latent variables

APP – appraisal of the recent past
    (range from negative to
    positive):

COM – competence (range from
    low to high):

RED – perceived reduction and
    restriction of life space
    (range from weak to strong
    reductions):

CHA – using chances (from less to
    more intensive):

FUT – quality of future time
    perspective (range from
    positive to negative):

SAT – satisfaction with everyday
    life (from low to high):

EVA – evaluation of present
    situation (from negative
    to positive):

Observed variables

21 – number of important events during the last year
39 – amount of perceived stress during the last year

18 – education
42 – WAIS score

47 – concern about reduction of chances and
    possibilities
49 – concern about restrictions of range of
    social contacts

45 – using chances and possibilities left

7 – dealing with finitude
40 – extension of future time perspective
41 – attitude toward future

44 – satisfaction with the change of work
    and rest in everyday life
34 – perceived uniformity of everyday life
35 – appraisal of everyday life as
    unpleasant/pleasant

4 – desire for correction of behavior
5 – evaluation of present age
6 – concern about general disappointment with life

Figure 9.6. Model for prediction of "evaluation of present situation" (sixth measurement, 1976/77). Standardized solution.

concern about restriction of the personal life space is connected to a narrow range (and a tendency to a more negative tone) of future time perspective. The more restricted and negatively toned the future time perspective, the more negative is the evaluation of the present situation. This result supports the emphasis on future time perspective as one of the main determinants of human behavior (Schreiner, 1969; Nuttin, 1985).

The intriguing negative path from "competence" to "using the chances left" raises the following questions: Does higher competence raise the level of aspiration and in this way forestall the enjoyment of small pleasures? Are subjects with a higher general level of aspiration and expectation more sensitive to shortcomings in life, which can be coped with more easily by the less-competent persons? Further analysis with other sets of variables will be needed to clarify this issue. If this negative influence of competence in general life satisfaction were valid, could both concepts be used in the definition of successful aging? There is another, more methodological explanation for this finding. Because we used only spontaneous utterances of this "theme of thoughts and feelings," it is possible that more competent subjects are too controlled and self-conscious to mention these "irrelevant" things.

The strongest path leads from "appraisal of the recent past" to "using chances left," and from here to "satisfaction with everyday life," and finally to "positive evaluation of the present situation."

Conclusion. This model apparently supports the use of global measures of life satisfaction at least in addition to more domain-specific ones. It should be noted, however, that the three variables defining the general evaluation of the present situation are "global" in very different directions: "Evaluation of the present age" (constituting the theme of most items of LSI scale) has the strongest connection with this general evaluation. "Desire for changes in one's life" touches a very general issue but is very specific in the direction of the question being asked. "Concern about general disappointment of life" is a summary statement by the interviewers about spontaneously expressed feelings and thoughts. From this point of view, the construct covers a broad range of experiences that are influenced by appraisals of the recent past, mainly in terms of experienced stress and crises, by perceived restrictions and chances, by the quality and scope of future time perspective – altogether a system of very specific experiences and cognitive representations. This is also true for the connection between "using chances" and "satisfaction with everyday life." These paths include constructs defined by sets of variables that are very specific in the domain for which satisfaction is to be assessed, but their combination covers a broad range. It can be concluded that global conceptualizations of life satisfaction always have to be based on concrete, situation-specific perceptions. This is the only way to attain valid measures for domain-specific as well as for global satisfaction.

Concluding remarks

From the principles of interactional personality psychology (Magnusson & Endler, 1977) we know about mutual influences between general attitudes toward dis/satisfaction with life and the appraisal of the situation or social role for which satisfaction is assessed. This suggests that in an analysis of the relationship between situation and satisfaction, one has to pay attention to response habits, identity styles, and the like as intervening between specific "objective" situations and the feeling of well-being or satisfaction. A similar conclusion was drawn by Carp and Carp (1984) and Whitbourne (1987).

In her review on personality development in adulthood and old age, Whitbourne (1987) developed a taxonomy displaying current research that tests the relationships between age, stressful life events, coping strategies, personality, health, and psychological well-being. Summarizing recent studies, she came to the conclusion that stressful life events have a negative impact on psychological well-being. Stressful life events and outcomes, however, are mediated by the individual's use of coping strategies. This is indeed the essential part of the paradigm we reflect with our models. The situations selected for our analyses are considered to represent different domains of everyday life, associated with a potential of stressful events such as daily hassles (Lazarus & Launier, 1978). In everyday life domains the individual is exposed to a series of events he or she has to cope with. Different strategies can be described in terms of the degree to which a "person–environment fit" is attained. The strategies can also be classified in terms of the social environment and of the patterns, styles, techniques, habits, and hierarchies leading to a balance of individual values, needs, beliefs, and expectations (see also Williams & Wirths, 1965). The view that psychological processes mediate between "objective" situational demands and individual responses is emphasized by cognitive theories of behavior and especially of coping as formulated by Lazarus and Folkman (1984) and Thomae (1970, 1987, 1988).

The main result of our analyses can be summarized as follows: Cognitive representations of specific aspects of the present situation are more effective in the explanation and prediction of behavior and feelings, such as well-being and satisfaction, than "objective" conditions, such as health as assessed by a physician, income, or education level. From this point of view, the analyses presented here give additional support to the cognitive theory of aging, according to which perception and evaluation of situations are more relevant for determining behavior than the objective situations.

NOTES

The authors thank Claudia Berg, Jane Janser, Michael Kavsek, Christian Rietz, and Anouk Zabal for their invaluable assistance and support in preparing this chapter.

1 Covariance structure analysis carried out with the LISREL VI (Jöreskog & Sörbom, 1986) computer program was used to evaluate both models and also the models in Figures 9.1–9.6. Covariance structure analysis allows a priori specifications of relations among unobserved, hypothetical constructs (referred to as *latent variables*). The latent variables are shown within circles; measured variables are shown within boxes. Each path connecting a latent variable to a measured variable represents a factor loading. It is significant if a given measured variable loads on one latent variable and not on the others. In our models, each latent variable is associated with at least one measured variable. The double-headed (curved) paths that interconnect the latent variables represent the correlations among those latent variables. The covariance structure approach to model fitting is a confirmatory one. The investigator specifies the form of the model to be fitted. In our analyses, the input of the computer program consists of a sample polychoric correlation matrix. Unweighted least squares procedure is used to estimate all of the model's unknown parameters. The goodness of fit index (GFI) indicates whether the model is a plausible representation of the data. The larger the value of this GFI, the better the fit. Maximum fit is indicated by GFI = 1.00. Not very much is known about the distribution of the GFI. Thus, caution must be exercised when using this statistic to evaluate goodness of fit.

REFERENCES

Adams, D. (1969). Analysis of a life satisfaction index. *Journal of Gerontology, 24,* 470–474.

Adams, J. (1971). Correlates of life satisfaction in old age. *Gerontologist, 13,* 64–68.

Atchley, R. C., & Miller, S. J. (1980). Older people and their families. *Annual Review of Gerontology and Geriatrics, 1,* 337–369.

Baltes, M. M. (1987). Erfolgreiches Altern als Ausdruck von Verhaltenskompetenz und Umweltqualität. In C. Niemitz (Ed.), *Der Mensch im Zusammenspiel von Anlage und Umwelt* (pp. 112–138). Frankfurt: Suhrkamp.

Baltes, M. M., & Baltes, P. B. (1986). *The psychology of control and aging.* Hillsdale, NJ: Lawrence Erlbaum.

Blume, O., Hauss, W. H., Kuhlmeyer, E., & Oberwittler, W. (1974). *Abschlussbericht der interdisziplinären Untersuchung über den Gesundheitszustand älterer Menschen* (MAGS Altenhilfe). Dortmund: Westfalendruck.

Brandtstädter, J. (1984). Personal and social control over development: Some implications of an action perspective in life-span developmental psychology. In P. B. Baltes & O. G. Brim (Eds.), *Life-span development and behavior* (Vol. 6, pp. 1–32). New York: Academic Press.

Burgess, E. W., Cavan, R., Havighurst, R. J., & Goldhammer, H. (1949). *Personal adjustment in old age*. Chicago: Science Research Associates.

Busse, E. W., & Maddox, G. L. (1986). *The Duke Longitudinal Studies of Normal Aging in 1955–1980*. New York: Springer.

Cantril, H. (1965). *Patterns of human concerns*. New Brunswick: Rutgers University.

Carp, F. M. (1975). Long-range satisfaction with housing. *Gerontologist, 15*, 68–72.

Carp, F. M., & Carp, A. (1983). Structural stability of well-being factors across age and gender, and development of scales of well-being unbiased for age and gender. *Journal of Gerontology, 38*, 572–581.

Carp, F. M., & Carp, A. (1984). A complementary/congruence model of well-being of mental health for the community elderly. In I. Altman, M. P. Lawton, & J. F. Wohlwill (Eds.), *Human behavior and environment. Vol. 7: Elderly people and the environment* (pp. 279–336). New York: Plenum Press.

Caspi, A., & Elder, G. H., Jr. (1986). Life satisfaction in old age: Linking social psychology and history. *Journal of Psychology and History, 1*, 18–26.

Coerper, C., Hagen, W., & Thomae, H. (1954). *Deutsche Nachkriegskinder*. Stuttgart: Thieme.

Diener, E. (1984). Subjective well-being. *Psychological Bulletin, 95*, 542–575.

George, L. K. (1981). Subjective well-being: Conceptual and methodological issues. In C. Eisdorfer (Ed.), *Annual review of gerontology and geriatrics* (Vol. 2, pp. 345–382). New York: Springer.

Hagen, W., & Thomae, H. (1962). *Deutsche Nachkriegskinder*. München: Barth.

Hagestad, G. (1986). Family. In G. Maddox (Ed.), *Encyclopedia of aging* (pp. 247–249). New York: Springer.

Havighurst, R. J. (1961). Successful aging. *Gerontologist, 1*, 4–7.

Havighurst, R. J. (1963). Successful aging. In C. Tibbitts & W. Donahue (Eds.), *Processes of aging* (pp. 299–320). New York: Williams.

Havighurst, R. J., Munnichs, J. M., Neugarten, B. L., & Thomae, H. (1969). *Adjustment to retirement: A cross-national study*. Assen: Van Gorcum.

Hoyt, D. R., & Creech, J. C. (1983). The Life Satisfaction Index: A methodological and theoretical critique. *Journal of Gerontology, 38*, 111–116.

Hoyt, D. R., Kaiser, M. A., Peters, G. R., & Babchuk, N. (1980). Life satisfaction and activity theory: A multidimensional approach. *Journal of Gerontology, 35*, 935–941.

Jöreskog, K. G., & Sörbom, D. (1986). *LISREL VI – Analysis of linear structural relationships by the method of maximum likelihood and least squares methods*. Uppsala: University of Uppsala.

Klemmack, D. L., & Roff, L. L. (1984). Fear of personal aging and subjective well-being in later life. *Journal of Gerontology, 39*, 756–758.

Kuypers, J. A., & Bengtson, V. L. (1973). Social breakdown and competence: A normal model of aging. *Human Development, 16*, 181–201.

Larson, R. (1978). Thirty years of research on the subjective well-being of older Americans. *Journal of Gerontology, 33,* 109–125.

Lazarus, R. S., & Folkman, S. (1984). *Stress, appraisal, and coping.* New York: Springer.

Lazarus, R. S., & Launier, R. (1978). Stress-related transactions between person and environment. In L. A. Pervin & M. Lewis (Eds.), *Perspectives in interactional psychology* (pp. 287–327). New York: Plenum Press.

Lehr, U. (1967). Attitudes toward the future. *Human Development, 10,* 230–238.

Lehr, U. (1969). *Frau im Beruf: Eine psychologische Analyse der weiblichen Berufsrolle.* Frankfurt: Athenäum.

Lehr, U. (1982). Social-psychological correlates of longevity. In C. Eisdorfer (Ed.), *Annual review of gerontology and geriatrics* (Vol. 3, pp. 102–147). New York: Springer.

Lehr, U. (1985). Erfolgreiches Altwerden als Thema von Entwicklungsberatung. In J. Brandtstädter & H. Gräser (Eds.), *Entwicklungsberatung unter dem Aspekt der Lebensspanne* (pp. 150–173). Göttingen: Hogrefe.

Lehr, U. (1987, July). Consistency and change in personality: Findings from the BOLSA. In D. Field (Chair), *Continuity in personality in the later years: Findings from four longitudinal studies.* Symposium conducted at the Ninth Biennial Meeting of the International Society for the Study of Behavioral Development, Tokyo.

Lehr, U., & Thomae, H. (1958). Eine Längsschnittstudie bei 30–40 jährigen Angestellten. *Vita Humana, 1,* 1–100.

Lehr, U., & Thomae, H. (1965). *Konflikt, seelische Belastung und Lebensalter.* Opladen: Westdeutscher Verlag.

Lehr, U., & Thomae, H. (1987). *Formen seelischen Alterns: Ergebnisse der Bonner Gerontologischen Längsschnittstudie.* Stuttgart: Enke.

Liang, J. (1984). Dimensions of the Life Satisfaction Index A: A structural formulation. *Journal of Gerontology, 39,* 613–622.

Liang, J. (1985). A structural integration of the Affect Balance Scale and the Life Satisfaction Index A. *Journal of Gerontology, 40,* 552–561.

Liang, J., & Bollen, K. A. (1983). The structure of the Philadelphia Geriatric Center Morale Scale: A reinterpretation. *Journal of Gerontology, 38,* 181–189.

Liang, J., Lawrence, R. H., & Bollen, A. (1986). Age differences in the structure of the Philadelphia Geriatric Center Morale Scale. *Journal of Psychology and Aging, 1,* 27–33.

Magnusson, D., & Endler, N. S. (1977). *Personality at the crossroads: Current issues in interactional psychology.* Hillsdale, NJ: Lawrence Erlbaum.

Medley, M. L. (1976). Satisfaction with later life among persons sixty-five years and older. *Journal of Gerontology, 31,* 448–455.

Nuttin, J. (1985). *Future time perspective and motivation.* Leuven: University of Leuven Press.

Okun, M. A. (1986). Life satisfaction. In G. L. Maddox et al. (Eds.), *Encyclopedia of aging* (pp. 399–401). New York: Springer.

Palmore, E. (1979). Predictors of successful aging. *Gerontologist, 19,* 427–431.

Palmore, E. (1981). *Social patterns in normal aging: Findings from the Duke Study.* Durham, NC: Duke University Press.

Palmore, E., & Kivett, V. (1977). Change in life satisfaction. *Journal of Gerontology, 32,* 311–316.

Pollak, O. (1948). *Social adjustment in old age: A research planning report.* New York: Social Science Research Council.

Rudinger, G., & Schmitz-Scherzer, R. (1976). Sample and methods. In H. Thomae (Ed.), *Patterns of aging: Findings from the Bonn Longitudinal Study of Aging* (pp. 12–19). Basel: Karger.

Ryff, C. D. (1986). The failure of successful aging research. *Gerontologist, 43* (Special issue), 37A.

Schreiner, M. (1969). *Zur zukunftsbezogenen Zeitperspektive älterer Menschen.* Unpublished doctoral dissertation, Universität Bonn, Bonn.

Schwarz, K. (1974). Voraussichtliche Entwicklung der Zahl älterer Menschen and ihre Lebenserwartung. In R. Schubert & W. Störmer (Eds.), *Schwerpunkte in der Geriatrie* (Vol. 3, pp. 17–19). Munich: Werk Verlag.

Shock, N. W. (1984). *Normal human aging: The Baltimore Longitudinal Study of Aging.* NIH Publication, No. 94-2450. Washington, DC: NIH.

Stock, W. A., Okun, M. A., & Benin, M. (1986). Structure of subjective well-being among the elderly. *Psychology and Aging, 1,* 91–102.

Thomae, H. (1968). Psychische und soziale Aspekte des Alterns. *Zeitschrift für Gerontologie, 1,* 43–55.

Thomae, H. (1970). Theory of aging and cognitive theory of personality. *Human Development, 13,* 1–16.

Thomae, H. (1983a). Perceptions of and reactions to life stress in old age. In E. Beverfelt (Ed.), *Aging: Living conditions and quality of life* (pp. 64–84). Oslo: Norwegian Institute of Gerontology.

Thomae, H. (1983b). *Alternsstile und Altersschicksale.* Bern: Huber.

Thomae, H. (1987). Conceptualizations of responses to stress. *European Journal of Personality, 1,* 171–192.

Thomae, H. (1988). *Das Individuum und seine Welt: Eine Persönlichkeitstheorie* (rev. ed.) Göttingen: Hogrefe.

Ward, R. A. (1985). Informal networks and well-being in later life: A research agenda. *Gerontologist, 25,* 55–61.

Whitbourne, S. K. (1987). Personality development in adulthood and old age: Relationships among identity style, health, and well-being. In K. W. Schaie & C. Eisdorfer (Eds.), *Annual Review of Gerontology and Geriatrics* (pp. 189–216). New York: Springer.

Williams, R. H., & Wirths, C. G. (1965). *Lives through the years.* New York: Atherton Press.

10 Risk and protective factors in the transition to young adulthood

BARBARA MAUGHAN AND LORNA CHAMPION

Change continues throughout the life cycle so that changes for better or for worse are always possible. It is this continuing potential for change that means that at no time of life is a person invulnerable to every possible adversity and also that at no time of life is a person impermeable to favourable influence.

John Bowlby, 1988

Introduction

The twin themes of consistency and change, continuity and discontinuity, lie at the heart of studies of human development. Both are ever-present possibilities, but some phases of the life course highlight the tensions between them with special clarity. Developmental transitions – times of greater than usual change, whether prompted by biological maturation, psychological growth, or changes in social roles and statuses – are among the most important of these. Such periods place often heavy demands on the individual for adaptation to new conditions but also hold within them the potential for new beginnings, opportunities to overcome earlier difficulties and to set out on new developmental trajectories (Emde & Harmon, 1984). Examining the processes that make for more and less successful negotiation of such transitions, that maintain vulnerabilities or protect against them at such periods, may thus constitute one fruitful approach to the study of successful aging.

Our aim in this essay is to consider risk and protective processes of this kind for one of the major transition periods in the life span: that marking the entry to adult life. From a developmental perspective, this period is one of central interest and importance. It involves changes in the great majority of an individual's social roles and relationships; introduces qualitatively new demands and responsibilites; and sets the foundations on which much later development will be built. Decisions made at this

296

stage, whether concerning education, career, or choice of life partner, may have a major influence on life chances and satisfaction for many years to come.

Our particular interest in this period lies in the role it may play in contributing to continuities or discontinuities between childhood adversities and individual functioning in adult life. To date, much research on these issues has been aimed at establishing predictable associations between defined childhood risks and a range of potential adult outcomes. This in itself is no simple task. Many childhood adversities overlap, making it difficult to isolate the independent contribution of individual factors, and it is already clear that any given early risk may be associated with a range of adult sequelae. To take two recent examples, Parker and Asher (1987) have confirmed associations between poor peer relationships in childhood and such varied later difficulties as dropping out of school, criminality, and adult psychopathology; and Holmes and Robins (1987) have demonstrated links between harsh discipline in childhood and both alcoholism and depression in adult life.

Where, as in these examples, such long-term associations can be established, they provide intriguing suggestive evidence for causal associations. But the links whereby such associations may be mediated across the intervening period of development are still relatively little understood. Our aim in this chapter will be to explore the role of the transition to adulthood as one possible source of such intervening links and as a "window" on some of the processes that may be involved. Two main questions will guide the discussion. First, how far and in what ways do risks and adversities encountered earlier in development continue to have an impact at this stage of the life course; and second, what evidence do we have that the changes of the early adult period can be supportive of new patterns of development and hold within them the potential to offset earlier disadvantage? We shall confine our focus to psychosocial risk and protective factors and attempt, by means of a selective, illustrative review of existing longitudinal findings, to highlight issues that require further clarification in future research. We begin, however, by commenting briefly on some general issues that arise in the study of risk and protective factors and by outlining some key features of the transition period to young adulthood.

Studying risk and protective factors

The study of risk and protective factors in development presents many challenges. Masten and Garmezy (1985) have recently reviewed these concepts, together with the related issues of stress, vulnerability, and resilience, in the context of research in developmental psychopathology, and Rutter (1985, 1987) has dealt more specifically with protective factors and mechanisms.

Both discussions highlight the conceptual and methodological complexities of research in this area. For any given outcome, such psychosocial risk or protective factors as are identified can often be seen as opposite poles of an underlying continuum, raising issues of the separability of the two concepts. When a range of differing outcomes is considered and a developmental dimension added to the picture, further complexities arise; it is not inconceivable, for example, that the same factor could show risk relationships with one outcome but protective associations with others and that the effects of each may vary with the developmental level and other characteristics of the individual involved. Stressors or adversities that constitute risks at one period of development may have protective effects at later stages, perhaps through the operation of "steeling" mechanisms or through their potential as learning experiences. An exclusive focus on *factors* in the sense of specific variables is thus likely to lead us into a quagmire of definitional problems; the eventual aim will be to elucidate the *processes* at each stage of development whereby such factors have their effects. In our present state of knowledge, it is rarely possible to do this with any certainty; many of the factors identified could plausibly be argued to operate through external social processes or internal psychological mechanisms, or indeed some combination of the two. In either case, establishing causal links will eventually require evidence from experimental or intervention research. To date, almost all evidence on possible risk or protective processes in psychosocial development derives from nonexperimental, longitudinal studies. For all these reasons, our interpretations will need to be appropriately tentative.

The transition to adult life

In exploring risk and protective processes in the transition to adulthood, we must begin with some general schema of the developmental changes typically taking place during this period and the likely pitfalls and possibilities that these may present. Despite differences in theoretical orientation, most writers who have proposed stage models of psychosocial development (see, e.g., Erikson, 1980; Havighurst, 1972; Levinson, Darrow, Klein, Levinson, & McKee, 1978) are in broad agreement on the main developmental tasks of the period. The passage to adulthood is characterized by the (often conflicting) demands of structure changing and structure building (Levinson et al., 1978): a progressive disengagement from childhood and adolescent identities and testing, exploration, and eventual commitment to new roles and relationships. Over a period of years, key choices and decisions may be made in a range of major life domains. If we consider three domains of particular importance at this period – those concerning work, personal relationships, and independence from the family of origin – it is clear that key transitional events, marking major role changes, are likely to occur in each area: completing education and both choosing and engaging in a career; leaving home and moving to independent living; embarking upon marriage or committed relationships; starting a family of one's own. In each case, such events may be the culmination of a more extended period of anticipation, planning, and experimentation with potential new roles, and the latest in a series of more minor, but nevertheless important, transitions: first date, first sexual relationship, first responsibility for managing finances, and so forth. The formation of adult life goals is a central concern of the period as a whole, and these goals can give a sense of direction and coherence, guide relative investments in each domain, and act as the benchmarks against which later achievements and progress can be assessed.

Like other transitional periods, this stage of the life course is one that makes heavy demands on the individual's adaptive resources and is likely to be associated with relatively high levels of stress. Calculated risks or hardships may be faced in the short term in the hope of long-term gains. Developments in one area of life may precipitate unanticipated changes in others. There is a need to plan developments within each separate domain but also to coordinate progress between them. More than at any earlier stage, there is the potential, and often the requirement, for the individual to play a consciously perceived role in shaping his or her development, determining long-term goals and more immediate courses of action, and selecting the environments, both interpersonal and physical, in which those plans will be played out. Decisions taken during this period lay the foundations for much adult development. Opportunities taken or passed by at this stage may have a major impact on the individual's possibilities for growth and satisfaction or risks of poor functioning for many years to come.

How then might we characterize "successful" or "optimal" progress through these transitions? As we shall see, research conducted to date offers a wide range of possible criteria, varying with the particular aims and focus of the studies involved. We offer no simple prescriptions here but suggest that at least two broad types of assessment need to be included. First, we require a focus on the transitional period itself and measures of individuals' progress through the change points involved. Certain childhood risk factors may, for example, predispose to particular patterns in the timing or sequencing of events, in the extent to which individuals are able to plan for them, or in the inner resources they bring to new demands and responsibilities. Our first concern will thus be to chart how far different groups negotiate transitional changes in characteristically differing ways.

Second, however, we require measures of the implications of such differing patterns for later adaptation, adjustment, and personal satisfaction. Particular types of early adult changes may, for example, set serious restrictions on later opportunities or increase the likelihood of later stressors, which in their turn will contribute to poor functioning in later life. The timing of outcome assessments at any phase of the life course characterized by change is crucial: We need to be sure that we are not simply picking up transient negative reactions or responses to temporary stressors that have no significant implications in the longer term. Later assessments are critical in evaluating the effects of a transitional phase, when the success of achievements will rest perhaps more centrally on implications for future development than on more immediate effects, and when these two types of assessment may well not coincide. Magnusson and Allen (1983) have elegantly demonstrated that individual differences in both the timing of key events and the rate of change during critical periods of development make assessments during those periods potentially unstable. To assess progress through, and the effects of, any transitional period, we need measures at points during the transition but also at some more stable point beyond it, when any initial problems of adjustment or adaptation should in general have been overcome. Following our focus on psychosocial development, such later assessments might include a variety of indicators. Poor outcomes would clearly be indexed by the development of disorder or serious social deviance, but we would also argue for the importance of including a wider range of measures of social functioning and of the individuals' perceptions of their own progress. The complexity of the tasks involved requires multiple types of assessment, in a range of key life domains: Work, relationships, parenting, and the individual's sense of self-worth are all appropriate areas in which to assess outcome.

To examine outcomes in this way and make links with earlier adversities we thus need longitudinal data with measures at a number of different time points: beginning in childhood, including measures of behavior or events during the transition, and concluding with assessments of functioning well beyond the end of the transitional period. To highlight protective mechanisms, studies of high-risk childhood samples are likely to be of greatest value (Rutter, 1987). Not surprisingly, studies satisfying all of these requirements are rare. Although we can learn a good deal from a focus on more limited elements of the sequence, the nature and complexity of the processes involved are demonstrated most persuasively by accounts spanning the whole period from childhood to adult life. We thus begin our discussion with a number of illustrative examples of this kind. Each takes differing childhood risks and adult outcomes as its focus and investigates intervening events in somewhat different ways; each shares, however, a concern to illuminate process and to specify the conditions under which both initial risks and potential protective factors had their effects.

Some studies examining process issues in the transition to adult life

Economic deprivation in childhood

We begin with Elder's influential analyses of data from the Berkeley and Oakland longitudinal studies (Elder, 1979, 1986). Using the potential that these two studies offered for both between- and within-cohort comparisons, Elder's central concern was to explore the relationships between social history and individual life history and the processes whereby macrosocial change can find expression in psychological functioning. The severe economic deprivation of the 1930s Depression constituted the initial childhood risk in both studies, and the availability of follow-up data to the time the cohort members were aged 40 made it possible to trace its continuing impact and the effects of intervening events well beyond the early adult period.

Members of these two cohorts, born just 8 years apart in the 1920s, experienced the impact of economic deprivation at differing points in their childhoods, and to differing degrees. These age variations, together with the nature of existing family relationships, had powerful mediating effects on assessments of their adjustment in adolescence: the degree of goal-directedness, sense of personal worth and initiative, and levels of social competence shown as they approached their adult lives. In the younger, Berkeley cohort, many of whose members faced economic hardship from early childhood onward, economic deprivation was associated with negative outcomes in adolescence only in families where parental relationships had been discordant before the Depression and where, in particular, there was a poor relationship between the child and the parent of the same sex. Because job losses and a sudden drop in family income often served to undermine the role of fathers, while strengthening that of mothers, the negative effects were greater for boys than for girls. Indeed, Elder suggests

that poor father–son relationships – characterized by hostility or indiffer-
ence, and often inconsistent discipline – were the crucial factors in
determining an incompetent sense of self in adolescence amongst boys
regardless of economic deprivation (Elder, 1979). Girls in this cohort, by
comparison, appeared protected by the high quality of relationships with
their mothers and the strong and positive role models provided by women
in these difficult times.

For the older, Oakland cohort, who experienced the Depression from
late childhood onward, the effects on adolescent self-competence were
reversed, boys faring better than girls. The explanation appeared to lie in
the respective roles available to adolescents in families facing severe
financial difficulties. For older boys, economic hardship often involved
taking on more adultlike responsibilities, so that deprivation was likely to
have been associated with experiences of mastery over adversity and
possibly with an enhanced sense of personal control. For the girls, by
contrast, domestic responsibility within the home increased, assigning
priority to a domestic career of marriage and parenthood.

The early stages of the studies thus emphasized the varying impact of
apparently similar risk factors for differing subgroups within these cohorts. Later follow-ups highlighted the effects of early adult experiences
for their subsequent development. The younger boys, indecisive and
passive in adolesence, were of greatest interest here. By mid-life, although
they continued to experience difficulties in some areas, adolescent ratings
of lack of self-competence were not predictive of similar ratings in adulthood: "By the age of 40, these men bore less resemblance to their
adolescent personality than to the self competence of equally successful
adults from relatively affluent families" (Edler, 1979, p. 48).

What determined this discontinuity? In brief, early adult opportunities
to gain independence from the family and to achieve a sense of personal
worth seem to have been crucial. Elder (1986) points to the major
importance of military service for this vulnerable group. A high proportion of the deprived boys entered military service, and most had done so
by the age of 21. Early entry to the military appeared to have been a
crucial factor in opening up new opportunities, which in their turn created
a series of protective effects. A number of elements may have been of
importance here. One would be the break from negative and difficult
family situations and the chance to achieve a sense of mastery in a range of
important and useful new skills. At the same time, appropriate and more
positive role models, previously lacking, were provided for these young
men. In addition, military service increased their later chances of going to
college and reversing often negative school experiences. College education
in itself, independent of military service, appeared to be important in

Table 10.1. *Military service and later life course: Berkeley cohort*

| | Military service | | |
| | | | Level of |
Later life-course measures	Veteran	Nonveteran	significance
Mean age at			
Education exit	25.0	22.0	**
First full-time job	21.7	19.9	**
First marriage	24.2	21.8	***
First child	26.2	22.7	***
Last child	33.0	32.2	
Educational level			
% postgraduate	23	15	
% college graduate	31	23	
% some college	30	19	
% less than college	17	42	
Early work life: 1945–1955			
Mean occupational status			
after education[a]	3.2	4.4	***
Later work life: 1956–1968			
Mean occupational status in			
1968	2.7	3.4	*

[a] 1 = high, 7 = low.
$*p < .10; **p < .05, ***p < .01.$
Source: After Elder, 1986.

improving later outcomes; in its absence, men from deprived origins experienced more instability in both work and marriage than the sons of nondeprived parents. Finally, both military service and entering college had the additional effects of delaying marriage and the start of family building, which further reduced the likelihood of negative outcomes among these vulnerable groups (Elder, 1986). The later timing of both these transitional events was associated with greater marital stability at mid-life. Table 10.1 illustrates the range of effects of military service on the Berkeley men's later lives.

For boys in the older cohort, who as a group had received more positive ratings of self-competence in adolescence, continuing opportunities in early adulthood were still necessary for positive later outcomes: Those from economically deprived working-class backgrounds who did not enter college ranked lowest on the utilization of skills and resources in adult life. Less information is available on adult outcomes for girls in either cohort;

it was clear, however, that deprived girls in both groups equaled or surpassed the nondeprived in terms of the social status of their partners by their late thirties, regardless of their own college achievements. Elder (1979) comments on the importance of two adult coping strategies (Pearlin & Schooler, 1978) that appeared to represent a positive legacy of childhood hardship: first, the use of "positive comparisons," whereby difficulties in adult life still compared favorably with the extreme hardship experienced in childhood; and second, "selective ignoring," the process of finding good in adversity and hence being able to manage it more effectively. Via all these differing routes, severe difficulties in childhood had nevertheless been followed by relatively positive functioning for many members of these cohorts in later adult life.

Institutional rearing

We turn now to a very different type of childhood adversity: extended periods of institutional care. Quinton and Rutter (see Quinton & Rutter, 1985; Rutter & Quinton, 1984; Quinton, Rutter, & Liddle, 1984; Quinton & Rutter, 1988) have reported findings from a prospective study of girls who were separated from their parents in early childhood following family breakdown and who spent the major part of their childhoods in residential care. A central concern of the adult follow-up in this instance was to assess the implications of an institutional upbringing for the women's own later skills as parents. This study again included measures collected in childhood and assessed outcomes in the twenties for the "ex-care" women and a comparison group drawn from the same socially disadvantaged inner-city area but who had been brought up within their own families.

Overall, the ex-care women showed poorer adjustment than the controls on all the early adult measures of outcome examined: general psychosocial functioning, an assessment of parenting, and the quality of marital relationships (see Figure 10.1 and Table 10.2). Although genetic factors were clearly likely to have played some part here, as were continuities from deviant behavior shown by the girls in childhood and adolescence, their later difficulties also seemed to reflect a series of more indirect linkages over time. Leaving care, they were likely either to return to discordant families or to face the transition to adulthood with little advice or support. They more often became involved in relationships to "escape" from their home situation, and risks of teenage pregnancy were increased. These factors, in their turn, contributed to the increased likelihood of their having unsupportive or deviant spouses and facing other environmental stressors in adulthood; under such circumstances (but not without them), their parenting was often poor.

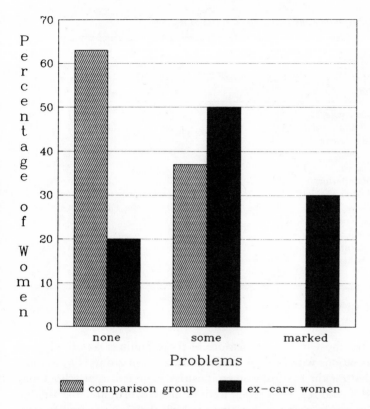

Figure 10.1. Ex-care women: overall psychosocial outcome (after Quinton & Rutter, 1985).

By no means all of the women, however, faced this particular conjunction of difficulties; about a third showed good outcomes in adulthood, which appeared to reflect a sequence of protective effects. First, positive school experiences were important for the ex-care women; they were associated with more constructive approaches to "planning" early adult transitions and with a more considered choice of marriage partner in particular (see Table 10.3); having a supportive or nondeviant spouse was then associated with later good parenting, even under otherwise adverse circumstances. Although this chain of more positive developments seemed to stem in many instances from positive experiences in the teens and the use of more adaptive coping strategies by these women, it was also clear that a supportive marital relationship had strong protective effects even when it appeared to have arisen independently of these earlier influences, without obvious planning.

Table 10.2. *Pregnancy and parenting histories of women*

Pregnancy and parenting histories	Ex-care women (%) ($n = 81$)	Comparison group (%) ($n = 42$)	Statistical significance χ^2	df	p
Those ever pregnant	72	43	8.50	1	.01
Those pregnant by 19 years	42	5	16.75	1	.001
Those who had surviving child	60	36	5.85	1	.02
Those with children	($n = 49$)	($n = 15$)			
Without a male partner	22	0	Exact test $p = .039$		
With any children ever in care or fostered	18	0	Exact test $p = .074$		
Experiencing temporary or permanent break-down in parenting	35	0	Exact test $p = .009$		
Living with father of all children	61	100	6.52	1	.02

Source: After Quinton & Rutter, 1985.

Perhaps the most interesting feature of these findings was the lack of similar associations with later outcome in the control group. The authors speculate that for the ex-care women, positive experiences at school may have played a vital role in creating feelings of self-worth and a sense that they could control events in their lives, which then contributed to their later more considered planning in terms of choice of marriage partner. For women in the control groups, experiences in their families would doubt-less have provided many other avenues for the development of feelings of self-worth; experiences at school might well have reinforced these but did not in themselves play any crucial role. For the ex-care group, however, such an external source of positive experiences may well have been necessary to *create* this more positive self-view, which then had major implications for the ways in which they approached their early adult lives.

Lack of parental care in childhood

Our final example also concerns women and lack of parental care in childhood. Early loss of a parent has received considerable attention as a major risk factor in childhood, especially in relation to possible links with adult psychiatric disorder (Birtchnell, 1980; Crook & Eliot, 1980; Ten-

Table 10.3. *Positive school experiences and planning for marriage*

	Positive experiences	
Planning for marriage	0/1 ($n = 49$) (%)	2 or more ($n = 22$) (%)
Planner	47	77
Nonplanner	53	23

Note: $\chi^2 = 4.51$, df $= 1, p < .05$.
Source: After Quinton & Rutter, 1985.

Table 10.4. *Percentage of women with current depression by quality of care and type of loss in childhood*

Type of loss	Lack of care (%)	Adequate care (%)
Death of mother	34 (13/38)	10 (4/40)*
Separation from mother	36 (12/33)	4 (1/28)*
Separation from father (no loss of mother)	50 (2/4)	12 (2/17)*
Death of father (no loss of mother)	0 (0/1)	0 (0/19)
No loss of parent	13 (1/8)	3 (1/37)
No loss of mother	21 (3/13)	4 (3/73)*

*$p < .01$. All other differences are not significant.
Source: After Harris, Brown, & Bifulco, 1986.

nant, Bebbington, & Hurry, 1980). The results of these studies have, however, proved inconsistent. We turn now to a retrospective study that attempted to resolve these inconsistencies by tracing intervening experiences that might account for varying adult outcomes (Brown, Harris, & Bifulco, 1986; Harris, Brown, & Bifulco, 1986, 1987).

The findings were important first in refining understanding of the source of the initial childhood risk; rather than loss of parent per se, it appeared that lack of adequate parental care following a loss was the crucial factor in creating later risk for psychiatric disorder (see Table 10.4). Harris et al. (1987) proposed that this lack of care affected both the inner and the outer resources of the women involved: It showed links with a sense of helplessness and low self-esteem and also with greater environmental adversity. These two avenues for effects are illustrated in a series of

speculative models of the causal process involved, one of which is repro-
duced in Figure 10.2.

The early adult period appeared to be the point at which these two
strands of effects, inner and outer, became "inextricably entwined" and
when the chain of negative effects could become crystallized into environmental "traps" that seriously elevate risk of depression in the face of later
stressors. Harris et al. (1987) liken the process to a conveyor belt "on
which people land at some crucial point, perhaps as they enter adulthood,
and are then carried forward to a future which only the luckier or more
agile can avoid by getting off" (p. 169). In terms of the women's external
life circumstances, premarital pregnancy appeared to constitute a critical
link in this process. Those who had experienced early loss of mother were
more likely to become pregnant before marriage (24% [33/139] vs. 10%
[9/86], $p < .05$). Premarital pregnancy then increased the likelihood of
other adult difficulties – early marriage and lack of marital support –
which in turn increased vulnerability to depression in women facing other
acute stressors (42% clinically depressed in the year before interview
among those who had been premaritally pregnant, 15% among other
women, $p < .001$). The ways in which women coped with early pregnancy
were thus central in reversing or perpetuating this negative spiral of
adversity: Adaptive coping was more prevalent in middle-class than
working-class women, and indeed the chain of adversities stemming from
early pregnancy showed much closer links for working-class than middle-
class groups. Middle-class women who did not cope effectively, however,
often experienced downward social mobility in addition to a raised
likelihood of depression. The immediate precursors of disorder could be
traced to particular conjunctions of later stressors; through these earlier
intervening linkages, early lack of care appeared to predispose to increased risks of social adversity in adult life, which were in turn associated
with an increased rate of clinical depression.

These brief vignettes – which do no more than hint at the rich detail of
the studies involved – exemplify the complex nature of the empirical and
theoretical models required to trace risk and protective mechanisms
across this period of the life span. Several features are immediately
apparent: the varied chains of linkages involved in the long-term associations of childhood adversity and adult outcome; the varying specificity of
those linkages for differing subgroups within each sample; and the range
of processes, social and psychological, that affect the individual's inner
and outer worlds and that can be invoked to explain them. We shall now
consider these issues in more detail, drawing on material not only from
these vignettes but also from the wide range of other studies that provide
related evidence, some also covering the full age span from childhood

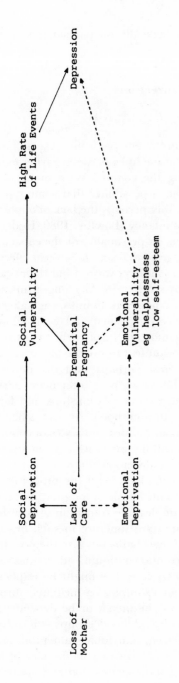

Figure 10.2. Inner and outer routes for effects of early loss of mother (after Brown, Harris, & Bifulco, 1986).

to adulthood, others focusing more specifically on particular stages or aspects of the processes involved.

Issues: Current findings and future directions

Sequential and indirect links

Perhaps the most striking general feature to emerge from these and other studies is the indirect nature of many of the links between earlier experience and later outcomes, emphasizing the complexity of many of the processes involved. Although it remains a possibility that some types of serious childhood adversity – most notably perhaps the lack of opportunity to establish selective attachments in infancy (Bowlby, 1980; Hodges & Tizard, 1989) – may have lasting effects on personality or the capacity to form relationships, much evidence suggests that any long-term effects of other childhood adversities may arise in indirect ways, from the negative chain reactions that initial stressors may set in train. Any long-term effects seem likely to be mediated by a series of shorter-term links, each affecting developments at the immediately succeeding stage and each allowing possibilities for the maintenance or reinforcement of earlier risks or for them to be offset. Developmentally relevant features of the picture change with time. Whereas family stresses and perhaps patterns of school achievement play a central part in childhood, peer influences exert an increasing impact in adolescence, and marital relationships and family and work opportunities are important in adulthood. At each stage, the individual's personal strengths and vulnerabilities and styles of coping or of relating derived from earlier stages will interact with current stressors and environmental supports to influence development.

Mapping the intervening links in such chains and the processes that mediate between them thus becomes a central task for longitudinal studies in this field. As is clear from these examples, the transition to adulthood marks what may be an especially important juncture in such linkages, with opportunities to break out of negative chains but also the possibility that childhood risks will be transformed into continuing adversities in the adult years. A number of different possible routes might be implicated here. Long-term associations might, for example, be mediated through disorder or deviance already evident in childhood; or be dependent on continuities – all too frequent in at-risk childhood groups – in adverse environmental circumstances; or arise from individual vulnerabilities set up in response to early stressors but only activated in the face of later adversity. We turn now to look at some of the factors that may contribute to the perpetuation or disruption of such negative chains.

Maintaining and breaking links with childhood adversity

Pretransitional resources. Our vignettes suggest that the resources that individuals can draw on as they approach the early adult period are likely to play a crucial part in maintaining or breaking links with previous adversity. Limitations in these resources – which would include individual dispositions and coping strategies, the availability of support and guidance in the immediate environment, and perceived as well as actual opportunities in the wider adult world – may be among the more important avenues whereby childhood risks become transmuted into adverse adult circumstances. By the same token, the new opportunities that may open up as young people enter adult life may respresent crucial sources of protective effects. In some instances, these may be achieved by actual breaks with past environments. Elder suggests that one of the more important functions that entry to military service served for the vulnerable Berkeley men may have been to create a sharp discontinuity from the stresses and restricted opportunities of their homes and family lives and to provide a range of new role models, skills, and aspirations. In a similar way, moving away from high-delinquency areas and presumably the influence of delinquent peers has been shown to be associated with reduced levels of offending in previously delinquent young men (West, 1982). In other instances, breaks from adverse circumstances may arise from individual strengths and coping strategies: The more considered planning of some ex-care women and adaptive coping with premarital pregnancy in Harris et al.'s (1987) study members, each did much to ensure that potential risks were not in fact perpetuated. Although the early adult period is clearly one during which important new opportunities can be opened up for previously at-risk individuals, it is equally clear that they need to approach these with openness and flexibility and with the capacities to take the best advantage of new relationships or experiences, if the potential of such opportunities is in fact to be realized.

Timing, sequencing, and synchronization of transitions. Turning next to the implications of events during the early adult period, the timing, sequencing, and synchronization of role changes and transitions may all constitute sources of both risk and protection. As we have seen, Elder (1986) argued that the delayed marriages of the relatively immature Berkeley men may have been central to their achieving stable and satisfying relationships in middle life. As a counterpoint to this type of pattern, early transitions and their effects on later life chances have attracted particular attention as possible risk factors for later development.

A variety of models might be proposed to account for such effects

(Brooks-Gunn, Petersen, & Eichorn, 1985): a "stage termination" model, whereby an early transition interrupts the completion of previous developmental tasks; a "goodness-of-fit" model (Lerner, 1985), whereby the individual may be too immature or unready to meet the demands of the new situation; a "preempting opportunities" model, whereby early transitions in one life domain effectively limit options in others; or a "deviance" model, whereby problems arise for those going through transitions early because they may be regarded, or regard themselves, as deviant from their peers. Neugarten (1979) argues that the life cycle is perceived as a set of norms covering both the events that should occur at different life stages and the boundaries for their most appropriate timing. Within any given setting, this internalized "social clock" identifies the expected stages of life transitions and will influence and interact with individual goals and plans. In Western societies, with the exception of the minimum age for completing education, for marriage, and for the start of such activities as drinking and voting, neither the timing nor the sequencing of early adult role transitions is institutionally prescribed but instead reflects relatively loose normative expectations (Featherman, Hogan, & Sørensen, 1984). But although the expected age ranges for most early adult transitions are broad, they are not infinitely elastic; both "off-time" events, occurring much earlier or later than is usual, and "non-events" (such as the failure to find work or the failure to establish committed relationships) may also, in addition to their real-world effects, have major implications for the individual's sense of self-worth, if they are perceived as seriously deviant from prevailing norms.

What constitutes an early or off-time transition must, of course, be assessed in the context of the particular sociocultural and historical circumstances relevant to any individual investigation. Cohort comparative studies provide graphic evidence of marked historical variations in the timing of transitional events over recent decades. Indeed, Baltes, Reese, and Lipsitt (1980) have suggested that of all phases of the life span, the early adult period may be the most subject to historical changes of this kind. The median time between starting work and first marriage, for example, fell dramatically, from 18 to only 8 years, for the generations of American men born between the turn of the century and the Second World War (Hogan, 1981). The expansion of educational opportunities and the continuing processes of urbanization and industrialization were the predominant influences, although more specific patterns of intercohort variability reflected unique combinations of historical circumstances: economic prosperity and depression, and the demands and possibilities of peacetime and wartime conditions. Technological advance, legislative change, variations in social provision, and, to take a pressing recent example, the spread of AIDS would be among other historically varying factors all likely to have a strong bearing on behavior or the timing of transitions at this stage. Alongside such historical factors, there is of course abundant evidence of social class gradings in the timing of many transition events within any given cohort and of consistent patterns of sex differences in both labor market participation and family formation. For women alone, British statistics on age at entry to childbearing have shown major social class variations since the 1920s, widening if anything over more recent years; by 1983, for example, over 17% of women married to men in social classes IV and V had their first child in their teens, whereas only 2% of their counterparts in classes I and II had done so (Joshi, 1985). Unqualified generalizations about typical patterns of transitional behavior will thus rarely be warranted; all such data need to be viewed in the context of the historical and sociocultural conditions that they reflect, and issues of this kind require careful attention at the stage of study design.

Early transitions. In the world of work, a large literature documents the links between length of schooling, educational qualifications, and later occupational status and earnings potential. Hogan (1981), in a large-scale study of American men entering the labor market from the 1920s onward, found that relatively early work transitions, depending more on family connections than educational attainments, had quite pronounced effects on occupational attainments and earnings early in men's careers, but that these largely dissipated by middle life. Relatively early marriage increased the probability of separation and divorce in earlier cohorts, but less markedly in more recent groups (perhaps because the availability of contraception reduced the frequency of enforced early marriages in later cohorts); where early marriage was also "out of sequence" with educational and occupational transitions, however, occurring while men were still completing their education and before they had started work, negative effects on both occupational and marital outcomes were compounded.

For women, early pregnancy, especially during the teens, has frequently been identified as a crucial linking factor between childhood adversity and continuing adult difficulties. Teenage mothers not infrequently come from large families where family relationships have been poor, and they themselves have performed poorly at school (Kiernan, 1980; Phipps-Yonas, 1980). They tend to marry men from similarly disadvantaged backgrounds. Early childbearing then not only limits future educational and career possibilities for women but may have similar effects for their spouses, forcing them to forgo occupational changes in the face of more immediate needs for financial support for the family (Hofferth & Moore, 1979). At somewhat later stages, both divorce and psychiatric problems show elevated rates among women who had their first child in their teens (Kiernan, 1980).

Such examples illustrate graphically the cumulative effects of early disadvantage and the pivotal role that experiences in the transition to adulthood can play in maintaining them. The most serious risks, as in these examples, seem likely to accrue from transitional changes in any one life domain that elevate the likelihood of continuing environmental adversities, that restrict options in other domains, or that deplete or place heavy stress on individual's personal coping resources or sources of external support. Early transitions and those that, like early pregnancy, may enforce moves in other areas – into marriage, home finding, and so forth – are among the most obvious of these. As Hogan (1981) argues, however, because previously disadvantaged or at-risk groups are the most likely to make such early transitions, it becomes important to assess whether transitional behavior largely acts to maintain prior disadvantage or makes an independent contribution to later outcomes, over and above any difficulties that might be anticipated anyway in such groups. In Hogan's own analyses, an independent contribution was indeed evident: early moves to work and marriage showed later deleterious effects independent of the impact of a variety of earlier background factors.

Although the effects of early transitions have attracted perhaps the greatest attention to date, childhood adversities may also predispose to poor adult functioning through quite different transitional routes. Farrington, Gallagher, Morley, St. Ledger, and West (1986a) examined the progress of a small group of boys from families at high risk for delinquency who nevertheless did not develop delinquent behavior in their teens. Most were withdrawn and isolated in childhood, and few showed good functioning in their early adult lives. The intervening years in these cases, however, had been marked by apparent avoidance of engagement in adult roles and delays in transitional moves, especially in the area of marriage. For this group, experiences of self-actualization in adulthood seemed limited not by early transitions but by unwillingness or inability to move into new roles and relationships.

Himmelweit and Turner (1982) provide suggestive evidence of yet other types of risk in a very different population, this time of able young men. For them, follow-ups in the midtwenties showed strong associations between depressive affect and upward occupational mobility, the most "successful" young men showing the lowest mood. The authors suggest that this may have reflected the "anomia of success," the lack of any continuing sense of purpose for a group that had already achieved its goals early in adulthood and so had few aspirations left to fulfill.

Such examples underline the importance of assessing a range of differing patterns of transition timing and their congruence with individuals' goals and aspirations in exploring potential risks for later functioning. As Rindfuss, Swicegood, and Rosenfeld (1987) have demonstrated, apparently disorderly patterns of transitions in nonfamilial roles – beginning work before completing education or moving in and out of roles such as homemaker – are much more common among recent cohorts than has been previously assumed. In a similar way, the implications of developments in one domain for likely progress in others cannot be taken for granted: "understanding the nature and importance of sequencing in the life course requires analyzing what the roles themselves mean and how they are causally linked" (Rindfuss et al., 1987, p. 799). As yet, we are only in the earliest stages of attempts to move into more complex assessments of this kind.

Early onset of problem behaviors. Magnusson, Stattin, and Allen (1985, 1986) and Jessor and Jessor (1977) have explored the issue of early transitions in the rather different context of the onset or frequency of problem behaviors – norm-breaking, drinking, drug use, and so on – in adolescence, and their effects on subsequent functioning. In the main, in general population samples, early onset of such behaviors appeared to carry no serious risks for later development; groups making transitions at different points tended to converge over subsequent years, with later maturers catching up and the differing time-of-onset groups becoming more homogeneous over time. By the age of 25, for example, there were no differences in alcohol use between girls who started drinking early or late in their teens (Magnusson et al., 1986) and only a slight tendency for early maturers to have been any more seriously involved in crime. They were still, however, differentiable in terms of educational qualifications, suggesting that early deviance may have had effects on attitudes to, and involvement in, schooling, with potentially limiting effects on later career opportunities. Such findings underline the heterogeneity of effects that may stem from particular transitional changes and the need to assess a wide range of outcomes, not simply those in the domain immediately involved, if the effects are to be detected.

In most respects, however, it appeared that early onset of such problem behaviors might be better seen in these instances as a means of approximating adult status than as reflecting deviance. Indeed, Silbereisen and

Eyferth (1986) argue that certain types of problem behavior – in particular, the use of substances such as alcohol or drugs – can serve a positive function during adolescence, enabling young people to cope with the short-term difficulties frequently faced in adapting to new roles and demands. Support for such a view can be found in prevalence figures for substance abuse in the general population (rather than in high-risk groups), where patterns are related less to chronological age than to normative life transitions. Yamaguchi and Kandel (1985), for example, found that marijuana use decreased or even stopped as a consequence of marriage or parenthood and that these transitions occurred later for users than non-users. When substance use does function in this way – as a means of mastering temporary age-typical difficulties in development – it may have few long-term negative effects.

These findings are, of course, in sharp contrast to those on the implications of the early onset of perhaps more serious deviance in childhood and early adolescence: conduct disorder, antisocial problems, and delinquency (Farrington, 1986; Loeber & Dishion, 1983; Robins, 1978, 1986). For problems of these kinds (which in general tend to show a sharp decline with the transition to adulthood), early onset has emerged as one of the more robust predictors of persistence into adult life. It is clearly of considerable importance that we gain a better understanding of why early onset of different types of problem behaviors in adolescence can have such differing consequences and what types of problems, or populations, are especially at risk of continuing such difficulties in more severe forms in adulthood.

Protective factors and processes

Turning next to the question of protective factors and processes, the early adult period, as our earlier vignettes exemplified, provides possibilities not only for the perpetuation of risks but also for major changes of developmental trajectory. Interrupting the sequence of negative chain reactions from earlier risks is, as we have seen, one important source of such changes. In addition, Rutter (1987) proposes that protective effects may frequently stem from the opening up of new opportunities and from the new relationships and experiences encountered in early adulthood that can enhance a sense of self-efficacy and self-esteem.

Elder's discussion of the benefits of military service for vulnerable young men is of particular interest here. He suggests that these positive effects may have arisen in a variety of ways: from the chance to develop new skills in the army that could be of later practical and symbolic importance, from the opportunities to expand horizons and aspirations through contacts with a much wider group of peers, from enhanced educational opportunities, and from delaying other transitions that these young men might otherwise have undertaken at a relatively immature stage. As in the case of risk mechanisms, these protective effects also appeared to cumulate over time, leading eventually – though often only after a period of somewhat disorganized functioning in the thirties – to satisfying work and home lives in later adulthood.

Similar arguments are advanced in the very different field of delinquency research; "opportunity" theories of crime (e.g., Cloward & Ohlin, 1960) posit that the new opportunities opening up to young people (especially perhaps the academically less able) as they move from school to the world of work may play a large part in explaining the drop in criminality in early adulthood, as more legitimate means for achieving status and satisfaction become available. In this connection, Farrington, Gallagher, Morley, St. Ledger, and West (1986b) have documented associations between offending and unemployment in the immediately postschool period. Rates of offending rose when young men were unemployed, but these risks were increased only for those with a preexisting tendency to offend; the positive benefits of employment may thus have been of particular importance for otherwise delinquency-prone young men. Rutter (1987) suggests that interaction effects of this kind are crucial in detecting protective processes; in many cases, the effects involved may only be evident in at-risk groups and reflect experiences that may be of little import for less vulnerable individuals. The role of positive school experiences in enhancing self-esteem and so leading to more adaptive coping for women brought up in residential care provides a further example of this kind. Finally, the supportive effects of new intimate adult relationships have emerged in a variety of studies as of major importance in enabling women to cope with later-life stressors.

Harris et al. (1987) suggested that only the luckiest or most agile members of their sample seemed able to get off the conveyor belt of adverse circumstances set in train by premarital pregnancy. The extent to which protective factors may reflect luck (external circumstances) or agility (individual characteristics) is of considerable importance. From an interactionist perspective, the answer must always lie in an admixture of the two, individual and environment being inextricably linked by constantly reciprocal influences. Even in the case of the major environmental discontinuities arising from entry to military service, Elder notes that some element of self-selection may have been involved, more vulnerable young men being more open to the attractions that army service held out. In the study of ex-care women, however, there were some pointers that protective effects might indeed arise independently of the individual: Positive school experiences increased the likelihood of planning even for girls who showed deviant behavior toward the end of their schooling, and supportive relationships exerted protective effects even when they had begun with little apparent planning. Although many factors important for protecting against risks at this and other stages of the life span may owe much to individuals' existing coping strategies, transitional experiences can clearly play a significant part in enhancing these.

How might these varying new opportunities have their effects? As we turn to consider the processes that both risk and protective factors may reflect, our discussion will inevitably be more speculative; existing research offers little guidance on the exact nature of the processes that may be involved, and many interpretations have perforce been made post hoc, most interestingly, as in the case of Elder's work on military service (Elder, 1986), by the study subjects themselves. Attempts to test competing hypotheses in studies of this kind are relatively rare, so that the data in general remain open to a number of plausible interpretations. We move on now to a consideration of some of the central issues in this area and to questions that will need to be addressed in future research, if our understanding of process is to be advanced.

Inner and outer worlds

As has been clear throughout, there is a need to consider effects of risk and protective factors on both the inner and the outer worlds of the individual. These two strands of possible effects are outlined explicitly in the Harris et al. (1987) models but are implicated, with differing emphases, in much other work. Childhood adversities appear both to elevate risks of continued environmental stressors and to increase inner vulnerability to them, whereas positive experiences may have their impact both through improved external conditions and through effects on the individual's sense of competence and worth. The inner worlds involved might be conceptualized in various ways and may involve a variety of cognitive processes: self-esteem (e.g., Harter, 1983), hopelessness (e.g., Beck, Rush, Shaw, & Emery, 1979), or the internal working models of relationships proposed by attachment theorists (e.g., Bretherton, 1985). For the ex-care women, positive school experiences were proposed as operating primarily through enhancing a sense of self-worth and competence, whereas the Depression hardships had their major initial impact by depleting just such inner resources. In the long term, some childhood adversities may strengthen individuals' coping skills; Macfarlane (1964), discussing later outcomes of men in the Berkeley Guidance study, points to the maturational value of some hardship experiences, in a manner akin to Elder's emphasis on the strategies of positive comparisons and selective ignoring used in adult life by many members of this cohort. Vaillant and Milofsky (1980), using Erikson's model of the life cycle (Erikson, 1963), emphasize the importance of inner resources in progress through the life course, while also addressing the ways in which external, environmental tasks such as forming intimate relationships and career building relate to these. The relationship between these two strands is viewed as a constantly interactive process; early gains in inner resources can be strengthened by later experience but can also be weakened by later adversity and are not impervious to negative external stresses at later points in the life cycle.

Although many studies acknowledge the likely importance, and interaction, of these two pathways, few attempts have yet been made to assess both directly in the same context. Consequently, although we know that some transition events that come early (such as pregnancy and marriage) are often indicative of poor outcome, we do not know exactly how these experiences have their impact. The same is true of positive, protective experiences: the development of new skills in adulthood, supportive marital relationships, and so forth. One central question here is whether such experiences have their effects primarily by improving the individual's external world, in the sense of reducing stressors, or by enhancing inner resources. If they operate primarily through the latter route, the presence of stress or adversity in the environment, at least in the short term, may be less crucial in influencing later outcomes. Both Elder and Vaillant suggest that positive outcomes in adult life are often preceded by considerable stress, turmoil, and adversity during the transitional period (Elder, 1979; Long & Vaillant, 1984). However, something is gained along the way that sustains these "at-risk" individuals and enables them to achieve a mainly positive outcome. What is gained is likely to be some sense of inner worth, understanding, integrity, and a belief that one is achieving one's goals in accordance with one's plans and expectations. This remains an area for speculation; it seems inevitable that the interaction between inner resources and outer experience is the crucial issue. At younger ages, transactional models, highlighting the reciprocal interplay of inner and outer worlds, have been proposed to account for the positive adolescent outcomes found among the highly disadvantaged Kauai children (Werner & Smith, 1982) and for the effectiveness, again assessed in the late teens, of some preschool intervention programs (Berreuta-Clement, Schweinhart, Barnett, Epstein, & Weikart, 1984). Increasing our understanding of how these two worlds interact and the types of inner resources of greatest importance at different stages of development is a vital task for future research.

Sex differences

Next, sex differences are clearly of importance in a variety of respects. Few studies have assessed both men and women; the most important domains of experience may be quite different for the two sexes in adulthood, as may the origins and exact types of inner resources crucial in promoting good outcome. Elder's work, for example, hints that women may be more protected by positive relationships with their mothers in childhood than are men and that college and work experiences may be more crucial for promoting a positive outcome in men than in women. Continuities may also be mediated by somewhat different routes; in a parallel follow-up of ex-care men, Rutter, Quinton, and Hill (1990) suggested that although marital support was as important for men as for women, continuities from childhood behavior difficulties were considerably more marked in men. As yet, however, evidence on such possible sex differences is extremely limited.

The importance of different domains of experience for the two sexes – to provide a simple distinction, work for men and marriage and family life for women – immediately draws attention to issues of historical time. The roles and expectations of girls and women have changed dramatically over the last 50 years. Today, it would no longer be sufficient or acceptable to assess the outcome of adult women in terms of the social status of their spouses. From an early age girls now expect to have employment and possibly a career. The opportunities to delay childbearing through the availability of contraception, together with changing educational and labor market options, have all radically altered the degree of choice regarding women's particular goals and plans during the early adult transition.

For the future, we need to consider how more recent historical events and changing views will have an impact on the expectations, options, and experiences of both girls and boys, men and women. One area of interest will be the extent to which investment and success in one domain of life can offset disadvantage in other areas and promote a positive outcome at a later stage. The protective effects of school experiences for the ex-care women suggest that positive experiences in one area may generalize in their positive impact to others; this view is supported for men by Vaillant and Milofsky's 1980 study, albeit at a much later point in the life course. Such issues clearly warrant further attention in future research.

Social relationships and social support

The study of social relationships, and more specifically of social support, is likely to provide one of the most fruitful avenues for the exploration of risk and protective processes. Individuals' styles of relating may play an important part in accounting for continuities in maladaptive functioning at different points in the life span. Kandel and Davies (1986) have charted links between dysphoric mood and lack of close relationships with parents in adolescence; in early adulthood, there appeared to be a carryover effect, with individuals reproducing in their marital relationships the types of interactions they had experienced earlier with parents, especially the parent of the opposite sex. Caspi, Elder, and Bem (1987) have explored similar issues in the context of the explosive temperamental style characterized by temper tantrums in childhood. Using path models, they tested two possible routes whereby such apparently maladaptive styles of relating might be perpetuated: cumulative continuities, in which the individual's dispositions systematically selected him or her into environments that, in their turn, reinforced the initial dispositions; and interactional continuities, where particular styles of interaction evoked reciprocal, maintaining responses from others, in the manner of the coercive spirals of negative family relationships described by Patterson (1982). Using data from the Berkeley Guidance study, evidence for both patterns was found. The effects were most pronounced for initially explosive boys from middle-class homes; for them, a chain of negative effects could be traced across the early adult period. Childhood tantrums predicted poor school achievements and truncated education; this, in turn, increased the likelihood of downward social mobility, and the explosive style of these men holding low-status, highly supervised jobs once again caused difficulties.

Not only styles of relating but the various types of support that relationships provide are clearly of central importance. Assessing the availability, quality, and type of an individual's social relationships and how these interact with defined risk factors at key transitional points in the life cycle presents an enormous challenge. Although there is a large literature on many aspects of social relationships, existing studies focus almost exclusively on either one period in the life span (childhood, adolescence, or adulthood) or on one type of social relationship (such as marital support or peer relationships). What is lacking is a clear conceptual framework for assessing a range of relationships using a life-span perspective. Attempting to formulate such a framework is beyond the scope of this paper; instead, our aim here is to highlight some important issues in examining the links between social relationships and other risk and protective factors.

First, there is a need to conceptualize social relationships in a way that can span the range of relational provisions that may be important for health and positive adjustment (e.g., Weiss, 1969, 1974). The literature on social support is informative here, as it defines a range of support functions that social relationships can provide and that may vary in importance at different stages of the life course: in childhood (Boyce, 1985), in adolescence (Barrera, 1981; Barrera & Ainlay, 1983), and in adulthood (Cohen & Wills, 1985). In conjunction with this, there is the need to consider the structure of the individual's social network (e.g., Greenblatt, Becerra, & Seafetinides, 1982) and, in particular, to study who, in the sense of their role relationships to the individual, can provide the various types of support necessary at different life stages. Parents or parent substitutes are likely to be of central importance in childhood, and marital partners will be important in adulthood. Peer relationships will be important at all stages (see Norris & Rubin, 1984). A range of other relationships, such as those with teachers in childhood and workmates in adult life, may also be relevant.

One central issue here is the extent to which different types of relationships can provide key support functions at different stages in the life course. If one type of relationship is lacking, such as that with parents or spouse, can similar functions be gained from significant others: close friends, professionals, or workmates? For those who are most at risk, are the most vital support functions provided at times when they may be most vulnerable, such as at times of stressful events, both normative and nonnormative? Transitional events throughout the period of interest, such as the onset of puberty, leaving school, starting work, unemployment, entering college, leaving home, marriage, and birth of first child, would all provide useful points at which to assess the effects of the availability of support across a range of different types of relationships and support functions. Until now, most studies have focused on one type of relational provision only. Although Elder (1986) suggests that the protective effect of military service for some deprived men may have been via the provision of a range of support functions obtained from a range of new types of relationships, this hypothesis was not tested directly.

Second, there are likely to be sex differences in the types of social support that are most protective for those at risk. Current research generally suggests that emotional support, including confiding, is particularly protective for adult women (Brown & Harris, 1978; Brown et al., 1986). However, intimacy and close ties, particularly with family members, may be less crucial protection for men (Billings & Moos, 1982; Henderson,

Byrne, & Duncan-Jones, 1981). In contrast, men may be more protected by the support functions of social companionship and help and support in task accomplishment (Cohen & Wills, 1985). This issue of sex differences in the complex links between social support and stress has not yet been investigated sufficiently, with most current evidence relating only to women. To examine sex differences in social support using a life-span perspective may be most fruitful in furthering our understanding of the links between stress, social relationships, and disorder.

Third, social relationships and the support they provide are not only a property of the external environment, or outer world; the individual needs to contribute certain skills and resources to achieve such relationships (Norris & Rubin, 1984). In the study of risk and protective factors, many aspects of these inner resources need to be considered. For example, what inner resources are required to establish successful relationships in early childhood? Do these early relationships then impart a number of stable inner resources such as self-esteem or a belief one is lovable that can then interact with outer resources to allow the individual to develop adaptive social relationships provided the appropriate others are there in the external world?

The person's perception of the adequacy of the relationships that are available to him or her is also of importance. This perceptual aspect needs to be examined across a range of the different role relationships the individual may have – with parents, friends, partner, and so forth (Power, Champion, & Aris, 1988). There is considerable research evidence that the individual's perception of the adequacy of key relationships is a more powerful predictor of mental health than the more objective measure of availability of relationships (Barrera, 1981; Henderson et al., 1981). Indeed, it is important to emphasize that most measures of social relationships that involve any form of self-report, including interviews, include a large element of the individual's own cognitive appraisal of what is or is not available to them in the outer world. Such cognitive appraisal will obviously refer to the individual's own cognitive structures, such as schema or mental models, which contain representations of knowledge acquired from earlier life experiences (Beck et al., 1979; Power & Champion, 1986). The role of early experiences in influencing the perception of social relationships in adult life is an area that is likely to be important in furthering our understanding of risk and protective processes in the transition to adult life.

Fourth, social relationships can clearly have negative as well as positive effects, contributing to risk as well as protection. In childhood, the impact of discordant parental relationships and divorce, especially for boys, has been documented in several studies (Elder, 1979; Hetherington, Cox, &

Cox, 1982). The review by Parker and Asher (1987) suggested that children who are actively rejected rather than neglected by their peers may be most at risk for disorder in adulthood. In adolescence, there is evidence that relationships with peers of certain types can have a negative effect on outcome in adult life. Magnusson et al. (1985) found that early-maturing girls were more likely to associate with older peers and were therefore more likely to break norms and be sanctioned less by these peers for such norm-breaking behavior. Research in criminality has consistently pointed to the role of peer influences on delinquency in adolescence and that breaks with delinquent subgroups may markedly reduce offending (Farrington, 1986; West, 1982).

In adulthood, some researchers have emphasized how even close social relationships may not always be positive or protective but can in some circumstances create stress rather than support (Belle, 1980; Wellman, 1981). Cohen and Wills (1985), in their comprehensive review of the relationship between stress and social support in adults, conclude that there is little evidence for a negative effect of social networks on symptomatology and that the provision of support functions is generally positive. However, this area has not been thoroughly researched. In examining outcome in early adulthood from a life-span perspective, we are interested in more broadly based assessments of psychosocial functioning than symptomatology alone. It may well be the case that some aspects of psychosocial functioning can be adversely affected by the availability of certain types of relationships, particularly those that increase the risk of stressful life events or encourage deviant or criminal behavior. This requires further study within the the context of a comprehensive approach to assess social relationships in conjunction with risk over the life span.

Some methodological considerations

We turn finally to a brief consideration of some of the methodological implications that flow from the issues raised in previous sections. Our discussion has centered heavily on studies spanning long time periods, and we have argued that such a long-term perspective, recognizing the developmental embeddedness of the early adult transition, is essential for a full understanding of the processes involved. Clearly, however, many designs other than prospective follow-ups can be of value here. Brown and his colleagues (1986) have elegantly demonstrated the role of retrospective approaches in testing specific hypotheses, and it is clear that although some measures would be difficult if not impossible to collect retrospectively, many important childhood indicators can be reliably assessed using retrospective methods (Robins et al., 1985). More focused investigations of delimited elements of the process or the "speeded up" longitudinal approaches employed by Jessor (1983) (covering extended chronological age spans through short-term studies of two or more cohorts of differing ages) can also be of major importance. Finally, as a number of our examples have powerfully illustrated, secondary analyses of existing data sets continue to generate important new insights.

Rutter and Pickles (in press) have recently offered a series of proposals for improving the quality of longitudinal data, all of which are applicable here. Among them, we would highlight the need in studying the effects of the wide-ranging changes of early adulthood, to include an equally wide range of measures of later outcomes. To date, much research has focused on functioning in specific role areas or on disorder or criminality in adulthood, often assessed at specific time points. As we have seen, however, developments in one life domain may well have implications for functioning in other areas, so that a restricted focus of this kind may be misleading. To chart the complex effects of risk and protective factors over this period, as wide a range of assessments as possible is desirable. Measures such as the recently developed Adult Personality Functioning Assessment (Hill, Harrington, Fudge, Rutter, & Pickles, 1989), which assesses functioning in a range of domains and over extended but standardized time periods, are likely to prove of particular value here.

Rutter and Pickles (in press) argue the need for "multiple data sources, sensitive and wide-ranging measures, an ability to disaggregate and recombine measures in different ways, and, above all, the possibility to test competing hypotheses." We conclude by adding further emphasis to this last point, which is crucial if we are to increase our understanding of the processes involved in making and breaking longitudinal linkages over time. As noted earlier, much of the research carried out in this area to date has been designed to generate, rather than to test, hypotheses. Both conceptually and statistically, it is now becoming increasingly possible to move on to the essential next stage, that of testing alternative models. Caspi et al., (1987) demonstrate the power of this approach using secondary analyses of existing data, and Patterson (1986) has described a range of differing performance models for assessing the development of antisocial behavior in boys, each of which allows for testing both cross-sectionally and longitudinally. Such approaches require explicitly causal models to be specified, outlining the processes assumed to be involved. They thus hold out the hope that our current suggestive interpretations of process will become increasingly refined and move from the realm of speculation on to increasingly certain ground.

Concluding remarks

As we have seen, existing research provides us with a variety of pointers to risk and protective factors in the transition to adulthood and many suggestive interpretations of the processes that these may signal. For the future, a process-oriented approach and as explicit as possible testing of alternative hypotheses seem likely to provide the most fruitful avenues for advance. Building on the base of existing findings, we have suggested a range of conceptual issues that require continuing clarification: the relative importance of inner and outer routes in mediating the effects of both risk and protective processes and the interactions and transactions between them; the varying effects of the timing and sequencing of transitional events; sex differences at all stages of the process; the implications of styles of relating and relationships; and the availability and functions provided by differing types of social support.

Although we have concentrated on one particular phase in the life span, it is clear that many of the issues that have arisen will find parallels at other stages. As our examples have illustrated, examining the ways in which risk and protective processes interact with the developmental tasks of early adulthood can do much to increase our understanding of the forces that shape more and less successful progress through this period. We feel confident that many similar insights will be gained from the application of this approach to other key points in the life span.

REFERENCES

Baltes, P. B., Reese, R. H., & Lipsitt L. P. (1980). Life-span developmental psychology. *Annual Review of Psychology, 31*, 65–110.

Barrera, M. (1981). Social support in the adjustment of pregnant adolescents. In B. Gottlieb (Ed.), *Social networks and social support* (pp. 69–96). Beverly Hills: Sage.

Barrera, M., & Ainlay, S. L. (1983). The structure of social support: A conceptual and empirical analysis. *Journal of Community Psychology, 11*, 133–143.

Beck, A. T., Rush, A. J., Shaw, B. F., & Emery, G. (1979). *Cognitive therapy of depression.* New York: Wiley.

Belle, D. (1980). Social ties and social support. In D. Belle (Ed.), *Lives in stress: Women and depression* (pp. 133–144). Beverly Hills: Sage.

Berreuta-Clement, J. R., Schweinhart, L. J., Barnett, W. S., Epstein, A. S., &

Weikart, D. P. (1984). *Changed lives: The effects of the Perry Pre-school Program on youths through age 19.* Ypsilanti: High Scope.

Billings, A. G., & Moos, R. H (1982). Social support and functioning among community and clinical groups. *Journal of Behavioural Medicine, 5,* 295–311.

Birtchnell, J. (1980). Women whose mothers died in childhood: An outcome study. *Psychological Medicine, 10,* 699–713.

Bowlby J. (1980). *Attachment and Loss. Vol. 3: Sadness and depression.* London: Penguin Books.

Bowlby, J. (1988). *A secure base: Clinical applications of attachment theory.* London: Routledge.

Boyce, W. T. (1985). Social support, family relations and children. In S. L. Syme (Ed.), *Social support and health* (pp. 151–173). New York: Academic Press.

Bretherton, I. (1985). Attachment theory: Retrospect and prospect. In I. Bretherton & E. Waters (Eds.), *Monographs of the Society for Research in Child Development, 50*(1–2, Serial No. 209).

Brooks-Gunn, J., Petersen, A. C., & Eichorn, D. (1985). The study of maturational timing effects in adolescence. *Journal of Youth and Adolescence, 14,* 149–161.

Brown, G., & Harris, T. (1978). *The social origins of depression: A study of psychiatric disorder in women.* London: Tavistock.

Brown, G. W., Harris, T. O., & Bifulco, A. (1986). The long term effects of early loss of parent. In M. Rutter, C. E. Izard, & P. B. Read (Eds.), *Depression in young people* (pp. 251–296). New York: Guilford Press.

Caspi, A., Elder, G. H., Jr., & Bem, D. J. (1987). Moving against the world: Life-course patterns of explosive children. *Developmental Psychology, 33,* 308–313.

Cloward, R. A., & Ohlin, L. E. (1960). *Delinquency and opportunity.* New York: Free Press.

Cohen, S., & Wills, T. A. (1985). Stress, social support and the buffering hypothesis. *Psychological Bulletin, 5,* 310–357.

Crook, T., & Eliot, J. (1980). Parental death during childhood and adult depressive disorders: A review. *Psychological Bulletin, 87,* 252–259.

Elder, G. H., Jr. (1979). Historical change in life patterns and personality. In P. B. Baltes & O. G. Brim (Eds.), *Life span development and behavior* (Vol. 2, pp. 118–159). New York: Academic Press.

Elder, G. H., Jr. (1986). Military times and turning points in men's lives. *Developmental Psychology, 22,* 233–245.

Emde, R. N., & Harmon, R. J. (1984). Entering a new era in the search for developmental continuities. In R. N. Emde & R. J. Harmon (Eds.), *Continuities and discontinuities in development* (pp. 1–11). New York: Plenum.

Erikson, E. H. (1963). *Childhood and society* (2nd ed.). New York: W. W. Norton.

Erikson, E. H. (1980). *Identity and the life cycle: A reissue.* New York: W. W. Norton.

Farrington, D. P. (1986). Stepping stones to adult criminal careers. In D. Olweus, J. Block, & M. Radke-Yarrow (Eds.), *Development of antisocial and prosocial behavior.* New York: Academic Press.

Farrington, D. P., Gallagher, B., Morley, L., St. Ledger, R. J., & West, D. J. (1986a). *Are there any successful men from criminogenic backgrounds?* Paper presented to the Society for Life History Research, Palm Springs, CA.

Farrington, D. P., Gallagher, B., Morley, L., St. Ledger, R. J., & West, D. J. (1986b). Unemployment, school leaving and crime. *British Journal of Criminology, 26,* 335–356.

Featherman, D. L., Hogan, D. P., & Sørensen, A. B. (1984). Entry into adulthood: Profiles of young men in the 1950s. In P. B. Baltes & O. G. Brim (Eds.), *Life-Span development and behavior* (Vol. 6, pp. 160–202). New York: Academic Press.

Greenblatt, M., Becerra, R. M., & Seafetinides, E. A. (1982). Social networks and mental health: An overview. *American Journal of Psychiatry, 138*, 977–984.

Harris, T., Brown, G. W., & Bifulco, A. (1986). Loss of parent in childhood and adult psychiatric disorder: The role of lack of adequate parental care. *Psychological Medicine, 16*, 641–659.

Harris, T., Brown, G. W., & Bifulco, A. (1987). Loss of parent in childhood and adult psychiatric disorder: The role of social class position and premarital pregnancy. *Psychological Medicine, 17*, 163–183.

Harter, S. (1983). Developmental perspectives on the self-system. In E. M. Hetherington (Ed.), *Handbook of child psychology: Vol. 4: Socialization, personality and social development* (pp. 275–385). New York: Wiley.

Havighurst, R. J. (1972). *Developmental tasks and education.* New York: David Mackay.

Henderson, S., Byrne, D. G., & Duncan-Jones, P. (1981). *Neurosis and the social environment.* Sydney: Academic Press.

Hetherington, E. M., Cox, M., & Cox, R. (1982). Effects of divorce on parents and children. In M. E. Lamb (Ed.), *Nontraditional families.* Hillsdale, NJ: Lawrence Erlbaum.

Hill, J., Harrington, R., Fudge, H., Rutter, M., & Pickles, A. (1989). The Adult Personality Functioning Assessment (APFA): An investigator-based standardized interview. *British Journal of Psychiatry, 155*, 24–35.

Himmelweit, H. T., & Turner, C. F. (1982). Social and psychological antecedents of depression: A longitudinal study from adolescence to adulthood of a non-clinical population. In P. B. Baltes & O. G. Brim (Eds.), *Life-Span development and behavior* (Vol. 4, pp. 315–344). New York: Academic Press.

Hodges, J., & Tizard, B. (1989). Social and family relationships of ex-institutional adolescents. *Journal of Child Psychology and Psychiatry, 30*, 77–97.

Hofferth, S. L., & Moore, K. A. (1979). Early childbearing and later economic wellbeing. *American Sociological Review, 44*, 784–815.

Hogan, D. P. (1981). *Transitions and social change: The early lives of American men.* New York: Academic Press.

Holmes, S. J., & Robins, L. N. (1987). The influence of childhood disciplinary experience and the development of alcoholism and depression. *Journal of Child Psychology and Psychiatry, 28*, 399–415.

Jessor, R. (1983). The stability of change: Psychosocial development from adolescence to young adulthood. In D. Magnusson & V. L. Allen (Eds.), *Human development: An interactional perspective* (pp. 321–341). New York: Academic Press.

Jessor, R., & Jessor, S. L. (1977). *Problem behaviour and psychosocial development.* New York: Academic Press.

Joshi, H. (1985). Motherhood and employment: Change and continuity in postwar Britain. In *Measuring socio-demographic change* (pp. 70–87) (Occasional Paper 34). London: British Society for Population Studies.

Kandel, D. B., & Davies, M. (1986). Adult sequelae of adolescent depressive symptoms. *Archives of General Psychiatry, 43*, 225–262.

Kiernan, K. E. (1980). Teenage motherhood – Associated factors and consequences – The experience of a British birth cohort. *Journal of Biosocial Science, 12*, 393–405.

Lerner, R. M. (1985). Adolescent maturational changes and psychosocial development: A dynamic interactional perspective. *Journal of Youth and Adolescence, 14*, 355–372.

Levinson, D. J., Darrow, D. N., Klein, E. B., Levinson, M. H., & McKee, B. (1978). *The seasons of a man's life.* New York: A. A. Knopf.

Loeber, R., & Dishion, T. (1983). Early predictors of male delinquency: A review. *Psychological Bulletin, 94*, 68–99.

Long, J. V. F., & Vaillant, G. E. (1984). Natural history of male psychological health. XI: Escape from the underclass. *American Journal of Psychiatry, 141*, 341–347.

Macfarlane, J. W. (1964). Perspectives on personality consistency and change from the Guidance Study. *Vita Humana, 7*, 115–126.

Magnusson, D., & Allen, V. L. (1983). Implications and applications of an interactional perspective for human development. In D. Magnusson & V. L. Allen (Eds.), *Human development: An interactional perspective* (pp. 369–387). New York: Academic Press.

Magnusson, D., Stattin, H., & Allen, V. L. (1985). Biological maturation and social development: A longitudinal study of some adjustment processes from mid-adolescence to adulthood. *Journal of Youth and Adolescence, 14*, 267–283.

Magnusson, D., Stattin, H., & Allen, V. L. (1986). Differential maturation among girls and its relations to social adjustment: A longitudinal perspective. In P. B. Baltes, D. L. Featherman, & R. M. Lerner (Eds.), *Life-span development and behavior* (Vol. 7, pp. 136–172). Hillsdale, NJ: Lawrence Erlbaum.

Masten, A. S., & Garmezy, N. (1985). Risk, vulnerability and protective factors in developmental psychopathology. In B. B. Lahey & A. E. Kazdin (Eds.), *Advances in clinical child psychology* (Vol. 8, pp. 1–52). New York: Plenum Press.

Neugarten, B. L. (1979). Time, age and life cycle. *American Journal of Psychiatry, 136*, 887–894.

Norris, J. E., & Rubin, K. H. (1984). Peer interaction and communication: A life-span perspective. In P. B. Baltes & O. G. Brim (Eds.), *Life-span development and behavior* (Vol. 6, pp. 356–391). New York: Academic Press.

Parker, J. G., & Asher, S. R. (1987). Peer relations and later personal adjustment: Are low accepted children at risk? *Psychological Bulletin, 102*, 357–389.

Patterson, G. R. (1982). *Coercive family process.* Eugene, OR: Castalia.

Patterson, G. R. (1986). Performance models for antisocial boys. *American Psychologist, 41*, 432–444.

Pearlin, L. I., & Schooler, C. (1978). The structure of coping. *Journal of Health and Social Behaviour, 19*, 2–21.

Phipps-Yonas, S. (1980). Teenage pregnancy and motherhood: A review of the literature. *American Journal of Orthopsychiatry, 50*, 403–431.

Power, M. J., & Champion, L. A. (1986). Cognitive theories of depression: A theoretical critique. *British Journal of Clinical Psychology, 25*, 201–215.

Power, M. J., Champion, L. A., & Aris, S. J. (1988). The development of a measure of social support: The significant others scale. *British Journal of Clinical Psychology, 26*, 349–359.

Quinton, D., & Rutter, M. (1985). Parenting behaviour of mothers raised "in-care." In A. R. Nicol (Ed.), *Longitudinal studies in child psychology and psychiatry*. New York: Wiley.

Quinton, D., & Rutter, M. (1988). *Parental breakdown: The making and breaking of intergenerational links*. Aldershot: Gower.

Quinton, D., Rutter, M., & Liddle, C. (1984). Institutional rearing, parenting difficulties and marital support. *Psychological Medicine, 14*, 107–124.

Rindfuss, R. R., Swicegood, C. G., & Rosenfeld, R. A. (1987). Disorder in the life course: How common and does it matter? *American Sociological Review, 52*, 785–801.

Robins, L. N. (1978). Sturdy childhood predictors of adult antisocial behaviour: Replications from longitudinal studies. *Psychological Medicine, 8*, 611–622.

Robins, L. N. (1986). The consequences of conduct disorder in girls. In D. Olweus, J. Block, & M. Radke-Yarrow (Eds.), *Development of antisocial and prosocial behavior* (pp. 385–415). New York: Academic Press.

Robins, L. N., Schoenberg, S. P., Holmes, S. J., Ratcliff, K. S., Benham, A., & Works, J. (1985). Early home environment and retrospective recall: A test for concordance between siblings with and without psychiatric disorder. *American Journal of Orthopsychiatry, 55*, 27–41.

Rutter, M. (1985). Resilience in the face of adversity: Protective factors and resistance to psychiatric disorder. *British Journal of Psychiatry, 147*, 598–611.

Rutter, M. (1987). Psychosocial resilience and protective mechanisms. *American Journal of Orthopsychiatry, 57*, 316–331.

Rutter, M., & Pickles, A. (in press). Improving the quality of psychiatric data: Classification, cause and course. In D. Magnusson & L. Bergman (Eds.), *Methodological issues in longitudinal research*. Cambridge: Cambridge University Press.

Rutter, M., & Quinton, D. (1984). Long-term follow-up of women institutionalized in childhood: Factors promoting good functioning in adult life. *British Journal of Developmental Psychology, 18*, 225–234.

Rutter, M., Quinton, D., & Hill, J. (1990). Adult outcomes of institution-reared children: Males and females compared. In L. Robins & M. Rutter (Eds.), *Straight and devious pathways from childhood to adulthood*. Cambridge: Cambridge University Press.

Silbereisen, R. K., & Eyferth, K. (1986). Development as action in context. In R. K. Silbereisen, K. Eyferth, & G. Rudinger (Eds.), *Development as action in context: Problem behaviour and normal youth development* (pp. 3–16). New York: Springer.

Tennant, C., Bebbington, P., & Hurry, J. (1980). Parental death in childhood and risk of adult depressive disorders: A review. *Psychological Medicine, 10*, 289–299.

Vaillant, G. E., & Milofsky, E. S. (1980). Natural history of male psychological health. IX: Empirical evidence for Erikson's model of the life cycle. *American Journal of Psychiatry, 137*, 1348–1359.

Weiss, R. S. (1969). The fund of sociability. *Trans-Action, 6*, 36–43.

Weiss, R. S. (1974). The provisions of social relationships. In Z. Rubin (Ed.), *Doing unto others* (pp. 17–26). Englewood Cliffs, NJ: Prentice-Hall.

Wellman, B. (1981). Applying network analysis to the study of support. In B. H. Gottlieb (Ed.), *Social networks and social support* (pp. 171–200). Beverly Hills: Sage.

Werner, E. E., & Smith, R. S. (1982). *Vulnerable, but invincible: A longitudinal study of resilient children and youth.* New York: McGraw Hill.

West, D. J. (1982). *Delinquency: Its roots, careers and prospects.* London: Heinemann.

Yamaguchi, K., & Kandel, D. B. (1985). On the resolution of role incompatibility: A life event history analysis of family roles and marijuana use. *American Journal of Sociology, 90,* 1284–1325.

11 Avoiding negative life outcomes: Evidence from a forty-five year study

GEORGE E. VAILLANT

Introduction

As we go through life we see vigorous, happy, generative octogenarians, and we wonder what were the relevant antecedents? A definitive answer is not possible. But if gerontology is to understand successful adaptation to aging as well as it understands unsuccessful aging, the parameters and antecedents of successful aging must be addressed.

To better understand successful aging, the longitudinal study of entire cohorts seems valuable for several reasons. First, aging must always be studied as a process, for aging conveys change; it has a past and a future. Second, longitudinal study is necessary to encompass premature death – a negative outcome to be avoided. Third, longitudinal study is also necessary in order to assess predictive validity, the closest we will ever have to a gold standard with which to assess value-laden judgments like relative success in life. For this reason, the present chapter will discuss a 45-year prospective longitudinal study of socially favored men. It will seek to identify the most promising predictors of successful late–mid-life adaptation among 204 Harvard College sophomores, followed since 1940.

As a means of assessing successful aging, the two outcome measures used in this chapter – *physical health* and *psychosocial adjustment* – will be organized around the seven-dimensional model of successful aging suggested by Baltes and Baltes earlier in this volume. With the passage of time, progressively diminished physical reserves are an inevitable part of aging, but the rate at which these diminished reserves occur is variable. One can be young or old for one's chronological age. Health and longevity are two different ways of assessing the multifaceted process associated with declining biological reserves. Thus, two of the dimensions of Baltes and Baltes (length of life and biological health) will be combined to create here one outcome variable: physical health.

Positive evidence of mental health provides a third dimension of successful aging. Mental health reflects the capacity to master stress; grief, conflict, and past failure. In addition, good self-care (Rowe & Kahn, 1987) and self-esteem, close correlates of mental health, often make the difference between being old and being sick.

Successful aging is also reflected by relatively sustained physical and mental vigor. Continued capacity for success at working and loving and good performance on age-appropriate tests and tasks are perhaps reasonable reflections of the fourth dimension that Baltes and Baltes call psychosocial efficacy.

Fifth, successful aging also requires that the individual regard the present period of life as somewhat more than satisfactory – ideally, the subjectively best period of one's life. Thus, life satisfaction is as important a dimension of successful aging as survival or the absence of biological morbidity.

These three dimensions – mental health, psychosocial efficacy, and life satisfaction – will be combined to create this chapter's second outcome variable: psychosocial adjustment.

Finally, successful aging must include maintaining optimal autonomy. Increasing physical limitations and the accelerated losses of loved ones are inevitable consequences of the passage of time. As individuals grow older, they must be adept at replacement and substutition. They must be prepared for growing yet older, for avoiding dependency where possible and accepting it when necessary. This process can be conceptualized as one of personal control, the sixth facet of successful aging suggested by Baltes and Baltes here and elsewhere (Baltes & Baltes, 1986). This last dimension of successful aging is still only minimally evident in the 65-year-old men to be discussed in this chapter. Very few are physically disabled and many, by virtue of education and occupation, still maintain community roles that permit leadership. Nevertheless, this paper demonstrates that choice of dominant styles of defense (coping) may be seen as one aspect of personal control.

There is a seventh dimension of successful aging that will be addressed only in passing. This dimension includes those tasks that individuals can do better after age 60 than before. These ill-defined processes come under headings like experience, wisdom, and "keepers of the meaning." Older individuals' skills often manifest increased capacity to conserve and transmit cultural heritage. Liberated from personal allegiances, older individuals are more likely to be trusted by both sides to mediate conflict. The mean age for genealogists, for high court judges, for church leaders, and for trustees is often beyond the retirement age for most occupations.

Methods and results

The sample

Successful aging, no matter how humanely defined, is a value judgment. So are the concepts of forward motion and velocity. All three – velocity, forward motion, and successful aging – depend on the vantage point of the observer. But if we wish to understand our own lives in time and space, these are nevertheless judgments worth making. What Leo Kass (1975), a research professor of bioethics, said of health can be applied to successful aging as well: "Health is a natural standard, a norm – not a moral norm, not a 'value' as opposed to a 'fact,' not an obligation but a state of being that reveals itself in activity" (p. 28). If successful aging is to be empirically validated, it needs to be looked at in terms of objective "activity."

Thus, physical health and psychosocial adjustment were assessed as two separate, if intercorrelated, outcome variables. Thus, on the one hand, this chapter will focus upon the antecedents of men remaining in excellent *physical health* at age 63 to 65. On the other hand, this chapter will also focus upon the antecedents of men who, at age 65, are still experiencing superior psychosocial adjustment as defined by life satisfaction *and* mental health *and* the clear ability to play *and* to work *and* to love.

The cohort that this chapter describes consists of a 10% sample of three consecutive college classes. The sample was created between 1940 and 1942 when the Harvard University Health Services under Arlie Bock, M.D., began a longitudinal study of Harvard College sophomores (Health, 1945).

The men were originally selected for intensive multidisciplinary study because their freshman health service physical examination had revealed no mental or physical health problems and their college deans saw the men as becoming promising adults (Health, 1945). This cohort, also known as the Grant Study, has been prospectively followed from age 18 to age 65, from 1940 to 1988 (McArthur, 1955; Vaillant, 1984). In college, the men received 20 to 30 hours of multidisciplinary assessment. The men were reinterviewed at age 25, at age 30, and again between ages 47 and 57. For 45 years or until their death, the men have also been followed by means of annual or biennial questionnaires. In addition, physical examinations have been obtained every 5 years. By design, important outcome ratings at each period have been made by raters blind to other ratings.

Of those 204 men originally in the sample, 6 dropped out in college, 5 died in combat in World War II, and 5 died young from deaths unrelated to identified mental illness. As indicated in Table 11.1, of the remaining

Table 11.1. *Attrition within the sample*

1940–42	204 19–20-year-old college sophomores selected for study
1968–70	188 still had complete data sets (10 died young and 6 drops)
1985	173 men still had complete data sets (13 had died and 2 had incomplete data sets)

188 middle-aged men who had complete data sets at age 47, 173 remained alive and active in the study until after age 60. Of the missing 15, 13 men died prior to age 60, and 2 had incomplete data sets.

Before discussing the findings, let me put the cohort into historical perspective. Born just after 1920, these men were adolescents during the Depression. Almost all saw active military service in World War II and on return benefited from high employment, a valuable dollar, and the American G.I. Bill, which virtually guaranteed these successful college students graduate education. Having forgotten the pacifism that many of them had shared in 1940 and 1941, these combat veterans were confronted – and often dismayed – by their "baby boom" children, who came of age in the 1960s, children who protested American military involvement in Vietnam, cohabited before marriage, and smoked marijuana. The men themselves were young enough to benefit from the secular trends of 1960–1980 toward middle-aged fitness and smoking cessation.

Among other longitudinal studies, the Oakland Growth Study cohort from the Institute of Human Development at Berkeley described by Glen Elder (1974) captures the historical times of these men well. But in contrast to Elder's cohort, their Harvard degrees gave the men of the Grant Study, whatever their social origins, a ticket of entry to the upper middle class.

Physical health

One of the great difficulties of longitudinal studies is halo effects. Thus, physical health, like all the major variables discussed in this paper, was assessed by raters blind to all other variables.

Approximately every 5 years the study obtained physical examinations from the men (preferably by an internist) including chest x-rays, routine blood chemistries, urinalysis, and an electrocardiogram. An internist, blind to psychosocial adjustment, rated these examinations on a 5-point scale of objective physical health. Table 11.2 illustrates the rating scale used for assessing our first outcome variable, physical health, at age 63. Table 11.2

Table 11.2. *Progression of illness in 188 men surviving until age 45*

Age (years)	Excellent health (%)	Minor problems (%)	Chronic illness (%)	Chronic illness with disability (%)	Dead (%)
25	96	4	0	0	0
40	80	17	2	1	0
50	48	35	13	2	2
63	22	42	22	4	10

Note: The table excludes the 6 drops and the 10 men who died before age 45. In quantifying relative physical health the following scale was used: excellent = 1; minor problems = 2; chronic illness = 3; disabled = 4; dead = 5.

also depicts the first two dimensions of successful aging, length of life and the progressive decline over time in the physical health of these men. As suggested by Fries (this volume), at this point in the men's lives morbidity, not mortality, is the dominant problem. At age 50, very few of the men had been chronically ill, but at 65 few are still completely well. Of the 188 men alive at age 45, only 41 men were still in excellent health at age 63 ± 1 (i.e., revealed no evidence of significant irreversible illness or physical defect). The men who fell into the category "minor problems" had experienced potentially progressive difficulties such as reversible hypertension, hypercholesterolemia, hearing loss, or moderate arthritis. The category "chronic illness" refers to illnesses that could be expected to be progressive, that would shorten life or significantly affect daily living. Examples are coronary thrombosis, diabetes, multiple sclerosis, and hypertension not fully controlled by medication. "Chronic illness with disability" includes men whose irreversible illnesses have led to significant restrictions in daily living.

Psychosocial adjustment

Table 11.3 combines three dimensions of successful aging into the second of this chapter's two outcome variables: psychosocial adjustment from age 50 to age 65. The American psychiatrist Roy Grinker pleaded for "operational referents" in order to make the concept of psychosocial health less metaphysical (Grinker, Grinker, Timberlake, 1962). Thus, Table 11.3 tries to provide such operational referents for three of the more general (or platonic) definitions of successful aging: life satisfaction, psychosocial efficacy, and mental health. But in so doing I must acknowledge that

Table 11.3. *Measure of outcome: Psychosocial adjustment from age 50 to 65*

Individual scale item (range) (only the most unfavorable category for each outcome is illustrated)	Psychosocial adjustment score			
	Best[a] $n= 37$ (%)	Middle $n = 99$ (%)	Worst $n = 37$ (%)	Interrater reliability[b] (%)
I. Psychosocial efficacy				
Early retirement (1–3 points)	3	25	46	.70
Career declined (1–2 points)	0	9	60	.47
Career not enjoyed (1–2 points)	0	15	70	.54
Less than 3 weeks' vacation[c] (1–2 points)	19	33	43	.64
Failed marriage (1–3 points)	0	34	57	.80
Few social activities (1–2 points)	54	62	92	.54
II. Mental health				
10 + psychiatric visits (1–3 points)	0	9	32	.87
Regular mood-altering drug use (1–3 points)	0	10	6	.78
5 + days of sick leave/year (1–2 points)	3	11	41	.55
III. Life satisfaction				
Observer-rated life dissatisfaction (1–5 points)	0	5	73	.60

[a]The group with the best psychosocial adjustment received scores of 10–12, the middle group ranged from 13 to 17, and the worst group from 18 to 26.
[b]Kendall's tau b was the statistic used.
[c]The only variable not significantly associated with the global outcome variable at $p < .001$.

assessing psychosocial health is more controversial and value-laden than assessing physical health. The scale used to assess psychosocial adjustment is set forth in Table 11.3. The scale closely follows the global measure designed to assess positive mental health at age 47 (Vaillant, 1975, 1979), but fortuitously the scale proves quite congruent with the criteria set forth by Baltes and Baltes in this volume. The points assigned to each item are indicated to the right of each item in Table 11.3. (A low score was favorable.) The first two items assess work. First, were the men still working full-time at 65 (1 point), had they cut back (2 points), or were they retired (3 points)? Second, were their occupational responsibilities after age 60 at least as great as they had been at age 50, or had the men become less effective?

Two items were chosen to reflect the men's ability to play. First, did they appear to regard work and/or retirement as enjoyable (1 point), was their enjoyment ambiguous (2 points), or did they regard their work or retirement as demeaning or boring (3 points)? Although in identifying overall psychosocial adjustment, the second item – presence or absence of an enjoyable 3-week vacation – did not seem as important at age 65 as it had at age 47, it was retained to maintain symmetry with the age 47 scale.

Two items in Table 11.3 assessed social relationships. On three occasions after age 50 the subjects, and on 2 occasions their wives, were asked a variety of scaled questions about both the stability and their enjoyment of their marriage. These scores were averaged, and cutting points were chosen to indicate a marriage that over the 15-year period of observation was consistently and mutually enjoyable (1 point); of ambiguous stability (2 points); clearly unhappy or terminated by divorce during the period or nonexistent for reasons other than widowhood (3 points). The item *no social activities* indicated that the individual did not engage in regular group activities with friends, for example, golf, bridge, or charitable enterprises. (However, the men were by no means as socially isolated as the rater's strict interpretation of this item makes it appear.)

The next three items reflect efforts to operationalize mental health. During the 15-year period from age 50 to 65, had the men never visited a psychiatrist (1 point), made 1–10 visits (2 points), or made more than 10 visits (3 points)? Second, during the same period, had the men never used mood-altering drugs (hypnotics, minor tranquilizers, antidepressants) (1 point), used them for less than 30 days (2 points), or used such medicine for more than a month (3 points)? Third, because at age 47 the number of days of sick leave taken each year had been more highly correlated with mental than with physical health (Vaillant, 1975, 1979), this item was retained. The cutting point was 5 or more days of sick leave a year.

Finally, each rater made a clinical assessment of the subject's own attitude toward his life between 55 and 65 and his expressed attitude toward growing older. An effort was made to discount the effects of either alcoholism or poor physical health per se. Greatest weight was given to the subject's own responses to the question asked at age 56 and again at age 64: Did he see the present decade as the happiest (1 point) or the unhappiest decade of his life (5 points), or was this decade intermediate in happiness relative to the rest of his life (3 points)? Although it may be argued that subjective happiness cannot be accurately measured by a simple 5-point scale, a simple, face-value measure may be the best we can hope for. Certainly, the enormous literature (e.g., Diener, 1984; Hoyt & Creech, 1983; Larson, 1978) on life satisfaction in the elderly suggests little evidence that complexity of measurement offers greater validity. Assessment of relative happiness will always reflect the crudest of approximations.

The points from the 10 items in Table 11.3 were summed to provide a 10–26 point assessment of psychosocial adjustment. The purpose was not to provide an arbitrary definition of successful aging but rather to provide an empirical rank ordering of the men. Clearly, the presence or absence of predictive validity of such a scale must be assessed at some later date. Nevertheless, Table 11.3 demonstrates that it was possible to identify 37 men who at 65 had experienced virtually none of the negative criteria. It was possible also to identify 37 men who had experienced negative outcomes in all three domains of life satisfaction, mental health, and psychosocial efficacy.

In order to make the ratings in Table 11.3, the independent raters had to integrate data from interview material and from seven participant questionnaires and two questionnaires completed by the wives; therefore, their judgments on individual items showed modest variation. Table 11.3 shows the interrater reliability for each item. Interrater reliability for the total measure was .72 (Kendall's tau). Cronbach's alpha for the entire scale was .69, but this is an inflated figure because the rater's estimate of life satisfaction, which in part was based on the other nine variables, was included as part of the global scale.

Table 11.4 looks at the intercorrelations between several of this chapter's operational dimensions of successful aging. In general, the individual facets of physical health, psychosocial efficacy, and mental health were only modestly associated with each other. Even the two global outcome variables of physical health and psychosocial adjustment correlated at only $r = .36$. By age 65, 51% of the men with the worst psychosocial adjustment had become chronically ill or had died, whereas poor health was present in only 16% of the best adjusters. However, there were only 16 men who were included both among the 41 men with excellent physical health *and* among the 37 men with the best psychosocial adjustment. Physical health, after all, reflects only one dimension of successful aging.

Table 11.4 examines other interrelationships of the psychosocial adjustment scale. Psychosocial adjustment assessed 15 years earlier showed a significant relationship with most of the items. The two exceptions were early retirement and long vacations. In this sample, early retirement was a relatively poor indicator of overall adjustment, and at age 65 the capacity to take enjoyable vacations no longer reflected the discriminative power that it had shown at age 47.

Two of the individual items, career/retirement enjoyment and tranquilizer use, were chosen for this table because they showed the highest

Table 11.4. *Intercorrelation of different dimensions of successful aging*

	Physical health, age 50–65	Psycho-social adjustment, age 47	Career/ retirement enjoyment, age 50–65	Mood-altering drug use, age 50–65	Observer-rated life satisfaction, age 50–65
I. Global Variables					
Psychosocial adjustment (age 50–65)	.36*	.51*	—	—	—
Physical health (age 63)	—	.23*	.13	.27*	.33*
II. Variables in Psychosocial Adjustment Scale (Age 50–65)					
Age at retirement	.13	.10	.31*	.15	19
Career success	.23*	.25*	.37*	.18	.47*
Career/retirement enjoyment	.16	.25*	—	.16	.50*
Length of vacation	−.01	.07	.16*	.02	.14
Marital satisfaction	.13	.38*	.16*	.23*	.33*
Social activities	.21	.21	.11	.10	.18
Psychiatric visits	.20	.34*	−.02	.42*	.12
Use of mood-altering drugs	.27*	.41*	.16	—	.37*
Sick days	.19	.17	.19*	.34*	.31*
Observer-rated life satisfaction	.33*	.36*	.50*	.37*	—

Notes: Spearman rho was the statistic used to calculate the correlations. For this table, all variables have been scaled as if the most favorable score was low (e.g., little mood-altering drug use correlates positively with little evidence of physical illness).
*$p < .001$.

correlations with the dimensions of psychosocial efficacy and mental health, respectively. Even these variables showed relatively weak inter-correlations with other variables when compared with life satisfaction. In short, observer-rated happiness showed greater correlations with every facet of late–mid-life aging than did present physical or mental health or prior global psychosocial adjustment.

Predictors of successful aging

Tables 11.5 and 11.6 look at different predictors of successful aging. Current physical health affected current psychosocial adjustment and was also affected by many of the predictor variables. For this reason, the

Table 11.5. *Correlation of significant antecedents with successful late–mid-life adjustment*

	Good physical health $n = 172^a$	Good psychosocial adjustment $n = 173^b$	Psychosocial adjustment controlling for physical health
Predictors, before age 20			
Ancestral longevity	.15*	.10	.06
Childhood environmental strengths	.27***	.25***	.17*
Closeness to siblings	.22**	.26***	.20**
College pulse rate	.09	.30***	.28***
Exercise in college	.14*	.22**	.18**
Predictors, before age 50			
Maturity of defenses (age 20–47)	.22**	.45***	.40***
Regularity of promotions	.15*	.28***	.24***
Use of mood-altering drugs	−.36***	−.47***	−.37***
Psychiatric visits	−.19**	−.37***	−.33***
Physiological symptoms with stress	.16*	.23**	.18*
Alcohol abuse before age 50	.28***	.27***	.17*

^{a}Health of one man unclassified.
^{b}To calculate the zero-order correlations in the same manner as the partial correlations in the right-hand column and in Table 11.7, the Pearson product moment coefficient was used rather than the Spearman rho.
*$p < .05$. **$p < .01$. ***$p < .001$.

association of antecedent predictor variables with psychosocial adjustment was calculated only after health at age 63 was partialed out.

In Table 11.5 ancestral longevity was estimated by computing the age at death of the subject's parents and four grandparents. Surprisingly, long-lived ancestors only weakly predicted good physical health at late mid-life, and psychosocial adjustment not at all. Indeed, even in a replication study on 90 of the now 75–79-year-old women in the Terman Study (Sears, 1984), ancestral longevity was only weakly correlated with vigorous late-life adaptation (unpublished data).

Assessment of childhood environmental strengths was provided by two independent raters blinded to the future but with access to all data gathered at age 18 on several facets of the men's childhoods. These data included several psychiatric interviews with the men and home interviews with their parents (Vaillant, 1974). Rater reliability was .71. Despite its

Table 11.6. *Theoretically important variables that did not predict outcome in late mid-life*

	Correlation[a] with	
	Physical health at age 63 n = 172	Adult adjustment at age 50–63 n = 173
Childhood social class	.01	.02
Stability, parental marriage	.05	.10
College scholastic aptitude	−.02	.07
Vital affect in college	.01	.06
Psychopathic in college	.03	−.08
Sociable in college	.02	.03
Not Correlated with Physical Health		
Childhood emotional problems	.05	−.14*
College psychosocial adjustment	.05	.15
Age 29 psychosocial adjustment score	.01	.21**
Not Correlated with Late–Mid-life Psychosocial Adjustment		
Ancestral longevity	.16*	.09
Number of octogenarians	.18**	.11
Death of a parent in childhood	−.15*	.03

[a]Spearman rho was the statistic used.
*p < .05. **p < .01.

crudity and its dependence upon subjective clinical judgment, the scale's predictive validity over three to four decades has been as robust as the best measures from reviews of other prospective studies (Kohlberg, La-Crosse, & Ricks, 1970). Over the years, the most powerful predictive subscales of the childhood environmental strengths scale were cohesiveness of the home and whether or not the boy's relationships with his mother and father were conducive to trust, autonomy, and initiative. However, what was particularly interesting to observe in Table 11.5 was that at age 65 the simple 0–2 subscale (2 = destructive relationship with siblings or no siblings, 1 = ambiguous data or no siblings, 0 = close to at least one sibling) proved as powerful a predictor of adjustment at age 63 as the full 20-point childhood environment scale or, for that matter, as any other variable assessed before age 30.

A low standing pulse during the men's college physical examination provided another predictor of successful late–mid-life adjustment. Previous work (Phillips, Vaillant, & Schnurr, 1987) has shown that for this sample this association was independent of physical fitness. We speculate that the predictive power of an elevated pulse rate may reflect social anxiety (see Kagan, Reznick, & Snidman, 1988).

Mental health between 30 and 50 was the best adult predictor of late – mild-life outcome. The number of psychiatric visits, the use of tranquilizers, and the presence of few physiological symptoms with stress between age 20 and age 50 (Vaillant, 1978) were significantly correlated with late–mid-life adjustment. None of the 21 men who were ever diagnosed as significantly depressed before age 50 (i.e., meeting *DSM-IIIR* criteria for either dysthymic disorder or major depressive reaction) fell in the top quartile of psychosoical adjustment at age 65. Previous studies have suggested that income is a powerful predictor of life satisfaction in old age (e.g., Diener, 1984). In future studies, it would be important to control for mental illness and alcoholism, which exert strong negative effects on income, before taking such findings at face value.

Table 11.6 illustrates that many potential predictor variables known to be important in adolescence and young adulthood were not associated with successful aging. For example, childhood social class (lower-middle to upper), stability of parental marriage, childhood parental loss, and college scholastic aptitude – variables often found to be associated with adjustment in young adulthood – were uncorrelated with long-term outcome. Similarly, extroverted personality variables estimated in college failed to predict adjustment in late mid-life (Health, 1945; Wells & Woods, 1946). For example, *sociable* (i.e., general ease in social relationships) correlated with good psychosocial adjustment in college ($r = .24$, $p < .001$) and at early mid-life ($r = .13$, $p < .05$), and *vital affect* correlated with adjustment in college ($r = .31$, $p < .001$) and in young adulthood ($r = .18$, $p < .02$). Perhaps most dramatic was the fact that the trait *psychopathic* (the psychiatrist's estimate of categorical psychological impairment in college), which correlated with global college adjustment ($r = -.35$) correlated only $r = -.04$ with poor adjustment in late mid-life. Clearly, people change over time.

Other variables in Table 11.6 were associated with either physical health or psychosocial adjustment but not both. Variables associated only with good late-life psychosocial adjustment included the absence of emotional problems in childhood, early adult psychosocial adjustment, and the more surprising association between college standing pulse and outcome (Phillips et al., 1987) shown in Table 11.5. Ancestral longevity assessed in a variety of ways was a better predictor of decline in physical health than of psychosocial adjustment.

Our numbers are so small and there is so much colinearity among the variables in Table 11.5 that modeling procedures are suspect. As a conservative solution, Table 11.7 identifies those variables that are able to

Table 11.7. *Unique variance of predictor variables in explaining physical health and adult adjustment at late mid-life*

	Partial correlation of each predictive variable, with the other five controlled, with	
	Physical health at age 63	Adult adjustment at age 50–65
Use of mood-altering drugs before age 50	−.39***	−.28***
Maturity of defenses (age 20–47)	.04	.32***
Childhood environmental strengths	.21***	.08
Alcohol abuse before age 50	−.16*	−.18*
Vigorous exercise in college	.11	.22**
Ancestral longevity	.07	.01

Note: $n = 164$ due to missing variables for some subjects.
*$p < .05$. **$p < .01$. ***$p < .001$.

explain unique variance once others are controlled. Thus, the correlation of each of the variables with outcome is examined by itself. The six variables chosen were selected on the basis of significant zero-order correlation and because they were relatively independent of other predictive variables. (For example, *psychiatric visits* was excluded because it correlated highly with tranquilizer use and reflected the same dimension of mental illness.) Tranquilizer use before age 50 provided the most robust and the most discriminating predictor of both physical and psychosocial outcome at age 65. This finding corroborates my clinical impression that presence or absence of significant depression was the best predictor of global psychosocial and physical health outcome. The reason for choosing mood-altering drug use as a variable rather than psychiatric diagnosis is that it could be objectively quantified and estimated without knowledge of other variables. Assessment of clinical depression could not be easily made as a blind judgment.

Ancestral longevity was a variable theoretically antedating both childhood environment and the use of tranquilizing drugs. Although in Table 11.7, once those other two variables were controlled, ancestral longevity failed to explain additional variance in physical health, to deny ancestral longevity a unique and significant etiological role is logically indefensible. A reasonable hypothesis might be that some of the variance explained by ancestral longevity is mediated through childhood environmental instability resulting from early parental death. However, the association of ancestral longevity and physical health was not reduced by controlling for parental loss in childhood.

Defense mechanisms

The fact that in Table 11.7, with the other five variables controlled, maturity of defense mechanisms accounted for 9% of the explained variance in late–mid-life psychosocial adjustment requires comment. By way of introduction, there are three broad ways of coping with stress. First, there are the ways in which an individual elicits help from appropriate others, for example, social support. Second, there are conscious cognitive strategies designed to make the best of a bad situation (Folkman & Lazarus, 1980). Third, there are unconscious adaptive mechanisms, often subsumed under the psychoanalytic term *ego mechanisms of defense* (Freud, 1937), that distort internal and external reality. For many years, this third type of coping, the "defense mechanism," has been deservedly unpopular in experimental psychology, due to difficulty in empirically verifying unconscious processes (Kline, 1972). However, the idea of "involuntary" adaptation has recently reentered the literature of cognitive psychology under such rubrics as "hardiness" (Kobasa, Maddi, & Kahn, 1982), "self-deception" and "emotional coping" (Lazarus, 1983), and "illusion" (Taylor & Brown, 1988). In recent years, experimental strategies for studying defense mechanisms have improved (Haan, 1977; Horowitz, 1986; Vaillant, 1986).

Some purposes of such "unconscious" mechanisms that can be inferred are, first, to keep affect within bearable limits during sudden changes in emotional life, for example, following acute object loss; second, to restore psychological homeostasis by postponing or deflecting sudden increases in biological drives; third, to attain a respite and to master changes in self image that cannot be immediately integrated, for example, puberty, major surgery, or promotion; and fourth, to handle unresolvable conflict with important people, living or dead. The use of such mechanisms usually alters the perception of both internal and external reality and often compromises other facets of cognition.

In the psychosomatic literature, so-called defense mechanisms are sometimes discussed under the term *denial* (Hackett & Cassem, 1974). However, as sunlight may be divided into distinct colors by a prism, just so the many mechanisms making up the denial mechanisms have been refracted by the author – and many psychoanalytically influenced investigators before him (Vaillant, 1971) – into differentiated mechanisms, some of which are more adaptive and developmentally more "mature" (Vaillant, 1976) than others. By maturity of defenses is meant the ratio between the frequency with which the men were noted to use so-called mature defenses like *suppression, sublimation, altruism,* and *humor* and the frequency with which they used "immature" defenses like *schizoid fantasy, projection, passive aggression, hypochondriasis,* and *dissociation* (denial of feeling) in situations of conflict. Rater reliability for the ratio of mature to immature defenses was .86 (Vaillant, Bond, & Vaillant, 1986).

However, a major difficulty in defining defenses is that there is no commonly accepted language. For example, within 50 miles of a single American city (San Francisco) there are currently six competing non-overlapping classifications used by six respected investigators (or pairs of investigators) of stress and coping (Block & Block, 1980; Folkman & Lazarus, 1980; Haan, 1977; Horowitz, 1986; Moos & Billings, 1982; Weinberger, Schwartz, & Davidson, 1979). Even in this volume, for example, Thomae and co-workers report an empirical assessment of conscious and unconscious efforts at adaptation that depends on a completely different nomenclature from the one used in this chapter.

However much readers may wish to dispute the terms used in this chapter in contrast to those in competing nomenclatures, the terms that I have used (*a*) have been widely used in the past within a highly developed theoretic framework (Vaillant, 1971), (*b*) have been defined in a mutually exclusive way (Vaillant, 1986), and (*c*) are defined in *DSM-III-R* (APA, 1988). In addition, this study's prospective design and independent rating of somatic health and defensive style lend some credibility to the value of distinguishing mature mechanisms from immature mechanisms. First, previous work had shown that maturity of defenses, even though derived from intrapsychic processes, correlates with multiple models of mental health at least as well as many other more widely accepted measures (Vaillant & Schnurr, 1988). Second, it may be that defenses can provide an explanation for the so-called invulnerability among the environmentally disadvantaged. For example, previous work (Vaillant 1983a, 1983b) suggests that maturity of defenses is only modestly affected by successful childhood and very little by social class. Third, as illustrated in Figure 11.1, adaptive choice of defense mechanisms may provide some kind of immunization against unsuccessful living.

Figure 11.1 contrasts the declining physical health of 79 men with relatively mature defenses with the declining health of 61 men with relatively immature defenses. (The men with intermediate defenses were excluded from the analysis.) Maturity of defenses was assessed on the basis of the men's adaptive style between age 20 and age 47 years. The bars of the graph show the percentages of men still in good health (*excellent* or *minor problems*) at the start of each 5-year period who became chronically ill or who died before the end of the 5-year period. It can be

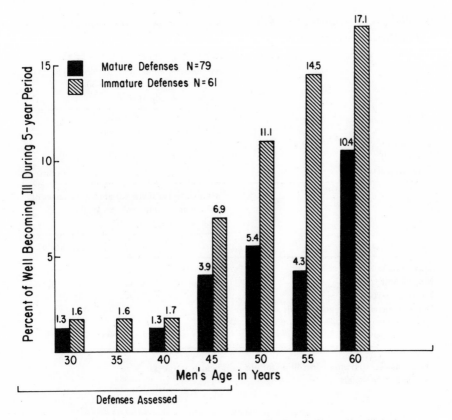

Figure 11.1. Association of maturity of defenses with the likelihood of becoming ill during sequential 5-year periods.

argued that poor health prior to age 50 may have affected the men's adaptive style as much as the reverse. However, for at least 10 years after the age of 50, the health of the men with mature defenses continued to deteriorate less quickly.

Unfortunately, the size of the data set provides too little statistical power to allow the estimated variance contributed by external manifestations of mental illness (e.g., clinical diagnosis, use of mood-altering drugs) to be dissected from the estimated variance contributed by the highly correlated style of inferred intrapsychic homeostasis (i.e., maturity of defense mechanisms). Although the possibility cannot be excluded that immaturity of defenses and vulnerability to anxiety and depression may simply reflect two sides of the same coin, such circularity can be used to argue the power of the concept.

Table 11.8. *Association of psychosocial adjustment during other periods of adult life with adjustment in late mid-life*

	Psychosocial adjustment at previous ages of the 37 men with the best age 50–65 psychosocial adjustment		
	Age 21	Age 29	Age 47
Top quartile	41%	49%	54%
Middle half	57%	38%	54%
Bottom quartile	3%	13%	11%
	Psychosocial adjustment at previous ages of the 37 men with the worst age 50–65 psychosocial adjustment		
	Age 21	Age 29	Age 47
Top quartile	27%	25%	8%
Middle half	51%	40%	27%
Bottom quartile	22%	35%	65%
Pearson correlation of adjustment at each earlier age period with age 50–65 adjustment[a]	$r = .16*$	$r = .29***$	$r = .44***$

[a]This was assessed after controlling for physical health at age 63.
$*p < .05.$ $***p < .001.$

Discontinuities

Table 11.8 illustrates that over time there was diminishing concordance of adult psychosocial adjustment with that in earlier time periods. At four points in the men's lives (age 21, age 29, age 47, and age 65) independent assessments were made of psychosocial stability. This global assessment was always the most powerful predictor of psychosocial adjustment at the next age period. With the passage of time, not surprisingly, clear shifts occurred that could not be explained by just chance variation.

That shifts in psychosocial adjustment occur was perhaps most dramatically illustrated by the following observation (Vaillant & Schnurr, 1988). Of the 188 men still active participants at age 47, only 16 men were consistently in the top quartile of adjustment. Eighty-seven of the 188 men in this cohort selected for mental health could have been described as psychiatrically impaired in college *or* at age 29, *or* at age 47, *or* at age 62, *or* by meeting the *DSM-III* criteria for alcoholism, *or* for some other *DSM-III*

Table 11.9. *Association of suppression and self-discipline before age 50 with successful aging at age 65*

	Physical health	Psychosocial adjustment	Psychosocial adjustment controlling for physical health
Suppression a major adaptive style before age 50	.8	.26***	.25***
Days sick leave from work before age 50	−.20**	−.26***	−.19**
"Practical and organizing" in college	−.01	.18**	.21**
"Well integrated" in college[a]	.11	.24***	.21**
Duration of college treadmill run	.12	.18*	.14
Pounds over ideal weight, age 50	−.13*	−.23**	.20**
Heavy smoker before age 50	−.19**	−.29***	.24***

[a]The definition of *well integrated* was "steady, stable, dependable, thorough, sincere, trust-worthy."
*$p < .05$. **$p < .01$. ***$p < .001$.

Axis I diagnosis. Only 10 of these 87 "impaired" men, however, fell in the bottom quartile of psychosocial adjustment at every point of observation.

Perhaps the two most important variables in causing shifts from good to poor psychosocial adjustment were the onset of poor physical health or alcoholism. Of the 12 men who were in the top quartile at age 29 and yet who were in the bottom quartile at age 65, seven had developed alcoholism and/or poor health.

The most important factor in men's psychosocial adjustment improving in late mid-life may have been the increasing importance of perseverance and self-control with mature adjustment. This speculation is based on the statistics shown in Table 11.9. As previously noted, college variables like being practical and organized became relatively more important and college personality variables like vital affect and sociability became less important with the passage of decades. Table 11.9 documents the association of earlier stoicism and self-discipline with good outcome in late mid-life. Space does not permit extensive discussion of the defense mechanism of suppression – the postponement but not repression of gratification, the capacity to see but not exaggerate the bright side – here, but the defense is discussed in detail elsewhere (Vaillant, 1977, 1986, in press). Men with good outcomes were more likely to have been thought "dependable" and "trustworthy" in college, have exercised vigorously, completed the treadmill run in college, and not stayed home from work with minor illnesses. In short, men who between 20 and 40 had appeared disappointingly dull were often enjoying life at 65 more than some of the men with a far more colorful youthful adult adjustment. The race, as Ecclesiastes and Aesop suggest, is not always to the swift.

Case history

Most men in the Grant Study sample are still too young to be at risk for the major negative outcomes of unsuccessful aging – mortality, institutional living, need for multiple aids to daily living, and conflictual dependence on others for basic needs. Only one of our subjects has experienced Alzheimer's disorder and no one has as yet been confined to a nursing home. But adaptation to these more melancholy aspects of aging must be addressed in any discussion of successful aging. For the concept of successful aging can be valuable if we see it as *process* rather than product. Indeed, the concept of successful aging will be demoralizing both to subject and to observer if successful aging is seen as being "better" than others or being healthy all of one's days.

Successful aging must also reflect vital reaction to change, to disease, and to environmental imbalance. Indeed, the contemplation of successful aging forces us to reflect upon human dignity. There is an old adage: Better to be an unhappy Socrates than a happy pig. One of the subjects in the study described in this chapter expressed the dignity of aging and mortality a little differently when he wrote, "What's the difference between a guy who at his final conscious moments before death has a nostalgic grin on his face, as if to say, 'Boy, I sure squeezed that lemon' and another man who fights for every last breath in an effort to turn time back to some nagging unfinished business? Damned if I know, but I sure think it's worth thinking about" (Vaillant, 1977, p. 357). Because the social sciences lack adequate metrics for assessing philosophers, happy pigs, and squeezed lemons, let me substitute a case history of a Grant Study member, Dr. Eric Carey (a pseudonym), who died young.

Dr. Carey began life as a gregarious member of a close family. Both his parents were social workers in the spirit if not the letter of the phrase; and as a 13-year-old, Dr. Carey, too, had made a commitment to a life of service to others. The general experience of the Grant Study has been that the Eriksonian (1959) tasks of intimacy, career consolidation, generativity, and keeper of the meaning are mastered in sequential order (Vaillant & Koury, in press; Vaillant & Milofsky, 1980). But if Dr. Eric Carey illustrates a life that violates such principles, there was no one else in our study quite like him. Indeed, Dr. Carey even violated the principle that good physical health per se has something to do with successful aging. For Dr. Carey is dead, but while dying he demonstrated a capacity to make meaning for himself and to keep meaning for others. Thus, his late-life psychosocial adjustment put him among the most successful outcomes. For Dr. Carey's life suggests that death and retirement by no means reflect failure, but that the capacity while alive to remain productive and generative provides pleasure and meaning.

Early on, Carey collected a sense of himself, consolidated it, and shared it with discretion throughout the 45 years that he revealed himself to the study. But all life events – and there were severe setbacks for this man – were moderated by his relationship to people, both on a personal and on a professional level. At age 23, when asked about his "fitness for his present work" (medical school), Dr. Carey wrote that "children fascinate me; I enjoy playing and working with them.... I get along well with children, enjoy taking the time to amuse them or circumvent their distrust of doctors; ... I'm patient enough to do with children what many other people do not have time nor patience to do." Dr. Carey described what a pediatrician does, but there was also a sense of self-content in his words. It was not just a career but the relationship and the skill in the relationship that came through. Later, at age 26, when Dr. Carey was asked what was stimulating or interesting about his career, he replied, "the opportunity for aid to children through increasing parental understanding" and that the meaning of his work was "to make a contribution to the community."

Not only had Dr. Carey begun the work of generativity young, he began the work of growing old early. At age 26 the not-yet-crippled Dr. Carey had already told the study his "philosophy over rough spots": "That no matter what personal difficulty I struggle with, others have survived worse; and that, fundamentally, there is a force of events which will carry us through even though at personal sacrifices."

At age 32 Dr. Carey developed poliomyelitis. Newly liberated from 6 months in an iron lung and knowing that he would never walk again, Dr. Carey responded as follows to the Thematic Apperception Test (TAT) card of a youth with a violin:

Here is a young boy who ... started out in college with brilliant prospects, a bright future but becomes disillusioned with life, morose, despondent ... and decides to end his life. He is apprehended in the process of jumping from a tall building. As he does so, he closes his eyes. Before them flashes a panorama of his past life, hopes, aspirations, sadness of ... failure, realizing then the agony of being cornered ... the despondency to end his own life.

He'll be examined by a psychiatrist and placed in a hospital for therapy. After months, his goals will be altered. After being in therapy a little longer, he'll get what he wants. He'll be able to be of use to society again, to go on to achieve that which ... in later years will be satisfying.

By age 35, cripplied by polio, Dr. Carey continued as both a pediatrician and a teacher. Confined to a wheelchair, he did not use his academic success as an excuse to withdraw from being a full-time clinician. His generativity was not derived from the old saw "those who can, do; those who can't, teach." Nor did his pleasure in teaching come from didactic instruction, from self-aggrandizing *telling*. His success as a teacher came from enabling others, from, as it were, giving the self away. I suspect that this process is vital to successful aging. Dr. Carey wrote that the nurses and the medical students he taught "seem to respond to increased participation and responsibility, in contrast to the passive roles they often play in our clinics." Later in the same questionnaire, he wrote of the fact that he worked as an active clinician from a wheelchair: "Others can get not only professional help but some measure of comfort from my carrying on as if nothing had happened." Mentorship means to show and to share, not merely to tell.

Almost 20 years later, the progressively crippled Dr. Carey again expressed the challenge of old age: "The frustration of seeing what needs to be done and how to do it but being unable to carry it out because of physical limitations imposed by bedsores on top of paraplegia has been one of the daily pervading problems of my life in the last four years." But 3 years later, at age 55, Dr. Carey answered his own challenge: "I have coped ... by limiting my activities (occupational and social) to the essential ones and the ones that are within the scope of my abilities."

At 57, although he was slowly dying from pulmonary failure secondary to 20 years of muscular paralysis, Dr. Carey wrote that the last 5 years were the happiest of his life. "I came to a new sense of fruition and peace with self, wife and children." He spoke of peace, and his actions portrayed it. During this time he had "let go" the stamp collection that had absorbed him for half a century; he had given it to his son. A year before his death, in describing to an interviewer his "risky anesthesia" and recent operation, Dr. Carey said, "Every group gives percentages for people who will die: 1 out of 3 will get cancer, 1 out of 5 will get heart disease – but in reality '1 out of 1 will die' – everybody is mortal."

At age 32, Dr. Carey had written of his work motivations: "to add an iota to pediatric knowledge, the sum totals of which may ultimately aid more than the patients I see personally." But it takes a longitudinal study to differentiate between real-life behavior and facility with pencil-and-paper tests. That Dr. Carey's words were not pious good intentions but rather intimations of immortality was confirmed by the fact that when Dr. Carey died, an endowment for a professorship in his name was raised to perpetuate his lifelong contribution to pediatrics. Throughout his life, his wife, his children, his colleagues, and his patients loved him.

Earlier I suggested that generativity and keeping the meaning were tasks to be mastered in the second half of life. But what do I mean by *keeping the meaning?* Generativity and its virtue, *care*, require taking care of one person rather than another (Erikson, 1959). Keeping the meaning and its virtue, *wisdom*, involve a more nonpartisan and less personal approach to others (Vaillant, 1977; Vaillant & Koury, in press). Wisdom, unlike care, means taking sides impersonally. The focus of keeping the meaning is on the collective products of humanity – the culture in which one lives and its institutions – rather than in the development of its children. Kotre (1984) separates the two components by observing that the targets of Eriksonian generativity must be *both* "the culture and the disciple, and the mentor must hold the two in balance" (p. 14). If the mentor puts too much into his mentees (i.e., "generativity"), "he neglects and dilutes the culture's central symbols. But if the preservation of culture is paramount [i.e., "keeping the meaning"] he makes anonymous receptacles of disciples" (Kotre, 1984, p. 14). I believe that Dr. Carey mastered both tasks.

Discussion and conclusion

Critique

The introduction to this chapter looked at some of the dimensions of aging that must be considered in designing a valid outcome measure for successful aging. In conclusion, it must be asked, have this chapter's outcome variables met reasonable epidemiologic criteria for validity? Several caveats need mention.

In trying to evaluate alleged causal connections between antecedent variables and outcome, it is important to assess whether or not appropriate competing risk factors have been controlled. In some instances this has been possible. For example, before antecedent variables affecting physical health could be suggested as also contributing to psychosocial adjustment, current phyiscal health had to be controlled (Table 11.5). However, in other instances this chapter has failed. For example, the relative causal contributions of childhood environment and maturity of defenses, two of the most interesting antecedent variables considered, remain unclarified.

In assessing potential causation, time relationships must be kept explicit. Predictive measures must be clearly separated in time from outcome measures. This has been achieved. Ratings of major variables were made by raters blinded to other data. All of the predictive measures in Tables 11.5, 11.6, and 11.7 were gathered before age 50 by raters blind to the future, and all outcome measures were gathered after age 50 by raters blind to the past.

Ultimately, in any study of life-span development, the dependent variables for one phase of life must become the independent variables for evaluating the next stage. Thus, the validity of this chapter's outcome measures must in part depend on their *ability to predict the future*. Put differently, how adequately might this chapter's definition of successful aging at late mid-life serve as an intermediate variable on the developmental path toward becoming engaged, vigorous, and happy octogenarians? Clearly, it is too soon to tell. Another criterion of an outcome measure is *replicability*. Replicability touches on one of the few real shortcomings of longitudinal research. Both cost and the vagaries of history make it not feasible to repeat a 40-year longitudinal study. My own strategy will be to try to examine the same measures in this chapter in secondary analysis of the Terman sample of women (Sears, 1984) and of an inner-city sample that has also been followed for 40 years (Glueck & Glueck, 1968; Vaillant, 1983b, 1986).

The external validity of our outcome variables may be criticized for reflecting *value judgments*. As an effort to correct for this, in the future I shall test the degree to which the outcome criteria used in this study are confirmed or refuted by results obtained from longitudinal study of gifted women and socially disadvantaged men. However, it is also important to reflect upon the utility of value judgment and not to judge such criteria too hastily. For example, many people would call classing divorce as a maladaptive outcome a value judgment, but almost everyone would agree that loving a spouse for a long period of time is a good outcome. Divorce – as an event – therefore can serve as a concrete negative indicator of the less value ridden but more difficult to measure good marriage. In many samples, golf, bridge, and participation in charitable endeavors would be a ludicrous measure of assessing capacity for sustained social activities with others. However, for the present sample such criteria may be adequate, for we are comparing members of a relatively homogenous sample with themselves.

A final criterion for an outcome variable is its *importance*. Too often social scientists measure the reliable rather than the meaningful. The reader must decide whether longevity, subjective happiness, and the value-laden assessment of working and loving are more or less "important" than outcomes reflected by more reliable and replicable pencil-and-paper assessments, for example, personality inventories.

Conclusion

Because there are no absolute answers, why should we bother to ask questions about succeful aging? The answer, of course, is that we know much about pathologic aging but only anecdotally about successful aging. Thus, even if the present findings are tentative and controversial, they may enhance knowledge.

Certainly this sample of 173 men was a biased one, and biased toward successful aging. The study members were white and male and they had been selected for good physical health and high academic achievement. Most men received some graduate education and had forged their occupational careers during a time of American economic growth and prosperity. They had access to good medical care, knowledge of good nutritional practices, and opportunity for exercise. Such homogeneity of background allows their lives to cast light on certain variables associated with late–mid-life aging, without interference from undue environmental adversity.

Perhaps the most striking finding was that absence of psychiatric vulnerability in young adulthood and absence of psychiatrist/tranquilizer utilization and depressive disorder were the most important variables predicting late–mid-life psychosocial adjustment. Other more obvious, potentially negative causal variables – shortened ancestral longevity, bleak childhoods, and alcoholism – appeared, if anything, more associated with physical decline. Still other variables, those in Table 11.8, that common sense might have picked as predictor variables were uncorrelated with outcome. Indeed, it was perhaps instructive that extensive exercise habits in college should predict psychosocial adjustment at 65 better than they did good health at 65 and that a warm childhood environment should predict late-life physical health better than it predicted happiness and vigor. If we are to understand successful aging, we must learn to expect such surprises and to conceptualize the mind and body as a whole.

NOTE

The preparation of this paper was supported by research grants K05-MH00364, MH39799, and MH42248 from the National Institute of Mental Health.

REFERENCES

American Psychiatric Association (1988). *DSM-III-R, Diagnostic and statistical manual of mental disorders*. Washington, DC: American Psychiatric Press.

Baltes, M. M., & Baltes, P. B. (Eds.). (1986). *The psychology of control and aging.* Hillsdale, NJ: Lawrence Erlbaum.

Block, J. H., & Block, J. (1980). The role of ego-control and ego-resiliency. In W. A. Collins (Ed.), *Development of cognition, affect and social relations: The Minnesota Symposium on Child Psychology* (Vol. 13, pp. 39–101). Hillsdale, NJ: Lawrence Erlbaum.

Diener, E. (1984). Subjective well-being. *Psychological Bulletin, 95,* 542–575.

Elder, G. H., Jr. (1974). *Children of the Great Depression. Chicago:* Chicago University Press.

Erikson, E. H. (1959). Identity and the life cycle. *Psychological Issues, 1,* 1–171.

Folkman, S., & Lazarus, R. S. (1980). An analysis of coping in a middle-aged community sample. *Journal of Health and Social Behavior, 21,* 219–239.

Freud, A. (1937). *Ego and mechanisms of defense.* London: Hogarth Press.

Glueck, S., & Glueck, E. (1968). *Delinquents and nondelinquents in perspective.* Cambridge: Harvard University Press.

Grinker, R., Grinker, R. R., Jr., & Timberlake, J. (1962). "Mentally healthy" young males (homoclites). *Archives of General Psychiatry, 6,* 405–453.

Haan, N. (1977). *Coping and defending.* New York: Academic Press.

Hackett, T. P., & Cassem, N. J. (1974). Development of a quantitative rating scale to assess denial. *Journal of Psychosomatic Research, 18,* 93–100.

Health, C. W. (1945). *What people are.* Cambridge: Harvard University Press.

Horowitz, M. J. (1986). *Stress response syndromes* (2nd ed.). Northvale, NJ: Jason Aronsen.

Hoyt, D. R., & Creech, J. C. (1983). The Life Satisfaction Index: A methodological and theoretical critique. *Journal of Gerontology, 38,* 111–116.

Kagan, J., Reznick, J. S., & Snidman, N. (1988). Biological bases of childhood shyness. *Science, 240,* 167–171.

Kass, L. R. (1975). Regarding the end of medicine and the pursuit of health. *Public Interest, 40,* 11–42.

Kline, P. (1972). *Fact and fantasy in Freudian theory.* London: Methuen & Co.

Kobasa, S. C., Maddi, S. R., & Kahn, S. (1982). Hardiness and health: A prospective study. *Journal of Personality and Social Psychology, 42,* 168–177.

Kohlberg, L., LaCrosse, J., & Ricks, D. (1970). The predictability of adult mental health from childhood behavior. In B. Wolman (Ed.), *Manual of child psychopathology* (pp. 1217–1284). New York: McGraw-Hill International Book Co.

Kotre, J. (1984). *Outliving the self.* Baltimore: Johns Hopkins University Press.

Larson, R. (1978). Thirty years of research on the subjective well-being of older Americans. *Journal of Gerontology, 33,* 109–125.

Lazarus, R. S. (1983). The costs and benefits of denial. In S. Breznitz (Ed.), *Denial of stress* (pp. 1–30). New York: International University Press.

McArthur, C. (1955). Personality differences between middle and upper classes. *Journal of Abnormal and Social Psychology, 50,* 247–254.

Moos, R. H., & Billings, A. G. (1982). Conceptualizing and measuring coping resources and processes. In L. Goldberger & S. Breznitz (Eds.), *Handbook of stress: Theoretical and clinical aspects* (pp. 212–230). New York: Free Press.

Phillips, K. A., Vaillant, G. E., & Schnurr, P. (1987). Some physiological antecedents of adult mental health. *American Journal of Psychiatry, 144,* 1009–1013.

Rowe, J. W., & Kahn, R. L. (1987). Human aging: Usual and successful. *Science*, *237*, 143–149.

Sears, R. R. (1984). The Terman Gifted Children Study. In S. A. Mednick, M. Harway, & K. M. Finello (Eds.), *Handbook of longitudinal research in the United States* (Vol. 1, pp. 398–414). New York: Praeger.

Taylor, S. E., & Brown, J. D. (1988). Illusion and well-being: A social psychological perspective on mental health. *Psychological Bulletin, 103*, 193–210.

Vaillant, G. E. (1971). Theoretical hierarchy of adaptive ego mechanisms. *Archives of General Psychiatry, 24*, 107–118.

Vaillant, G. E. (1974). Natural history of male psychological health, II: Some antecedents of healthy adult adjustment. *Archives of General Psychiatry, 31*, 15–22.

Vaillant, G. E. (1975). Natural history of male psychological health, III: Empirical dimensions of mental health. *Archives of General Psychiatry, 32*, 420–426.

Vaillant, G. E. (1976). Natural history of male psychological health, V: The relation of choice of ego mechanisms of defense to adult adjustment. *Archives of General Psychiatry, 33*, 535–545.

Vaillant, G. E. (1977). *Adaptation to life*. Boston: Little Brown.

Vaillant, G. E. (1978). Natural history of male psychological health, IV: What kinds of men do not get psychosomatic illness. *Psychosomatic Medicine, 40*, 420–431.

Vaillant, G. E. (1979). Natural history of male psychological health: Effects of mental health on physical health. *New England Journal of Medicine, 301*, 1249–1254.

Vaillant, G. E. (1983a). Childhood environment and maturity of defense mechanisms. In D. Magnusson & V. Allen (Eds.), *Human development: An interactional perspective* (pp. 343–352). New York: Academic Press.

Vaillant, G. E. (1983b). *The natural history of alcoholism*. Cambridge: Harvard University Press.

Vaillant, G. E. (1984). The study of adult development at Harvard Medical School. In S. A. Mednick, M. Harway, & K. M. Finello (Eds.), *Handbook of longitudinal research in the United States* (Vol. 2, pp. 315–327). New York: Praeger.

Vaillant, G. E. (1986). *Empirical studies of ego mechanisms of defense*. Washington, DC: American Psychiatric Press.

Vaillant, G. E. (in press). Repression in college men followed for half a century. In J. Singer (Ed.), *Repression: Defense mechanism and personality style*. Chicago: University of Chicago Press.

Vaillant, G. E., Bond, M., & Vaillant, C. O. (1986), An empirically validated hierarchy of defense mechanisms. *Archives of General Psychiatry, 43*, 786–794.

Vaillant, G. E., & Koury, S. H. (in press). Late midlife development. In G. H. Pollock, & S. I. Greenspan (Eds.), *The course of life*. New York: International Universities Press.

Vaillant, G. E., & Milofsky, E. S. (1980). Natural history of male psychological health, IX: Empirical evidence for Erikson's model of the life cycle. *American Journal of Psychiatry, 137*, 1348–1359.

Vaillant, G. E., & Schnurr, P. (1988). What is a case? A forty-five year followup of a college sample selected for mental health. *Archives of General Psychiatry, 45*, 313–319.

Weinberger, D. A., Schwartz, G. E., & Davidson, R. J. (1979). Low-anxious, high-anxious and repressive coping styles. *Journal of Abnormal Psychology, 88*, 369–380.

Wells, F. L., & Woods, W. L. (1946). Outstanding traits: In a selected college group with some reference to career interests and war records. *Genetic Psychological Monographs, 33*, 127–249.

12 Developmental behavioral genetics and successful aging

NANCY L. PEDERSEN AND
JENNIFER R. HARRIS

Introduction

There is no consensus as to what the term *successful aging* means. A number of behavioral scientists operationalize the definition in terms of indicators of successful aging, such as life satisfaction (Butt & Beiser, 1987; Rudinger & Thomae, this volume) or development-related control beliefs (Brandtstädter & Baltes-Götz, this volume). Others have proposed models or strategies for aging "successfully" (e.g., Baltes & Baltes, this volume; Featherman, this volume), whereas biomedical researchers have addressed the effects of "successful" or "optimal" aging on life expectancy and morbidity (Fries, this volume). The distinction between successful and usual aging propposed by Rowe and Kahn (1987) highlights the consequences of the interaction between extrinsic and intrinsic factors in aging.

Regardless of one's theoretical orientation or preference of definitions, the term *successful aging* serves as a useful heuristic device for stimulating research and discussion. Many approaches to successful aging are compatible with a developmental behavioral genetic perspective, especially in the extent to which they emphasize variation and plasticity. Furthermore, they point out interesting phenotypes or phenomena for study. Because the role of intrinsic and extrinsic factors presented in the definition by Rowe and Kahn directly addresses a primary concern of behavioral genetics (i.e., etiology of individual differences) we have chosen to emphasize their orientation to the topic in the introduction to this chapter. Examples from other perspectives on successful aging will be included in the remaining sections. Our intention is to present a general discussion of the interface between behavioral genetics and successful aging. Due to the scope of the topic, we will restrict ourselves to broad issues rather than present a detailed description of behavioral genetic methodology.

Extrinsic and intrinsic factors in aging

The role of extrinsic factors is central to the distinction between successful aging and usual aging made by Rowe and Kahn (1987). In their conceptualization of successful aging, extrinsic factors "play a neutral or positive role," whereas in usual aging, these factors "heighten the effects of aging alone" (p. 143). Much of the decline or loss previously attributed to the aging process may be explained in terms of extrinsic factors. Implicit to this definition is the concept that successful aging represents intrinsic aging or, at best, aging in which extrinsic factors result in improvement or enhanced function.

In this schema, it is important to differentiate the meaning of intrinsic from genetic. Intrinsic processes are those inherent to (inseparable from) aging itself; however, they may arise from both genetic and environmental effects. Thus, as described in the following, processes that are intrinsic to aging may or may not be inherited. In addition, characteristics that are inherited may or may not show genetic variation.

Genetic material can be involved in intrinsic aging processes in a number of ways (Johnson, 1988). Thousands of genes may have relevance for the pathobiology of aging (Martin, 1979), but few genes may control the rate of aging (Cutler, 1975). Temporal genes, which are "turned on or off" at specific times, may be involved in the timing of specific age-related events (Farrer, 1987; Paigen, 1980). Other genes may have differential effects at different stages, as described in the late-acting deleterious gene hypothesis, where aging is the result of pleiotropic genes that have good effects early in life but become harmful later in life (Williams, 1957). Some theories of aging (e.g., Hart & Trosko, 1976) point to the influence of genetic redundancy in the aging process, and others are concerned with insufficiency of repair systems, where aging results from the accumulation of somatic damage (Kirkwood, 1981) or unrepaired DNA lesions (for a review see Tice & Setlow, 1985). It is not clear whether age-related declines in repair mechanisms, which may be intrinsic to the aging process, reflect information encoded in the DNA, environmental effects, or the interaction of genetic and environmental effects. Despite the involvement of genetic material, both genetic and environmental mechanisms are probably important to intrinsic aging processes.

One often forgotten point about the influence of genetic factors on phenotypes is that inherited characteristics may or may not show genetic variability. Thus, characteristics intrinsic to the aging process that may be under genetic control may not contribute to variation in aging. In inbred strains of mice that should be genetically homogeneous, phenotypic variability arises from environmental differences. For example, the significant variability in life span and life expectancy reported for completely inbred, homozygous strains (Johnson & Simpson, 1985; Mayer & Baker, 1985; Sprott, 1983) can be attributed to environmental sensitivity. Another example is the well-documented finite growth potential of euploid fibroblast-like populations in vitro (Hayflick, 1965; Hayflick & Moorhead, 1961; reviewed by Norwood & Smith, 1985). Even if the limiting mechanism is genetically regulated, there may not be any genetic variability, and all observable variation would reflect environmental effects.

Extrinsic factors for aging need not necessarily be limited to those with a strictly environmental etiology. Life-style, habits and psychosocial factors may all show some degree of genetic influence. The behavioral genetic literature is replete with evidence of genetic variation for personality traits and psychosocial behaviors (for a review see Henderson, 1982). Recent developments in the field indicate that experience is directed by genotypes (Scarr & McCartney, 1983) and that individuals' perceptions of their environment are heritable (Plomin, McClearn, Pedersen, Nesselroade, & Bergeman, 1988). Thus, both genetic and environmental factors may be influencing both intrinsic and extrinsic aspects of aging (Figure 12.1).

Variability and successful aging

One of the general conclusions that can be garnered from longitudinal aging studies is that relatively few individuals follow the pattern of age changes predicted from the assessment of averages (Dannefer & Sell, 1988; Shock, 1985). Rather, variation is pervasive and a primary concern for the conceptualization of successful aging (Baltes & Baltes, this volume; Rowe & Kahn, 1987). Unlike approaches that emphasize the description of average values for a trait, the study of successful aging necessitates the examination of individual differences because the focus is on the factors contributing to heterogeneity. Developmental behavioral genetics (DBG) utilizes quantitative genetic methodology to examine these individual differences from a developmental or gerontological perspective.

The aim of this paper is to discuss the concept of successful aging from a DBG perspective. DBG techniques are designed to identify and to estimate the importance of genetic and environmental factors as they affect the phenotype of interest (for a general introduction, see Plomin, DeFries, & McClearn, 1989). Observed variation is parceled into a linear combination of genetic variation (V_G), environmental variation (V_E), their interaction ($V_{G \times E}$), and the covariance term (Cov_{GE}). Some of these components can be parsed more finely: V_G can be subdivided into additive and nonadditive components, and V_E can be decomposed into shared environ-

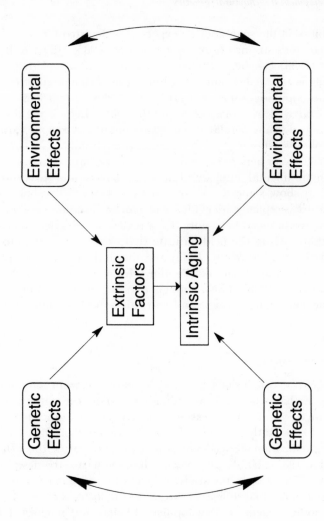

Figure 12.1. Influences of genetic and environmental factors in extrinsic and intrinsic aspects of aging.

mental affects (E_S) that contribute to familial resemblance and nonshared environmental effects (E_{ns}) that contribute to differences among family members. Error variance is included in the E_{ns} parameter. Various analytic procedures can be employed to yield estimates of these components, which are sample statistics representing population parameters. It should be noted that the $V_{G \times E}$ term represents interaction in terms of analysis of variance and should not be confused with interactions in individual development.

As applied to the study of successful aging, DBG can be used to assess the extent to which extrinsic and intrinsic aspects of aging are influenced by genetic and environmental differences. Given that aging is a dynamic process for which intrinsic aspects can be modified in various ways by different extrinsic factors, the a priori expectation is that the relative roles of genes and environment for aging phenomena will show developmental changes. A better understanding of the effect of our genetic substrate on the expression of the aging process can be achieved when DBG findings are combined with molecular genetic advances. Knowledge of the etiology of extrinsic factors in the aging process may enable more rational application of preventative and therapeutic measures.

Some considerations in behavioral genetic studies of successful aging

Definition of the phenotype

Obviously, an essential aspect of DBG studies is the choice of phenotypes. Are we interested in aging as the phenotype or phenotypes in aging individuals? A variety of phenotypes in numerous systems should be examined as there is "little evidence for the existence of a single factor that regulates the rate of aging in different functions in a specific individual" (Shock, 1985, p. 740). Depending on the design, either levels, patterns, duration in state, transitions, or rates may be considered as phenotypes. Both objective measures such as blood pressure or glucose levels and subjective measures such as life satisfaction or locus of control could be included as phenotypes. Even the concepts of reserve capacity and adaptability, if measurable, may be of interest.

Although the terms *successful aging* and *usual aging* represent an important conceptual distinction, differences in their interpretation may affect the selection of populations and phenotypes for study. To the extent that the term *successful* implies position on a distribution, it is tempting to shift one's focus from the actions of extrinsic factors to a simpler categorization of the population into successful and nonsuccessful agers. From a DBG point of view it may be better to apply the terms *successful* and *usual* subsequent to the analysis of extrinsic and intrinsic aspects rather than prior to the onset of a study.

Although categorization of the population might be helpful for some purposes, it limits the scope of the research questions and the generalizability of results. Several elegant designs that provide estimates of genetic influence on the expression of dichotomous traits have been developed within the field of genetic epidemiology (e.g., Emery, 1986; Morton & Chung, 1978). These designs, however, do not utilize the wealth of information provided by the variation within groups. Furthermore, if the population is artificially divided into successful versus nonsuccessful agers, emphasis is placed on class membership rather than on the effect of extrinsic factors on the aging process.

Alternatively, methods are available for assessing heritability of continuous traits in samples identified by the membership of one or more family members at the extreme of a distribution (DeFries & Fulker, 1985). Thus, a population of successful agers and their relatives (successful and nonsuccessful agers) could be identified, and the importance of genetic and environmental effects for any number of quantitative traits could be assessed. This approach is based on hierarchical multiple regression techniques that are difficult to expand to the multivariate case, in which the relationship among measures is of primary interest. Furthermore, this and other techniques that are dependent on dichotomizing the population do not lend themselves well to longitudinal designs because of their dependence on selection of probands at a specific time point. When followed longitudinally, a number of the subjects identified as "successful" at the outset of a study will decline in performance, and the distribution of these subjects may resemble a "usual" sample of the elderly with time. The generalizability of the results is thus dependent on the choice of measures involved in the initial selection of probands. Valuable information about important associations between phenotypes and extrinsic effects may have been masked by the selection process. If the sample is not truncated by selection, conclusions can be drawn about aging in the population as a whole rather than restricted to the description of a segment.

The study of quantitative measures in the population as a whole (without categorization by rank) is the basis of behavioral genetic analysis. Levels, changes, and rates can be phenotypes (Eaves, Long, & Heath, 1986; Hewitt, Eaves, Neale, & Meyer, 1988; McArdle, 1986; Plomin & Nesselroade, in press). Examples of interesting phenotypes include functional capacity, markers of aging, and extrinsic psychosocial effects. Not only can these phenotypes be analyzed univariately, but the associations among measures can be examined for genetic and environmental influences in the covariation among variables. For example, does a correlation between cognitive ability and forced vital capacity in older subjects reflect a group of environmental factors that affects both traits or a common set of genetic mechanisms? Shared genetic effects may be the basis for the observed association between survival and cognitive functioning reported by Jarvik and Bank (1983).

Cross-sectional designs

The choice of phenotypes to be studied is naturally limited by the type of study design. As in all developmental studies, measures of change can be examined only when data are collected at more than one time point. In cross-sectional studies, the degree of genetic and environmental influence for univariate measures or the multivariate relationships among these measures can be determined in the population ignoring or controlling for the possible effects of age. Such results describe the importance of genetic and environmental effects without specifying the importance of gender, age, or cohort.

Questions about the genetic and environmental etiology of successful aging are really questions about the etiology of age variation. There are several possible patterns of effects that may describe changes in the variance architecture of individual differences. For example, if the phenotype displays aged heterogeneity in which individual differences increase significantly, then it is possible to determine whether this added variation is genetic, environmental, or both. Comparative modeling techniques may be used to test for equality of the genetic and environmental parameters over time or age.

Alternatively, the phenotype may not be characterized by aged heterogeneity, but the relative importance of genetic and environmental influences may vary with age. Within a modeling framework, this could be tested by specifying invariance of the genetic and environmental proportions of variance. The presence or absence of significant age differences in parameter estimates can be established; however, these differences may reflect history-graded effects, intrinsic age changes, or both. This type of analysis in the Swedish Adoption/Twin Study of Aging (SATSA) suggests that there are very few measures for which the importance of genetic effects differs by age-group.

Longitudinal designs and the study of change

Several aspects of stability and change can be explored within the framework of a longitudinal behavioral genetic study. First, changes in the relative contributions of genes and environments to instrinsic and extrinsic aging processes can be estimated. In other words, is the proportion of genetic variation for a phenotype the same, or does it differ across occasions of measurement? Hints about such changes garnered from cross-sectional work can be confirmed or refuted in a longitudinal design. Along these lines, age changes mirrored age differences for the relative role of genes and environment for a measure of chronic illness (Harris, 1988).

Apart from assessing changes in the relative contributions of genes and environments at each occasion, it is possible to estimate stability of genetic (or environmental) effects. These estimates, called genetic (or environmental) correlations, indicate the extent to which the same genes (or environments) are operating at different occasions. The genetic correlation may be high (indicating genetic stability) or low (indicating genetic change) regardless of the heritability at those time points. For example, genetic change occurs when senescent genes, related to deterioration or decline, become activated later in life. Similarly, new extrinsic factors may come into play, thereby altering the overall variance structure of individual differences in aging.

Structural change, where the patterning of the relationships among many measures varies, represents a third type of change. If we consider a pleiotropic case, in which the same genes contribute to the variation in several phenotypes, then the relative proportion of genetic variance that is common to these phenotypes (i.e., loadings on a common genetic factor) may vary across time.

The fourth aspect of change that can be examined is related to the phenotype and is represented by relative or absolute change scores. Behavioral genetic analyses of change scores address the importance of genetic effects on aging parameters such as rate and duration. The emphasis is on the genetic contribution to change in the phenotype rather than change in the relative genetic contribution or changes in the genetic effects operating (Plomin & Nesselroade, in press).

Several path analytic models have been developed to describe how genetic and environmental influences on a trait might operate over time. Plomin and DeFries (1981) propose a model that includes separate latent genetic and environmental factors at each of the occasions of measurement. Genetic and environmental correlations are represented by the paths across time connecting these latent factors. In a more complex model (Eaves et al., 1986; Hewitt et al., 1988), the correlation between a particular trait measured at two times may be due to a persistence of genetic influences, a persistence of environmental influences, or to persistence at the level of the phenotypic trait itself. Occasion-specific effects that do not contribute to continuity may be operating as well. Other method-

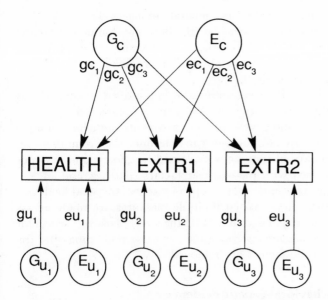

Figure 12.2. Examples of a path analytic model for genetic and environmental effects on a primary phenotype and measurable extrinsic factors.

ologists have presented analytic designs based on the simplex model (Boomsma & Molenaar, 1987) or latent-variable growth curve models (McArdle, 1986). Choice of a model is of course dependent on the study design and the nature of the data set.

Extrinsic factors and intrinsic aging in behavioral genetic designs

Figure 12.2 depicts one example of the nexus of relationships between genetic and environmental influences, extrinsic factors and intrinsic processes in aging. Let us presume that we can measure a characteristic that may change with age, for example, physical health (HEALTH), and extrinsic effects that may be related to the primary phenotype (EXTR1, EXTR2). These effects may be measures of the physical environment, such as exposure to infectious agents or accidents, or may be descriptive of the individuals' psychosocial environment, such as life-style, diet, and personality. For each of the measures (HEALTH, EXTR1, EXTR2) some of the variation is accounted for by common genetic and environmental factors (latent traits G_c and E_c) and some by genetic and environmental factors unique to the measure (latent traits G_u and E_u). Genetic influences, represented by the latent trait G_{u1}, may affect one's susceptibility to disease, and unmeasured environmental influences (latent trait E_{ul}) may also be important for physical health. Both environmental factors (latent trait E_u) and genetic factors (G_u) may account for the extrinsic effects; however, for measures of the physical environment, the path from the latent trait G_u is probably 0.

The model can be used to determine the importance of genetic and environmental influences unique to the primary phenotype physical health (paths g_u and e_u) and genetic and environmental influences unique to the extrinsic factors. In addition, one can determine the extent to which variation in the primary phenotype is explained by genetic and environmental variation shared with the extrinsic factors (paths g_c and e_c).

In this heuristic example, the phenotype of interest, physical health, is measured at one time point. When multiple measures are made across time, the model can be expanded to include the study of change scores for physical health. Changes intrinsic to aging are those remaining after the changes due to extrinsic factors are removed.

Developmental behavioral genetic evidence

Although considerable methodological advances are being made in the field of developmental behavioral genetics, as witnessed in special issues of *Child Development* (1983) and *Behavior Genetics* (DeFries & Fulker, 1986), little information is available on elderly individuals, and no studies as yet have specifically reported on successful aging (Plomin, 1986). Only one behavioral genetic study thus far has published longitudinal results on an elderly sample of twins (Kallmann & Sander, 1948; Jarvik & Bank, 1983). To our knowledge, only two other studies of aging twins are currently under way: SATSA (McClearn et al., 1986) and the Minnesota Twin Study of Adult Development (McGue & Hirsch, 1987). Other studies of adult twins and family studies have contributed to the development of analytical strategies and provided important data on life-span development (DeFries & Fulker, 1986). However, these studies fall outside the scope of this article because aging per se and successful aging in particular were not examined.

New York State Psychiatric Institute study of aging twins

In 1946, Kallmann and Sander (1948, 1949) organized a study of twins who were at least 60 years old and were residents of New York State. The sample consisted of 1,603 index cases of twins who were followed every 2 years to determine the role of heredity for morbidity and longevity. Identical twins (MZ) were consistently more concordant than fraternal twins (DZ) for specific diseases (Jarvik & Bank, 1983). Genetic effects for longevity were confirmed by smaller MZ than DZ intrapair differences (Falek, Kallmann, Lorge, & Jarvik, 1960).

Several findings have relevance to issues of extrinsic factors in aging that have been discussed here. The expression of traits that presumably represent aging (such as grayness and thinning of the hair, the configuration of baldness, senile wrinkle formation, the extent of general enfeeblement, and deficiencies of the eyes, ears, and teeth) may be largely controlled by inherited factors. Extrinsic environmental influences (such as residence in the country or the city, profession, marital status, and life-style) did not modify twin similarity in either appearance or age of onset for age-related traits.

In order to study genetic influences on normal behavioral aging, a subsample of intact pairs (75 MZ and 45 DZ) was selected for psychometric evaluation. The measures included digit span, digit symbol, similarities and block design from the Wechsler–Bellevue intelligence test, a vocabulary test from the Stanford–Binet, and a tapping test for eye–hand coordination. Genetic influences in intellectual abilities were evidenced by smaller MZ than DZ intrapair differences for all of the measures.

Retests were conducted about 1 year after the initial evaluation and again in 1955 (26 MZ and 10 DZ pairs) and 1967 (13 MZ and 6 DZ pairs). The findings were consistent with other reports that performance decreases on speeded cognitive tasks but is stable on nonspeeded tests until the age of 75. There was a more rapid rate of decline between the second and third test occasions, at ages 73–85, than between the first and second test occasions, at ages 65–73, on some of the psychological tests. Thus, aging not only affects traits differentially, but its effect on the same trait can vary across ages.

Longitudinal pairwise analyses showed that except for the digit symbols, the average intrapair differences converged for the MZ and DZ twins, which implies that genetic factors become less important. After 21 years the DZs actually were more similar than the MZs on the digit span test (Jarvik & Bank, 1983). Although interpretations must be treated cautiously because the sample size was greatly diminished at the last time of measurement, it is interesting that the SATSA found a similar pattern of converging twin similarity in both the cross-sectional and the longitudinal results for a measure of health among the twins reared together (Harris, 1988). Jarvik & Bank (1983) posit that this pattern is partially explained by the longitudinal design itself because the DZ pairs who are least similar for traits related to survival drop out of the sample. This hypothesis was supported by blood group data that indicated that the DZ pairs who remained in the sample were more similar than those who died or stopped participating.

This type of sample attrition has important implications for behavioral genetic research on aging. Results that show little difference in similarity for MZ and DZ twins would normally be interpreted as evidence for considerable environmental variation. However, if the phenotypes under investigation are correlated with survival, then the genetic and environmental effects on these phenotypes are conditional upon a sample selected for concordant survival. Indeed, there are several reports of a positive correlation between intellectual capacity and survival, and this association is often present several years before death (Berg, 1985; Jarvik & Bank, 1983). Thus the real importance of genetic effects may be masked by this sampling effect, which itself may be due to genetic factors for vitality and survival.

Swedish Adoption/Twin Study of Aging

The SATSA is a comprehensive, multiphase study of gerontological behavioral genetics based on the powerful adoption/twin design. The sample is comprised of twins from the population-based Swedish Twin Registry (Cederlöf & Lorich, 1978) who were separated at an early age and reared apart and a sample of control twins reared together matched on gender and date, and country of birth. Most of the pairs were born prior to the Second World War. Dates of birth range from 1886 to 1956; however, the distribution is skewed; 75% were born before 1925.

The study began in 1984 with a two-part questionnaire mailed to 591 intact pairs of reared-apart twins, 627 intact pairs of reared-together twins, and 418 single surviving twin individuals. The questionnaires included items on health, functional capacity as measured by activities of daily living, health-related behaviors (such as tobacco, alcohol, and coffee consumption and drug use), personality and attitudes, current and childhood environment (including psychosocial and socioeconomic aspects), and work environment and history. Following the questionnaire phase, a subsample of the twins participated in telephone interview assessment of cognitive abilities and received in-depth personal examination by nurses, including nutritional and neurological status, functional capacity, vital capacity, and cognitive abilities. The first longitudinal follow-up of the questionnaire phase, at a 3-year interval, has recently been completed, and longitudinal follow-up of the personal testing began in January 1989. Thus far, cross-sectional analyses of the first phase of SATSA have been completed, and by linkage with twin registry data, longitudinal analyses of a subset of the SATSA data are also possible. Further details concerning SATSA and the sample of twins reared apart are reported by McClearn, Pedersen, Plomin, Nesselroade, Friberg, and DeFaire (1989); Pedersen, Friberg, Floderus-Myrhed, McClearn, and Plomin (1984); Pedersen, Plomin, McClearn, and Friberg (1988); and Plomin, Pedersen, McClearn, Nesselroade, and Bergeman (1988).

The first analyses in SATSA were concerned with assessing the relative contribution of genetic and environmental variance for a number of traits. At this stage, conclusions can be drawn about phenotypes in aging individuals rather than aging as a phenotype. These analyses revealed that genetic factors are of importance for most measures of personality, physical and mental health, life satisfaction, stature, alcohol and coffee consumption, and perceptions of the environment in this sample of adult and elderly twins (McClearn et al., 1989). These findings are consistent with those based on younger samples; both genetic and environmental factors contribute to individual differences for these measures. In a number of cases, however, the relative importance of genetic influences (heritability) is somewhat less than that reported in samples from an earlier portion of the life span. It is not possible at the present time to determine whether the differences in the estimates reflect age differences, reflect sample differences, or are a result of the adoption/twin design, which provides estimates of genetic influence unbiased by shared family environment.

The presence of age differences in genetic and environmental parameters has also been examined in SATSA by comparing the fit of models that constrain the estimates to be equal across age-groups with the fit of models in which parameters are estimated separately for each age-group. Two important results have been revealed: There are very few phenotypes for which heritability differs across age-groups (defined by 10-year age-bands), and when there are age differences, they do not follow any single pattern (McClearn et al., 1989). Of the 21 personality scales examined for cross-sectional age differences, only two showed significant age effects: a locus of control subscale describing the sense of personal control over the direction of one's own life (LIFE DIRECTION) and a mental health subscale of depression. On the other hand, there were significant age differences for measures of physical health (the number of chronic illnesses or organ system disorders – SUMILL – and perception of one's own health – SRHEALTH) (Harris, Pedersen, McClearn, Plomin, & Nesselroade, 1989). Significant age effects were also found for one of the four health-related behaviors, coffee consumption.

Environmental influences unique to the individual became relatively more important in the older age-groups for both LIFE DIRECTION and SRHEALTH. For SUMILL, the proportion of genetic variation increased until the oldest age-group, for which it decreased. Environmental influences, especially those causing family members to resemble each other (shared family environment), were of greater relative importance in that age-group. For coffee consumption, a nonlinear pattern was seen: Genetic factors accounted for a greater proportion of the variation in the youngest and the oldest age-groups. The patterns of twin similarity for depression did not conform to quantitative genetic expectations in all of the age-groups and interpretation is obscured.

The phenotypes that exhibited significant age differences in heritability were not necessarily the same phenotypes for which total variation differed by age-group. For example, 6 of the 21 personality measures displayed aged heterogeneity while the relative proportions of genetic and environmental influences remained stable. For 11 of the measures, total variation was stable across the age-groups. Although these findings are constrained by the general limitations of a cross-sectional design, they illustrate important relationships between mean differences, variance differences, and the etiology of these differences. Mean values differ in the absence of variance differences; total variance can differ, yet the relative contributions of genetic and environmental effects to the variance can remain the same. Even if the relative proportion of genetic variance is consistent across groups, one cannot conclude that the same genetic or environmental factors are operating in the different groups.

Although longitudinal data are not yet available from SATSA, some longitudinal analyses have been made possible by linking SATSA data to those in the Swedish Twin Registry. Data on extraversion and neuroticism in 1973 are available for twins born in 1926–1958, and data on illnesses in 1963 and on health-related behaviors such as alcohol and coffee consumption in 1967 are available for the twins born in 1886–1925. The preliminary results, based on the comparison of simple cross-correlations (Plomin & DeFries, 1981) and presented in Tables 12.1–12.3, demonstrate some of the types of stability and change that can be assessed in DBG studies. The relative importance of genetic and environmental factors for the five phenotypes at two points of measurement is reported in Table 12.1. In general, genetic influences account for 17%–51% of the variation in these measures at Time 1. Nonshared environmental effects (i.e., those unique to the individual) are substantial and explain 32%–66% of the variation. In contrast, sharing the same family environment plays a relatively minor role except in coffee and alcohol consumption, for which it explains about 25% of the variance. The overall

Table 12.1. *Summary of genetic and environmental influences at two time points*

Measure[a]	Total genetic variation		Genetic correlation	Shared environmental variation		Nonshared environmental variation		Environmental correlation
	Time 1[b]	Time 2[c]		Time 1[b]	Time 2[c]	Time 1[b]	Time 2[c]	
Extraversion (295 pairs)	.51 =	.50	.84	.04 =	.03	.45 =	.47	.36
Neuroticism (293 pairs)	.34 =	.33	.66	.00 <	.17	.66 >	.51	.42
Coffee consumption (298 pairs)	.17 <	.37	.64	.23 >	.13	.60 >	.50	.61
Total alcohol consumption (310 pairs)	.44 =	.39	.93	.24 >	.16	.32 <	.45	.56
Illness (367 pairs)	.37 <	.48	.99	.00 =	.00	.63 >	.52	.56

[a]Extraversion and neuroticism for twins born 1926–1958. Other measures on twins born 1886–1925.
[b]Date of measurement for extraversion and neuroticism is 1973; for coffee and alcohol consumption, 1967; and for illness, 1963.
[c]Date of measurement is October 1984.

picture for Time 2 is similar to Time 1; however, shared environmental effects have emerged for neuroticism.

A comparison of the first two columns in Table 12.1 reveals that for two of the measures, coffee consumption and illness, the relative importance of genetic effects changes across time. Genetic factors become more important with increasing age. For the other measures, genetic factors account for the same proportion of variation at the two measurement occasions. Some aging paradigms emphasize the increased role of genetic factors with age, whereas others propose that the accumulated effects of individual experiences become relatively more important (Baltes, Reese, & Lipsitt, 1980). However, the findings here reveal that neither genetic nor environmental effects consistently increase or decrease in their contribution to variability with age. Rather, the patterning of changes in these effects is specific to the phenotype being studied.

The genetic and environmental correlations indicate the stability of the genetic and environmental factors operating at the two time points regardless of their relative importance at each occasion. Environmental correlations are less than the genetic correlations for these measures. The high genetic correlations for extraversion, alcohol consumption, and illness suggest that nearly all of the genetic effects operating at the first time point are operating at the second time point. This is particularly interesting for the illness measure, for which the *relative* importance of genetic effects changes. This can be contrasted with the smaller genetic correlation for neuroticism, for which there is less genetic stability between 1973 and 1984 despite the fact that the relative importance of these factors does not differ across time.

Table 12.2 describes genetic and environmental contributions to phenotypic stability. Whereas the genetic correlation (Table 12.1) indicates the extent to which genetic effects are stable across time, the results in Table 12.2 indicate the proportion of phenotypic stability attributable to genes or environments. For example, 36% of the phenotypic correlation for coffee consumption ($r = .45$) is due to genetic factors, whereas the genetic correlation of .64 reveals that many of the same genetic effects are operating at both time points.

Finally, relative change itself was analyzed for the five measures. The preliminary findings, reported in Table 12.3, indicate the extent to which genetic and environmental factors contribute to change. Very little of the total variation in change scores is attributable to genetic effects. These results parallel the pattern of results for the genetic correlations; measures for which the genetic correlation is high (i.e., for which there is considerable genetic stability) are the measures for which genetic factors are unimportant for change across time. On the whole, environmental in-

Table 12.2. *Summary of genetic and environmental influences on stability*

Measure[a]	Phenotypic correlation	Contribution to stability	
		Genetic	Environmental
Extraversion	.60	70%	30%
Neuroticism	.50	44%	56%
Coffee consumption	.45	36%	64%
Total alcohol consumption	.71	54%	46%
Illness	.76	55%	45%

[a]Extraversion and neuroticism for twins born 1926–1958. Other measures on twins born 1886–1925.
Note: Sample sizes are the same as in Table 12.1.

Table 12.3. *Summary of genetic and environmental influences on change scores*

Measure[a]	Genetic variation	Shared environmental variation	Nonshared environmental variation
Extraversion	0–13	0	.87–1.0
Neuroticism	.13–.18	.18–.19	.64–.68
Coffee consumption	.15–.19	.15–.16	.65–.70
Total alcohol consumption	0–.10	.16–.22	.74–.78
Illness	0	0–.04	.96–1.0

[a]Extraversion and neuroticism for twins born 1926–1958. Other measures on twins born 1886–1925.
Note: Sample sizes are the same as in Table 12.1.

fluences unique to the individual are primarily responsible for variability in change. In summary, in this sample of elderly adults genetic factors are generally stable across time, their relative importance is stable or, if anything, increases across time, and they contribute more to phenotypic stability than to change.

Conclusion

Behavioral genetic study of aging in general and successful aging in particular can provide important insights into the etiology of individual differences throughout the life span. Identifying the role of genetic and environmental factors in producing heterogeneity in aging is but one step in understanding what is intrinsic to aging and how extrinsic factors affect the aging process. Once these relationships are clarified, the meaning of the concept of successful aging will become more apparent. At present, the concept is useful for stimulating exploration of the full range of variation in aging and encourages study of the possibility of optimizing the capacity and well-being of older individuals. A number of suggestions can be made for future research agendas. Expanding existing gerontological studies with behavioral genetic designs by including information on relatives will provide opportunities to study further the nature of individual differences in the elderly. Considerable advances have recently been made in behavioral genetic methodologies and analyses. Such efforts should be encouraged and applied when possible to existing as well as planned data sets. Finally, much can be gained by continuing the discussion of successful aging and applying a multidisciplinary approach to its study.

Summary

This paper has discussed several issues associated with the DBG study of successful aging. Although the notions of *intrinsic* and *extrinsic* are integral aspects of the concept of successful aging, they must be kept distinct from ideas of what is inherent, genetic, malleable, and environmental. Intrinsic aging processes may be inherited but may not show genetic variation. Traits that have a genetic etiology are not immutable; on the contrary, identification of genetic mechanisms often is a first step in developing rational therapies. Characteristics that show predominantly genetic variation are not necessarily stable, and stable characteristics are not necessarily genetic. Furthermore, both genetic and environmental differences can contribute to the expression of extrinsic factors. Thus, usual aging, in which extrinsic factors "heighten the effects of aging alone," may reflect both genetic and environmental influences; successful aging, in which extrinsic factors "play a neutral or positive role," is not necessarily "genetic." The challenge for DBG researchers is to delineate the degree to which genetic and environmental variation is important for extrinsic factors affecting aging individuals and for characteristics intrinsic to aging.

The definition of successful aging has a number of implications for DBG studies. The choice of phenotypes and study design and the degree of generalizability hinge upon this definition. Restriction of interest to "successful agers" has wide-ranging consequences for the types of analyses that may be performed: Studying a subgroup restricts variation and limits generalization. If the study of successful aging is to include longitudinal aspects, the full range of variation in the aging process must be examined to enable the study of continuity and change.

Finally, data from two studies of aging in twins are presented to illustrate some of the phenotypes and designs that can be utilized and the conclusions that can be drawn. Although the sample from the New York State Psychiatric Study of Aging Twins (Kallmann & Sander, 1948) is too small to provide definitive evidence for the role of genetic and environmental factors in the aging process, interesting phenomena are reported that highlight the importance of genetic effects for longevity. The study also indicates that the expression of traits that presumably represent intrinsic aging, such as grayness and thinning of the hair, senile wrinkle formation, and the extent of general enfeeblement, may be largely controlled by inherited factors. DZ twins who remained in the sample over a 21-year period were more similar with respect to both cognitive and blood group data than pairs in which one or both had died. These results suggest that genetic factors for vitality or survival may influence sample attrition and hence may affect interpretation of longitudinal behavioral genetic studies.

The SATSA presents a promissory note for addressing issues of relevance to behavioral aging in general and successful aging in particular. Cross-sectional analyses performed thus far indicate that age differences in heritability are phenotypic specific and that these age differences may or may not parallel age differences in variability. Preliminary longitudinal results for a number of measures illustrate stability in the relative importance of genetic effects and continuity in which genetic or environmental factors may be operating. Genetic effects are of minimal or no importance to variability in relative change scores.

NOTE

This paper was written with the support of the MacArthur Foundation Research Network on Successful Aging and of the National Institute of Aging (AG-04563). SATSA is an ongoing study performed at the Department of Environmental Hygiene of the Karolinska Institute in collaboration with the Research Center for Developmental and Health Genetics in the College of Health and Human Development at The Pennsylvania State University.

REFERENCES

Baltes, P. B., Reese, H. W., & Lipsitt, L. P. (1980). Life span developmental psychology. *Annual Review of Psychology, 31*, 65–110.

Berg, S. (1985, July). *Intelligence and terminal decline.* Paper presented at the XIII International Congress of Gerontology, New York.

Boomsma, D. I., & Molenaar, C. M. (1987). The genetic analysis of repeated measures. I. Simplex models. *Behavior Genetics, 17,* 111–123.

Butt, D. S., & Beiser, M. (1987). Successful aging: A theme for international psychology. *Psychology and Aging, 2,* 87–94.

Cederlöf, R., & Lorich, U. (1978). The Swedish Twin Registry. In W. E. Nance, G. Allen, & P. Parisi (Eds.), *Twin research: Part C. Biology and epidemiology* (pp. 189–195). New York: Alan R. Liss.

Cutler, R. G. (1975). Evolution of human longevity and the genetic complexity governing aging rate. *Proceedings of the National Academy of Sciences USA, 72,* 4664–4668.

Dannefer, D., & Sell, R. R. (1988). Age structure, the life course and "aged heterogeneity": Prospects for research and theory. *Comprehensive Gerontology B, 2,* 1–10.

DeFries, J. C., & Fulker, D. W. (1985). Multiple regression analysis of twin data. *Behavior Genetics, 15,* 467–474.

DeFries, J. C., & Fulker, D. W. (1986). Multivariate behavioral genetics and development: An overview. *Behavior Genetics, 16,* 1–10.

Eaves, L. J., Long, J., & Heath, A. C. (1986). A theory of developmental change in quantitative phenotypes applied to cognitive development. *Behavior Genetics, 16,* 143–162.

Emery, A. E. H. (1986). *Methodology in medical genetics.* London: Churchill Livingstone.

Falek, A., Kallmann, F. J., Lorge, I., & Jarvik, L. F. (1960). Longevity and intellectual variation in a senescent twin population. *Journal of Gerontology, 15,* 305–189.

Farrer, L. A. (1987). Genetic neurodegenerative disease models for human aging. *Review of Biological Research in Aging, 3,* 163–189.

Harris, J. R. (1988). *The etiology of individual differences in health and anthropometric measures: A developmental study of adult twins.* Unpublished doctoral dissertation, Pennsylvania State University.

Harris, J. R., Pedersen, N. L., McClearn, G. E., Plomin, R., & Nesselroade, J. R. (1989). *Age differences in genetic and environmental influences for health from the Swedish Adoption/Twin Study of Aging.* Manuscript submitted for publication.

Hart, R. W., & Trosko, J. E. (1976). DNA repair processes in mammals. *Interdisciplinary Topics in Gerontology, 9,* 134–167.

Hayflick, L. (1965). The limited *in vitro* lifetime of human diploid cell strains. *Experimental Cell Research, 37,* 614–636.

Hayflick, L., & Moorhead, P. S. (1961). The serial cultivation of human diploid cell strains. *Experimental Cell Research, 25,* 585–621.

Henderson, N. D. (1982). Human behavior genetics. *Annual Review of Psychology, 33,* 872–883.

Hewitt, J. K., Eaves, L. J., Neale, M. C., & Meyer, J. M. (1988). Resolving causes of developmental continuity or "tracking." I. Longitudinal twin studies during growth. *Behavior Genetics, 18,* 133–151.

Jarvik, L. F., & Bank, L. (1983). Aging twins: Longitudinal psychometric data. In K. W. Schaie (Ed.), *Longitudinal studies of adult psychological development* (pp. 40–63). New York: Guilford Press.

Johnson, T. E. (1988). Genetic specification of life span: Processes, problems, and potentials. *Journal of Gerontology: Biological Sciences, 43*, B87–92.

Johnson, T. E., & Simpson, V. J. (1985). Aging studies in *Caenorhabditis elegans* and other nematodes. In V. Cristofalo (Ed.), *CRC handbook of cell biology of aging* (pp. 481–495). Boca Raton, FL: CRC Press.

Kallmann, F. J., & Sander, G. (1948). Twin studies on aging and longevity. *Journal of Heredity, 39*, 349–357.

Kallmann, F. J., & Sander, G. (1949). Twin studies on senescence. *American Journal of Psychiatry, 106*, 29–36.

Kirkwood, T. B. L. (1981). Repair and its evolution: Survival versus reproduction. In C. R. Townsend & P. Clow (Eds.), *Physiological ecology: An evolutionary approach to resource use* (pp. 165–189). Oxford: Blackwell.

Martin, G. M. (1979). Genetic and evolutionary aspects of aging. *Federation Proceedings, 38*, 1962–1967.

Mayer, P. J., & Baker, G. T., III. (1985). Genetic aspects of Drosophila as a model system of eukaryotic aging. *International Review of Cytology, 95*, 61–102.

McArdle, J. J. (1986). Latent variable growth within behavior genetic models. *Behavior Genetics, 16*, 163–200.

McClearn, G. E., Pedersen, N. L., Plomin, R., Nesselroade, J., Friberg, L., & DeFaire, U. (1986). The Swedish Adoption/Twin Study of Aging (SATSA): A program of research in gerontological genetics. *Gerontologist, 26*, 83A.

McClearn, G. E., Pedersen, N. L., Plomin, R., Nesselroade, J. R., Friberg, L., & DeFaire, U. (1989). *The Swedish Adoption/Twin Study of Aging: Individual differences in personality.* Manuscript submitted for publication.

McGue, M., & Hirsch, B. (1987). *Twin study of normal aging.* Minneapolis: University of Minnesota.

Morton, E. N., & Chung, C. S. (1978). *Genetic epidemiology.* New York: Academic Press.

Norwood, T. H., & Smith, J. R. (1985). The cultured fibroblast-like cell as a model for the study of aging. In C. E. Finch & E. L. Schneider (Eds.), *Handbook of the biology of aging* (pp. 291–321). New York: Van Nostrand Reinhold.

Paigen, K. (1980). Temporal genes and other developmental regulators in mammals. In T. Leighten & W. F. Loomis (Eds.), *The molecular genetics of development* (pp. 419–471). New York: Academic Press.

Pedersen, N. L., Friberg, L., Floderus-Myrhed, B., McClearn, G. E., & Plomin, R. (1984). Swedish early separated twins: Identification and characterization. *Acta Geneticae Medicae et Gemellologiae, 33*, 243–250.

Pedersen, N. L., Plomin, R., McClearn, G. E., & Friberg, L. (1988). Neuroticism, extraversion and related traits in adult twins reared apart and reared together, *Journal of Personality and Social Psychology, 55*, 950–957.

Plomin, R. (1986). *Development, genetics, and psychology.* Hillsdale, NJ: Lawrence Erlbaum.

Plomin, R., & DeFries, J. C. (1981). Multivariate behavioral genetics and development: Twin studies. In L. Gedda, P. Parisi, & W. E. Nance (Eds.), *Twin research: Part B. Intelligence, personality, and development* (pp. 25–33). New York: Alan R. Liss.

Plomin, R., DeFries, J. C., & McClearn, G. E. (1989). *Behavioral genetics: A primer* (2nd ed.). New York: W. H. Freeman.

Plomin, R., McClearn, G. E., Pedersen, N. L., Nesselroade, J. R., & Bergeman, C. S. (1988). Genetic influence on childhood family environment perceived retrospectively from the last half of the life span. *Developmental Psychology, 24,* 738–745.

Plomin, R., & Nesselroade, J. R. (in press). Behavioral genetics and personality change. *Journal of Personality.*

Plomin, R., Pedersen, N. L., McClearn, G. E., Nesselroade, J., & Bergeman, C. S. (1988). EAS temperaments during the last half of the life span: Twins reared apart and twins reared together. *Psychology and Aging, 3,* 43–50.

Rowe, J. W., & Kahn, R. L. (1987). Human aging: Usual and successful. *Science, 237,* 143–149.

Scarr, S., & McCartney, K. (1983). How people make their own environments: A theory of genotype → environment effects. *Child Development, 54,* 424–435.

Shock, N. W. (1985). Longitudinal studies of aging in humans. In C. E. Finch & E. L. Schneider (Eds.), *Handbook of the biology of aging* (pp. 721–743). New York: Van Nostrand Reinhold.

Sprott, R. L. (1983). Genetic aspects of aging in *Mus musculus:* January 1981–February 1982. *Review of Biological Research in Aging, 1,* 73–80.

Tice, R. R., & Setlow R. B. (1985). DNA repair and replication in aging organisms and cells. In C. E. Finch & E. L. Schneider (Eds.), *Handbook of the biology of aging* (pp. 173–215). New York: Van Nostrand Reinhold.

Williams G. C. (1957). Pleiotropy, natural selection and the evolution of senescence. *Evolution, 11,* 398–411.

Name index

Subject index